YOUR METABOLISM MAKEOVER

Your Metabolism Makeover

The Clean Eating Way to Lose the Weight for Good
with More Than 150 Delicious Recipes

Wendy Bazilian, DrPH, RD, and the editors of **Prevention**

RODALE.

Portions of this book were previously published by Rodale Inc. as *Eat Clean, Stay Lean* and *Eat Clean, Stay Lean: The Diet*

© 2017 by Rodale Inc.

Photographs © Rodale Inc.

Printed in the United States of America

Rodale Inc. makes every effort to use acid-free ∞, recycled paper ♻.

Photographs by Mitch Mandel/Rodale Images

Back cover recipe photos (*left to right*): Chicken Pot Pie (page 174); Spinach-Artichoke Dip (page 251); and Lemon-Raspberry Cheesecake (page 243)

Book design by Yeon Kim

Library of Congress Cataloging-in-Publication Data is on file with the publisher.

ISBN 978-1-62336-923-1   Direct mail hardcover

2   4   6   8   10   9   7   5   3   1

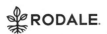

We inspire health, healing, happiness, and love in the world.
Starting with you.

Contents

PART 2

YOUR METABOLISM MAKEOVER: THE RECIPES

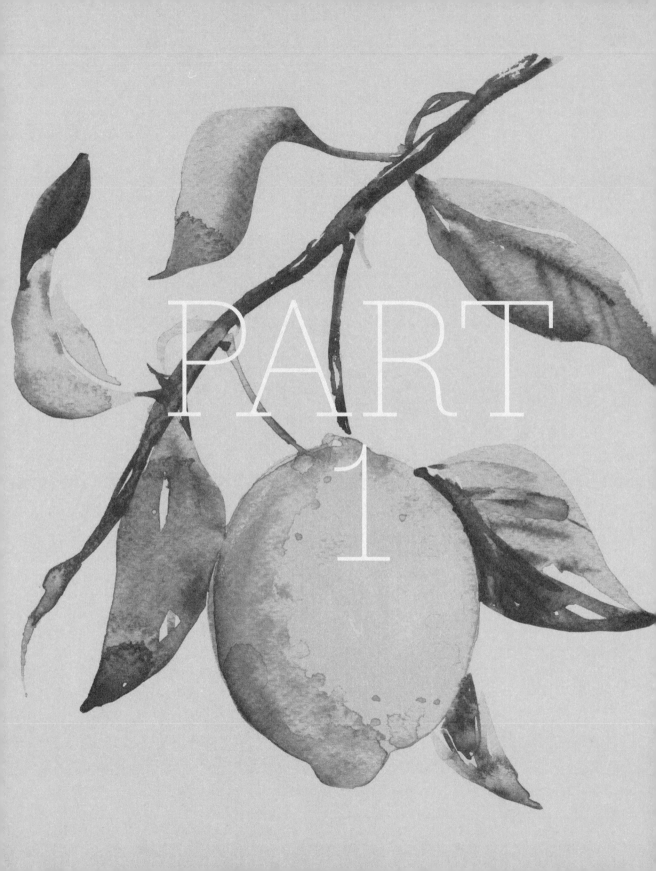

PART

1

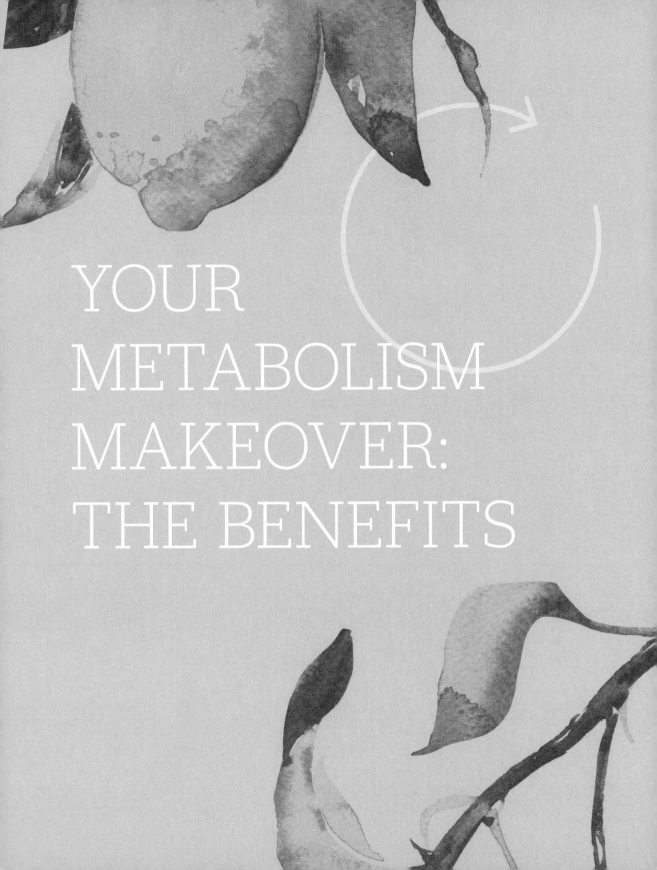

YOUR METABOLISM MAKEOVER: THE BENEFITS

MAKE OVER YOUR METABOLISM *with* Clean Eating

LET'S GET STRAIGHT TO THE POINT: Most diets are really only designed to be temporary. Sure, they might promise that you can stick with them forever. But in reality, all of those crazy rules and restrictions practically guarantee that they'll be impossible to stick with for the long term. If you've dieted before, you're used to hearing endless nos and barely any yeses. You're used to eating in a way that's inconvenient instead of one that fits into your life. You're used to tons of hard work that often ends in disappointment. Aren't you tired of that?

Since you're reading this book, we're willing to bet that the answer is yes. It's time to try something new to boost your metabolism and lose weight. It's time to try something that makes you feel good. It's time to try something that really works—because it supports your metabolism in fundamental ways that promote weight loss and help you maintain a healthy weight for life.

It's time to learn how clean eating is the basis of the *Your Metabolism Makeover* plan.

What Is Clean Eating?

You may have heard the term before, but what exactly does it mean? Clean eating is a way of life that can help you boost your metabolism, lose the weight, and keep it off for good—plain and simple. When you eat clean, you choose whole or minimally processed foods that are made from real ingredients, rather than choosing their highly processed counterparts. These clean foods look (and taste) like they came from the ground, or the farm, or the ocean, or maybe even someone's kitchen—not from a factory or a science lab. Think fresh fruit and nuts instead of a sugary granola bar. Organic roast chicken instead of frozen, breaded, chickenlike strips. A whole egg and vegetable omelet instead of a fast-food breakfast sandwich. Even homemade chocolate chip cookies instead of the kind that come in a box. You get the idea! Basically, it's how your grandparents ate before manufactured food took center stage.

If you're used to eating the standard American diet, the idea of giving your diet a makeover might feel a little overwhelming. But it's actually pretty easy to get the hang of. And once you do, it doesn't feel like you're doing anything weird or different or difficult. It just becomes a new way to eat. When you follow the *Your Metabolism Makeover* plan, you're giving your body the fuel it needs and the nutrients it craves. You're not constantly scrutinizing calorie counts, not cutting out food groups, and not depriving yourself of the things that you love. Clean eating allows you to feel your best. And it's the most effective way to boost your metabolism and get lean—and stay that way for life.

MEET THE NONDIET DIET

If you've tried other diets before, you might be wondering whether clean eating is truly all that different. It is. In fact, it's the complete and total opposite of every restrictive, gimmicky, run-of-the-mill diet out there. That's because eating clean doesn't just help you achieve a healthy weight—it also makes you *feel* good, so keeping it up to keep the pounds off is easy. Instead of trying to follow one hundred different rules, you follow just one basic principle: Choose real foods over their packaged, processed counterparts whenever possible.

Of course, you have to keep your portions in check. And of course, you have to enjoy things like clean desserts in moderation. In order to lose weight, both of those things are absolute musts. But eating clean, whole foods makes doing those things a lot easier, because *clean foods are what your body was designed to run on*. They're designed to fill you up so you don't want to keep eating and eating and eating. They're designed to help your blood sugar stay steady, so you're less susceptible to sugary cravings. They're designed to help you feel your best, so you have the energy to be active and keep making smart choices. It sounds pretty great, right?

NO RESTRICTIONS, NO GUILT

Most traditional diets work by doing one of two things. Some limit the types of foods that you're allowed to eat, such as by cutting out carbs or only allowing raw fruits and veggies. Others say that it's completely fine to eat anything you want—from doughnuts to Doritos—as long as you stay within your allotted (read: stingy) calorie budget. Both of these methods might work for a couple of weeks, or maybe even for a couple of months. But eventually you get tired of, say, never getting to eat bread or constantly feeling hungry because you're stuck eating too-tiny portions. At that point, it's totally natural to start dreaming about all of the delicious foods that have been off-limits. Eventually, your cravings get the best of you, and you find yourself at the table with a half-eaten pepperoni pizza and an empty pint of chocolate fudge ice cream thinking, "I messed up big time. Now what?" By then, you may feel so guilty that you end up abandoning your diet altogether and going back to

My Metabolism Makeover

* * *

"I've tried diets before, and nothing would happen. So I didn't expect this to work. Then I started seeing the numbers on the scale moving down. You've got to try eating clean, because it's easy, and you don't have to say, 'I can't eat this' or 'I can't go to that restaurant.' It's really very simple."

—RICHARD M.

Can you really eat anything? If it's made from real ingredients, yes. But let's exercise some common sense: There are some clean foods that are great to eat all the time and some that you need to save for once in a while in order to lose weight. For instance, it's better to make buttery steak and mashed potatoes with warm, homemade apple crisp for dinner the exception, rather than the rule—even if the steak is grass-fed and the apple crisp is made with rolled oats and unrefined sugar. (Though deep down you already knew that, right?)

But here's the thing: When you stop looking at food in terms of good things you can have and bad things that are never allowed—especially if you're in weight-loss mode—you might find that you actually start daydreaming about those formerly forbidden foods less often. This might seem hard to believe now, but trust me, it can—and most likely will—happen! In fact, among people actively trying to lose weight, studies show that even the thought of having to restrict certain foods can trigger overeating. And when it comes to not feeling deprived and achieving a healthier weight, that means everything.

your old ways. You regain the weight that you lost and maybe even pile on a few extra pounds. Sound familiar?

Here's how the *Your Metabolism Makeover* plan is different. When you commit to eating real food, nothing is off-limits. You don't have to cut out any category of food. You don't have to say no when you're invited to a restaurant or party because you're worried that the stuff on the menu won't work with your eating plan. With clean eating, there's almost always an option—even when the food being served isn't under your control. You don't have to subject yourself to eating pre-portioned diet meals or weighing and measuring every bite of food that goes into your mouth for the rest of your life. It's really freeing!

Naturally, portion sizes still matter. Food has calories whether it's clean or not, and there's no way around it: You have to eat less—and therefore take in fewer calories—in order to lose weight. But trimming portion sizes is much easier when you take the clean route. Clean foods deliver nutrients that help you stay full longer, so you're not hungry and cranky all the time. Plus, they make you feel like you're eating a lot, so you're less likely to feel deprived. Think about a sweet, crunchy apple. It has around 95 calories, which is similar to the number of calories in one little candy snack treat—you know, the tiny ones you give out on Halloween. But the apple makes you feel like you're eating more because it's bigger, and also because you spend more time chewing each bite. By the time you're done eating an apple, you feel like you're done eating, period. When you're done eating that snack bar? Chances are, you just want to grab another one.

DELICIOUS SATISFACTION—GUARANTEED

One of the biggest reasons that people abandon their diets is because the food just doesn't taste that good. And to make matters worse, it isn't very filling. After all, how many times can you eat a bunless, low-cal turkey burger or fat-free mac and cheese for dinner before you start dreaming about something better? Clean foods are fresh, vibrant, and unadulterated, so they naturally pack more flavor than their bland, processed counterparts. That means that when you get up from the table, you aren't hit with an overpowering urge to raid the pantry for a snack. (Not so sure yet? Check out the mouthwatering recipes and meal ideas starting on page 99.) In all, a delicious approach to eating is one that's easy to stick with. And by filling up on clean foods, you'll rev your metabolism so that you'll burn more of what you eat.

Rest assured, this is more than just a nice-sounding theory. Science shows that when you eat foods that are bursting with flavor, you'll probably eat less overall. In one *Flavour* journal study, researchers measured subjects' hunger and fullness levels while they ate a basic bowl of tomato soup. On another day, researchers measured the subjects' hunger and fullness levels again while the subjects ate a more flavorful tomato soup made with chile peppers. Unsurprisingly, the subjects said they liked the more flavorful soup better. But that didn't lead them to want to eat more of it. Instead, they decided that they were satisfied sooner.[1]

Of course, the takeaway isn't that you need to add chile peppers to everything you eat. (Unless you want to, of course.) It's that foods with more flavor—like fresh, clean fare—leave you more genuinely content with your meal, so you're less likely to want to keep noshing and noshing and noshing. While portion control is always important, eating clean will likely lead you to eat more food

> My Metabolism Makeover
>
> * * *
>
> **"Every day, I've had the opportunity to sit down to eat fresh, delicious food. The recipes are easy to follow, and I love all of the new whole grains I've been introduced to. In the evenings, I have a gourmet dinner to sit down to—and I'm the cook!"**
>
> —ALMARIE K.

bursting with the nutrients that your body is craving—and you'll enjoy your food even more.

A WAY OF LIFE THAT WORKS

When you're on a diet, you're constantly in a fight. You're fighting to maintain crazy food restrictions that don't fit your real day-to-day life. You're fighting the urge to scarf down a chocolate chip muffin instead of a yucky packet of artificially sweetened instant oatmeal. (Two equally poor options.) And you're fighting the urge to eat, period, because you're hungry all of the time. No wonder diets don't work—after a while, most of us give up out of sheer exhaustion. To top it off, these restrictions will also slow your metabolism.

There's no fighting in eating clean, which is why it's so easy. Instead of food being the enemy, it becomes the thing that nourishes your body and satisfies your hunger. Instead of living in a vacuum of prepackaged meals and diet snacks that force you to eat differently than everyone around you, you can make eating clean work anytime, anywhere. You're just eating the way you were designed to eat—and reaping the benefits of improving your metabolism and feeling stronger, more energized, and leaner. That's pretty easy to do, well, forever!

Fuel Your Metabolism

In fact, the very foods that many people turn to while "dieting"—artificial sweeteners and processed low-calorie meals and snacks—set you up for weight gain by leaving you hungry, addicted to junky processed-food ingredients, and prone to putting on pounds! In this chapter, you'll discover the research-backed evidence that shows that there are several ways processed foods can mess up your body's ability to maintain a healthy weight. And you'll discover the science behind clean eating—and how these foods get your metabolism back on track.

Metabolism means your body's ability to burn calories around the clock . . . and so much more. Your daily calorie expenditure is what experts call your resting metabolic rate, and it is based in large part on the amount of muscle you possess. But your metabolism also controls your weight in other profound ways. At least a dozen hormones are in charge of hunger, after-meal satisfaction, and cravings. Brain chemicals such as dopamine play important roles in cravings, too; that's one reason the fat, sugar, refined carbohydrates, and salt in processed foods can be so addictive. And a growing stack of research is revealing that what we eat every day affects the types of bacteria living in our digestive systems—and that these bacteria also influence weight and food choices.

HOW PROCESSED FOODS MESS UP YOUR METABOLISM

Loaded with calories but nearly devoid of the natural vitamins, minerals, and other nutrients your body needs for optimal functioning, processed foods are everywhere. We spend three-quarters of our food budgets on packaged and processed edibles,[2] and we buy more and more of them in places like convenience stores, where there's rarely a piece of fresh fruit or a carrot to be found. Manufacturers and stores lure us in with free samples, coupons, and eye-catching packaging designed by marketing gurus to make us (and our kids) reach for the boxes and bags on the shelves. Meanwhile, food scientists work hard to give these man-made edibles the perfect color and texture, based on consumer surveys. (Crunchy, crispy textures have been big sellers in recent years, in everything from candy to processed potatoes.)[3]

There's nothing natural or nice about them. To make matters worse, highly processed foods are engineered to be addictive—so you keep on eating, eating, eating and buying, buying, buying. Studies show that refined carbohydrates, sugar, fat, and salt all activate the reward system in your brain, prompting it to pump out megadoses of the pleasure hormone dopamine.[4] Dopamine, FYI, is the same hormone that your brain releases in response to highly addictive drugs like cocaine.[5]

Processed foods also mess with your metabolism in shocking ways that can promote weight gain. They trick your brain into wanting more and more. They reset your hormones so you never feel full. And they can trigger dramatic blood sugar surges and crashes, unleashing cravings that hit long before it's time for your next meal. Here are the traps that lure us into choosing highly processed foods, plus a discussion of what science has to say about them and weight control.

Trap #1: Refined carbohydrates. From white bread and white rice to pizza crusts and many breakfast cereals, crackers, and rolls, too many of the grains in our diets are missing all of the stuff that makes natural, whole grains great for your weight. When a grain is refined, it's stripped of nearly 90 percent of the micronutrients from its original form. Refined carbs contain virtually no fiber because the hulls of otherwise healthy grains, such as wheat and rice, are stripped away. Gone, too, is the smidge of good fat and treasure trove of vitamins, minerals, and phytonutrients from the real grain's kernel.

What's left? White starch that works against your metabolism. Refined carbohydrates don't do a good job at making you feel satisfied because they lack fill-you-up fiber. And alone they jack up your blood sugar, setting you up for a blood sugar crash that fuels cravings.

Your body is superefficient at squirreling away extra blood sugar as fast as it can—and at making you grab even more because you get hungry so fast. That made sense in cave-people days, when a honey-filled beehive was a rare treat. Today, carb-rich food is always on hand—in your pantry, office vending machines, in craft shops and hardware stores, and seemingly at every meeting, party, and church event we attend.

Refined carbs are metabolic time bombs. Along with that quick rise in blood sugar comes "a sequence of hormonal and metabolic changes that promote excessive food intake," according to one small but well-designed study of refined-carb eating in obese teenagers, published in the journal *Pediatrics*.[6] You may not be a teen any longer, but your adult body still works in pretty much the same exact way. Compared to healthier, cleaner meals, such as eggs and fruit or fiber-packed steel-cut oats (meals that had less of a negative effect on blood sugar), the one highest in refined carbs (highly processed instant oatmeal) kept hunger levels highest for the next 4 hours. As a result, the study volunteers who had the processed breakfast ate more throughout the day. Blood tests revealed that after the blood sugar rush, levels of important fuels (blood sugar and fatty acids) dropped. It was as if they were practically starving, so their bodies demanded more food.

Trap #2: Added sugars. Imagine eating $\frac{1}{2}$ cup of sugar every single day. Impossible? It's the reality for most Americans, who munch an average of 23 teaspoons' worth of added sweeteners every 24 hours, according to the nonprofit health watchdog group Center for Science in the Public Interest. That's 78 pounds of added sweeteners per year, which is equivalent to $15\frac{1}{2}$ five-pound bags of sugar![7] It's a disaster for your metabolism, your waistline, and your body weight.

Half of the added sweeteners in our diets comes from soda and other sugary drinks. Another one-fourth, not surprisingly, comes from candies, desserts, and sweet toppings, such as maple-flavored syrup and chocolate sauce. If you're trying to get sugar out of your life, you know to steer clear of that stuff. But here's the shocking part of the added-sugar story: The other one-fourth hides out in foods where you might not expect to find them or might

BOTTOMS UP!

When it comes to filling up faster and steering clear of junky snacks, plain old water might be your secret weapon. Research published in the journal *Obesity* found that dieters who downed 16 ounces of water before each meal for 12 weeks lost 3 more pounds than those who skipped the extra sips. The reason why is brilliantly simple: Having all of that liquid in your belly means that you need less food to feel full.

not realize that there's so much of them, such as ketchup, bread, breakfast cereals, and dairy products.[8] Altogether, added sweeteners make up 13 percent of the calories most Americans eat in a day—that's a whopping 235 calories if you're eating 1,800 calories a day![9]

But the problem isn't just calories. The natural sugars found in real fruit, minimally processed whole grains, and unsweetened dairy products are absorbed more slowly by your body because they come packaged with fiber, protein, and fat. In contrast, added sugars show up in many foods that don't put the brakes on the absorption of sugar into your bloodstream. They're often packaged with refined carbohydrates and in foods that lack fiber or much protein. Eating these processed foods launches your body onto a metabolic roller coaster as your blood sugar soars, then crashes when the hormone insulin pulls all that sugar into your cells and your bloodstream calling for more. As a result, your blood sugar plummets, leaving you feeling tired and cranky and ultimately craving another fix from the cookie jar.

Added sugars fool your metabolism in other ways, too. Researchers from the Harvard T. H. Chan School of Public Health note in a 2011 review in the journal *Current Opinion in Clinical Nutrition & Metabolic Care* that "liquid carbohydrates," like that big, sugary iced tea from the drive-thru or that fancy grande coffee drink from your favorite coffee shop, aren't as filling as solid carbs. You feel hungry afterward despite all of the calories you just sipped, and you're more likely to overeat later because the calories just didn't register with your brain.[10]

About 29 pounds of the added sweeteners we down each year come from high-fructose corn syrup (HFCS), which may stir up extra metabolic trouble.[11] Don't get us wrong—even healthy-sounding sugars such as honey, fruit concentrates, agave, and cane sugar mess with your metabolism while piling up calories and packing on pounds. But a growing amount of research suggests that HFCS may pose extra dangers. Unlike table sugar, which has a 50-50 mix of fructose and glucose, the form of HFCS used in drinks is 55 percent fructose.

(Glucose makes up 42 percent, and other sugars comprise 3 percent.)[12] "The digestion, absorption, and metabolism of fructose differ from those of glucose," explain leading American obesity experts Barry M. Popkin, PhD, professor, department of nutrition, University of North Carolina at Chapel Hill, and George A. Bray, MD, professor of medicine at the Louisiana State University Medical Center in New Orleans in a paper in the *American Journal of Clinical Nutrition*.[13] Compared to glucose, fructose doesn't stimulate the release of as much of the satisfaction hormone leptin. Fructose also fails to reduce levels of the hunger hormone ghrelin. It's a metabolic double whammy that leaves you craving more, contributing to weight gain.[14]

Trap #3: Saturated fat. Despite the headlines blaring that bacon, butter, and fat-marbled steaks "are back," too much saturated fat is still a very bad idea for your waistline. An impressive comparative Swedish study[15] tells the tale: Forty people munched three to four high-fat muffins a day made with either saturated fat or polyunsaturated fat (from sunflower oil, a heart-healthy fat) for 7 straight weeks. One dropped out, and another told a reporter, "Let's just say I won't be interested in muffins again for a while!"

Afterward, Uppsala University researchers not surprisingly found that all of the study volunteers gained weight as they had been designed to, so that researchers could measure what type and where fat was deposited. (You would, too, after consuming an extra 750 calories a day!) But the saturated-fat group put on more body fat than the sunflower group, including twice as much of the dangerous deep belly fat that wraps around internal organs. Both groups also put on more muscle, but the muscle gain was three times greater in the polyunsaturated-fat (sunflower) group. That's a nice bonus, because muscle cells burn calories around the clock, keeping your metabolism going strong.

Trap #4: Salt. Salt has no calories, but it's a metabolic "enabler" that can make you pack on pounds by literally tricking you into eating more and more fat. (Remember that familiar potato chip advertising slogan, "Bet you can't eat just one"?)

In an eye-opening study from Australia's Deakin University, 48 people ate lunches of macaroni and tomato sauce spiked with various amounts of salt and fat.[16] They ate 11 percent more food and more calories when salt levels were highest. And when fat and salt were both ramped up, people ate 60 percent more calories. Most troubling: People in the study who were naturally sensitive to the taste of fat overate when food was salty—even though they would normally eat less fat than other people.

No wonder a 2013 study of 20,856 adults published in the *European Journal of Clinical Nutrition* found that people whose diets contained the most salt were 18 percent more likely to be obese, compared to people who ate the least salt.[17] Among the 5,025 kids and teens also in the study, those eating high-salt foods had 78 percent greater odds of being obese.

Taking the salt shaker off your table can help you cut back, but added salt is the tip of the iceberg. More than 75 percent of the sodium in the typical American diet comes from processed foods plus meals and snacks purchased from fast-food places and restaurants, according to the Centers for Disease Control and Prevention.[18]

MORE METABOLISM BUSTERS: ADDITIVES AND OTHER CHEMICALS

Processed foods are also packed with chemicals that negatively impact your metabolism. Here's a list of some of the main culprits you'll steer clear of by eating clean.

- **Artificial sweeteners.** Zero-calorie and ultra-low-calorie artificial sweeteners aren't the solution if you want to get sugar out of your diet. More than 10 years of research shows that these chemicals mess up metabolism in astounding ways. No wonder one 749-person study from the University of Texas Health Science Center at San Antonio found that those who guzzled the most diet sodas over $9\frac{1}{2}$ years packed on almost three times more belly fat than those who rarely sipped these drinks.[19] And another study by the same researchers found that the biggest fans of diet drinks were almost twice as likely to become overweight or obese as those who skipped these sips.[20]

  Artificial sweeteners do your metabolism wrong in an astounding number of ways. For starters, according to a 2014 paper in the respected journal *Nature,* they negatively impact the bacteria living in your digestive system in ways that seem to alter metabolic pathways and thus potentially contribute to weight gain.[21] Low-cal sweeteners such as saccharin, sucralose, acesulfame potassium, aspartame, and the combination of erythritol plus aspartame have also been shown in lab studies to reduce calorie-burning after meals, reduce the release of the appetite-controlling gut hormone GLP-1 (short for glucagon-like peptide 1), increase fasting blood sugar levels, and boost weight and body fat gain.[22]

- **Emulsifiers.** These compounds are found in everything from mayonnaise and salad dressings to ice cream and cream cheese because they keep ingredients mixed together and help prevent them from separating. They're considered safe by the FDA, but two of them—polysorbate 80 and carboxymethylcellulose (CMC)—were shown in a recent Georgia State

University study to negatively affect bacteria in the digestive system in ways that boosted inflammation and obesity-related metabolic syndrome, as well as further harm their health.[23] The study was done with mice, but the scientists arrived at the same results a year later in a lab study that re-created these conditions in the human digestive system.

- **Preservatives.** The widely used preservatives sodium sulfite and sodium benzoate reduced the release of the "I'm full" hormone leptin called in a recent study from Austria's Innsbruck Medical University.[24] The researchers say this response could also contribute to obesity.

- **Obesogens.** Researchers suspect that these toxins in our food increase body fat, dial up hunger, and slow your metabolism. A triple threat! Compounds used to produce conventional foods— such as artificial hormones and the fungicide triflumizole—seem to trigger the body to store more fat, as seen in recent research in mice.[25, 26] In a 2012 report in the journal *Environmental Health Perspectives*, researchers from the US National Toxicology Program noted that pesticides used to grow food, as well as chemicals like bisphenol A (BPA, found in some hard plastics and in can linings) and phthalates (found in some plastic food containers), may also promote obesity and diabetes when they leach from packaging into food.[27]

BURN MORE CALORIES WITH CLEAN FOOD

Want to rev your metabolism? Turn to clean foods like protein, fruits, veggies, and delicious seasonings to give your body's natural calorie-burning engine a welcome nudge in the right direction.

Processed foods don't support your body's optimal metabolic rate. These factory-made foods and beverages deprive you of important vitamins, minerals, phytochemicals, healthy fats, and other compounds that your cells need in order to function at their peak. In addition, refined carbs, gobs of fat, and sugar-laden foods and drinks are just not very "thermogenic," meaning that your body doesn't have to burn very many calories to digest and convert them into energy.

Ah, but protein is a thermogenic superstar: It turns up your thermostat, requiring more energy to burn. During digestion, your body burns nearly three times more calories digesting protein than it does burning carbohydrates and ten times more than it does burning fat![28] In one study from Arizona State University East, published in the *Journal of the American College of Nutrition*, thermogenic rates were twice as high after higher-protein meals than after meals higher in carbohydrates. The researchers note that this digestion-fueled metabolic boost can last for 4 to 5 hours after you eat, and they estimate that this advantage could increase calorie burn by up to 90 calories per day.[29] In a similar study from the Athens University Medical School in Greece, published in the journal *Metabolism,* a higher-protein meal increased "diet-induced thermogenesis" nearly three times greater compared to a meal packed with fat.[30]

The good news? We're not talking about over-the-top, gigantic portions of protein. You'll never have to chew your way through a giant slab of meat without a fruit, veggie, or yummy whole grain in sight! Getting the right amount of protein, as you will with the strategies and recipes in this book, is all it takes.

But wait—you may be asking yourself, "Why not just eat a drive-thru bacon cheeseburger or a couple of slices of sausage pizza to boost thermogenesis?" You could. Protein is protein. But that can and will backfire. Clean protein—like lean poultry, fish packed with healthy omega-3 fatty acids, low-fat Greek yogurt, nuts, and fiber-filled legumes—delivers additional metabolic benefits that support a healthy weight. These include higher satisfaction levels after eating, a curb on cravings, less fat storage, and even happier "gut bugs"—the bacteria in your digestive tract that help control weight, appetite, and body fat distribution. Compare *that* to the downsides of burgers and other not-so-clean proteins. They come with unwelcome levels of saturated fat, refined carbs (in burger buns, pizza crusts, etc.), and a boatload of additives that toss all sorts of monkey wrenches into your metabolic machinery.

Eating enough protein also provides your muscles with the building blocks they need to stay dense and strong. That's a huge metabolic help because muscle cells burn calories around the clock. And like everyone else, you're battling the natural, age-related loss of muscle density that can torpedo your metabolism—unless you take action. Experts estimate that adults lose about 1 percent of muscle mass every year in middle age. Between 40 and 50, that could mean the loss of 10 percent of your muscle mass—and a 3 to 6 percent drop in your metabolism.[31] But eating enough protein at every meal (instead of skimping at breakfast and lunch and then overdoing it at dinner, as so many Americans do) helps maintain precious muscle density.[32]

Meanwhile, protein isn't the only thing that plays a role in revving your metabolism. Clean foods are full of nutrients that can increase your calorie burn. Here are some great examples you can add to your diet today.

- **Nuts.** Munching a small handful of almonds can increase calorie burn by about 15 percent for a few hours after you eat. Peanuts can increase it up to 40 percent, according to a Purdue University review in the *Journal of Nutrition*.[33]

- **Citrus, strawberries, broccoli, and bell peppers.** These juicy, crunchy goodies deliver a big dose of vitamin C. Research suggests that having healthy vitamin C stores can help your body burn 30 percent more fat during a session of moderate-intensity exercise than those with low vitamin C. Researchers from Arizona State University East note in their study paper in the *Journal of the American College of Nutrition* that people low on C may have more trouble losing body fat as a result.[34]

- **Apples, blueberries, and raspberries.** These and other colorful fruits and veggies brim with flavonoids—anti-inflammatory plant compounds that have also been shown to help with weight control. The reasons? Flavonoids have been linked with lower weight gain over time and, in some cases, even with an uptick in energy expenditure.[35] And in weight-loss studies, people who ate plenty of fruits and veggies as part of meal plans designed to keep blood sugar low and steady maintained a higher round-the-clock metabolic rate than people who ate foods that make blood sugar soar.[36]

- **Garlic and red peppers.** Turn up the sizzle, turn up the burn! Capsaicin, the ingredient that gives hot peppers their tongue-tingling zing, has been shown to increase metabolism after a meal, according to a number of studies.[37] And garlic has also been shown to boost calorie burn while simultaneously turning down fat production in mice.[38] Think a slice of processed white bread can do any of that stuff? Sorry, not a chance.

- **Green tea, coffee, and cold water.** These healthy sips could increase metabolism a little, research suggests. In fact, sipping green tea regularly was shown to help overweight men lose nearly a pound and a half in just 6 weeks, according to a study published in the *British Journal of Nutrition*.[39] A 2016 University of Minnesota study of 937 women saw decreased tissue fat in those consuming green tea extract.[40] And, caffeine (found in coffee and black tea) can boost metabolism by nearly 5 percent, according to a 2011 review of the research by scientists from Maastricht University in the Netherlands.[41] Sipping cold water may increase calorie burn by a little more than 4 percent, according to a 2006 study in the *Journal of Clinical Endocrinology and Metabolism* conducted by researchers from the University of Fribourg in France.[42] Alone, cold water won't make you lose weight, but it could be one factor as a recent University of Minnesota survey of 9,528 American adults research revealed that one in three adults was dehydrated. And dehydrated people were 60 percent more likely to be obese compared to those who were drinking plenty of fluids every day.[43]

MAKING THE MOST OF GREEN TEA'S METABOLISM BENEFITS

It's easy to reach for bottled green tea in a convenience store or at the supermarket. But according to a recent analysis by the private, independent testing Web site ConsumerLab.com, you'll get a bigger benefit if you brew your own.[44] And according to a report in the *New York Times,* the company found that loose tea yielded cups of green tea with the highest levels of epigallocatechin gallate (EGCG)—the beneficial compound in green tea.[45] But inexpensive green tea in bags also produced respectable levels when brewed. In contrast, some bottled green teas had little to no EGCG but did contain plenty of sugar. That's not a clean drink! Another option: Try matcha, a powdered green tea extract that's convenient and high in EGCG. Follow the label directions and enjoy a cup or two a day. Add a squirt of fresh lemon juice, and you'll get an even bigger boost: Consuming EGCG with something acidic, like citrus, helps your body absorb up to five times more of the fat burner, according to research conducted at Purdue University.[46]

LEARN HOW TO LOVE CLEAN FOODS

If you're used to the addictive, over-the-top flavors of processed foods, the idea of black bean soup or an apple with peanut butter might seem sort of . . . blah. That'll change as your taste buds adjust to fresh foods that aren't loaded with sugar, salt, and unhealthy fats—promise. But if you're not quite there yet, here are some tips to help get you hooked on clean fare faster.

1. **Forget how you felt as a kid.** Maybe you haven't let a certain vegetable slip past your lips since elementary school but you've repeatedly heard that it delivers multiple benefits and could help you lose weight. Though it can sometimes be tough to reconcile your feelings with the facts, now might be the time to give long-hated foods another try. Your taste buds are more sensitive to bitter flavors when you're young, so even though Brussels sprouts might have tasted like lawn clippings when you were 10, your adult self might actually like them. Preparation is so important, too. The broccoli of your childhood might have been mushy and bland—but cooking it differently today might yield a completely different result. (Ready to give it a go? Try the Roasted Broccoli with a Kick on page 202.)

2. **Surround yourself with healthy stuff.** French people aren't born loving snails and Japanese people don't come into this world craving sushi. Instead, they come to like those foods because they're a regular part of the environment, according to findings published in the journal *Appetite*. Instead of buying more boxed mac and cheese or chicken fingers, get into the habit of stocking your kitchen with whole wheat pasta and organic chicken. As you get used to having the clean stuff around, you might find yourself wanting it more often.

3. **Take small steps.** If the thought of eating plain raw red pepper strips is unappealing, don't do it. Start by pairing them with something

STORE LESS BELLY FAT!

Belly fat. Muffin top. Love handles. By any name, fat around your midsection is the most dangerous kind of all. A waistline measuring 35 inches or more for women and 40 inches or more for men is likely a hideout for visceral fat—the kind inside your abdomen that wraps around internal organs, lodges in your liver, and sends a boatload of health-threatening, inflammation-boosting compounds into your bloodstream. (It can also make you feel shy about showing up at a pool party in your bathing suit, tucking your shirt into your jeans, or buying a form-fitting dress for a special occasion.)

Clean foods clean up your metabolism so that your body stores fewer calories as belly fat. When 130 people followed a higher-protein or higher-carb eating outrageously delicious, like homemade ranch dressing. After a while, you might decide to start dunking them in something a little more nutrient-dense, like hummus or the Lemony Rosemary White Bean Dip on page 252. And if that's where you decide to stay, no problem. If you still don't like plain raw red pepper strips, you don't have to eat them.

4. **Appeal to your sweet tooth.** Take advantage of the fact that humans are hardwired to crave sugar. Instead of trying to choke down raw or steamed vegetables, try roasting them to bring out their natural sweetness and make them more palatable. You might not think a cauliflower floret could ever truly taste like candy, but when it gets caramelized and crispy, it really can.

5. **Go for the fancy stuff.** Research published in the *Journal of Sensory Studies* found that people who paid $8 for a buffet lunch reported being more satisfied with their meals than those who only paid $4, even though both groups ate the same exact fare. Why? Because sometimes we're shallow, and we automatically think that cheaper food is going to be lower quality. When possible, spend the extra couple of bucks on organic green leaf lettuce from the farmers' market instead of that so-so bunch at the corner store. Chances are it's a fresher, overall better choice than the droopy bunch flown in from who-knows-where. Thanks to your built-in selectivity, you might trick yourself into thinking the pricy stuff is pretty delicious.

6. **Make sure you're actually hungry.** Before you bother sitting down to that beet and quinoa salad, check in with your appetite. Why? Because when your stomach's really rumbling, you'll be way more willing to eat whatever's in front of you—even if it's a big bowl of vegetables. (For much more on how to read your body's hunger cues, check out Chapter 4.)

plan for 4 months, University of Illinois researchers found that both groups lost about the same amount of weight—about 18 pounds. But the people who ate meals higher in protein dropped 22 percent more fat, including belly fat.[47] And when researchers from the US Army Research Institute of Environmental Medicine checked up on the diets and waistlines of 23,876 Americans, they found that those who ate more protein weighed less and had slimmer waistlines.[48]

Protein is especially important when you're trying to lose weight. Pound for pound, on a high-carb diet, the weight you lose is about 65 percent fat and 35 percent muscle; bump up the protein and you improve that ratio to 80 percent fat, 20 percent muscle. Adding exercise could make it an even better 90 percent fat, 10 percent muscle, experts note.[49]

Every element of clean eating works to keep you slimmer. Take monounsaturated fats (MUFAs). The luxurious, clean MUFAs found in avocados, nuts, olive and canola oils, and (oh yes!) dark chocolate keep belly fat at bay. And in a fascinating Spanish study, 59 people followed one of three eating plans—high in carbohydrates, high in MUFAs, or high in saturated fats. Calorie levels were set so no one lost weight. But after 4 weeks, the carb group gained belly fat while the MUFA group saw theirs shrink.[50]

Dairy and other calcium-rich foods lend a hand, too. When 171 people got either 1,050 milligrams of calcium and 300 IU of vitamin D daily or a placebo for 16 weeks in a Massachusetts General Hospital study, the calcium-plus-D group lost two to ten times more visceral fat.[51] It's better to get calcium from foods such as dairy, calcium-enriched dairy alternatives, legumes (such as white and navy beans), spinach, kale, and turnip greens instead of relying too much on supplements, which may encourage the formation of calcium deposits in artery-choking plaque. Meanwhile, dairy packs another benefit: Types with some fat, such as low-fat milk or a small amount of flavorful cheese, deliver conjugated linoleic acid (CLA). A 2015 review in the *Journal of the International Society of Sports Nutrition* suggests that this fatty acid can help reduce belly fat.[52] CLA levels may be higher in milk (and beef) from grass-fed cows, too.[53]

Soluble fiber—found in delicious clean-food treats like sweet, juicy pears, hearty steel-cut oats, and satisfying barley—also banishes belly fat. Getting 10 grams a day (the amount you'd get if you had a small apple chopped up in your morning oatmeal, another small apple as a snack, lunchtime chili containing ½ cup of pinto beans, and a large helping of green peas at dinner) translated into a 3.7 percent decrease in visceral fat in a recent Wake Forest Baptist Medical Center study of 1,114 people. Those who also got moderate-intensity exercise two to four times a week bumped up belly-fat loss to 11 percent.[54] Soluble fiber may work its magic by turning off hunger and cravings, leaving you satisfied without overeating or oversnacking, the researchers note.

Everyday choices, whether you're dieting or not, can make a big difference in your waist. When Tufts University researchers analyzed the health records of 2,834 women and men, they found that people who ate the most whole grains had the least visceral fat, and those who munched the most refined grains had the most.[55] And in a Danish study that tracked 22,570 women for 5 years, study participants who ate more processed foods, which are full of simple sugars, refined carbs, and processed potatoes, saw their waistlines expand, too.[56]

Meanwhile, cruciferous vegetables such as kale, broccoli, and cabbage contain a beneficial compound called indole-3-carbinol (I3C). Research in the journal *Nutrition* on obese mice suggests that I3C may fight against the storage of excess body fat.[57]

CONQUER HUNGER, OVEREATING, AND CRAVINGS

On every level, highly processed foods are *designed* to make you overeat and still crave more. They light up reward centers in your brain that are also activated by mood-altering drugs. Their by-products sneak around systems in your brain and body designed by Mother Nature to tell you when you're full and can stop eating. They're manufactured with precisely the textures and flavors you long for. And they deliver processed ingredients that lead to weight gain while depriving you of nutrients that support health and a healthy weight.

The flip side: Clean foods can give you freedom from overeating.

Clean foods are *everything* that processed foods are not. Yes, simply avoiding processed food lets you avoid all sorts of overeating traps. But clean eating takes satiety—that good feeling of lasting fullness—to a whole new level. Research shows that eating clean activates and rebalances key appetite-control hormones. It flips metabolic switches built into your body and brain to tell you when you've eaten enough and also to help keep you from thinking about food for hours after a meal. (Just compare how you feel midmorning after having a doughnut for breakfast versus after a bowl of berries, walnuts, and Greek yogurt!)

Of course, it's possible to overeat clean foods and have *those* calories get stored as fat, too. But honestly, that's much harder to do when you're eating clean. After all, when you've finished that apple or bowl of bean soup or beautiful piece of grilled fish, you know you're satisfied! Here are five powerful ways clean foods work with and enhance your metabolism to stop hunger, crush cravings, and control overeating.

#1: Lower, steadier blood sugar. Your body breaks down the carbohydrates in grains, fruits, dairy, and even vegetables for blood sugar. Clean foods like whole grains and fresh produce are packed with fiber that slows down the rate of absorption of sugar (glucose) into your bloodstream. Along with protein and healthy fats, all that fiber maintains blood sugar at lower, steadier levels for hours after your meal, too. You don't get the spikes and dips that lead to hunger and cravings. No wonder making a single dietary change—eating at least 30 grams of fiber a day, double the American average—resulted in people effortlessly losing as much as 6 pounds in one year[58] in one recent University of Massachusetts Amherst study.

#2: More in your stomach. Clean foods—especially lean proteins, whole grains, beans, fruits, and vegetables—are less energy-dense than many processed foods. That means you can eat a larger volume for fewer calories and feel more physically full. When 20 overweight volunteers taking part in a Medical University of South Carolina study switched to higher-fiber diets featuring either a daily 1½ cups of beans or extra produce and whole grains for 4 weeks, both groups *felt more satisfied and less hungry,* even though they were taking in 300 fewer calories a day compared to their regular diets. And they lost more than 3 pounds apiece.[59]

The researchers measured satisfaction with a 15-point questionnaire that challenged volunteers to get real about their desire to eat. They rated how much they agreed or disagreed with statements like, "I just can't keep myself from eating snacks between meals" and "Sometimes I feel like food controls me rather than the other way around." Volunteers felt more in control of their eating after going high-fiber—dramatic proof that clean eating can change your food life for the better.

And here's an interesting factoid—and an added perk for fiber: When your stomach fills with food, which activates "stretch receptors" in the stomach that send a message to your brain that you've probably had plenty to eat. Solid foods with texture like fresh fruits and veggies can help make that happen. However, there's also some evidence that too much high-fat food may interfere with this important "I'm full" mechanism,[60] so keep your foods high in fiber and texture with moderate fat.

#3: A better balance between hunger and satisfaction hormones. At least a dozen different hormones play roles in the complex ballet that decides when you're hungry and when you're full. These include ghrelin, the hunger hormone that rises sharply just before meals, and leptin, the "I'm full and happy" hormone that overweight people may develop a resistance to, leaving them feeling hungry despite having eaten a big meal.[61] A growing stack of research shows that smart food choices, like those you'll make when you eat clean, can help regulate these powerful compounds.

For example, eating lean protein at breakfast helps increase fullness, reduce ghrelin, and keep energy high and hunger at bay all day.[62] That's why the *Your Metabolism Makeover* program recommends starting the day with lean protein. And it may be an important reason why women who ate 35 grams of protein (equal to about 5 ounces of cooked Alaskan salmon, 1 cup of cottage cheese with ¼ cup of raw pumpkin seeds and fruit, or 1 cup of low-fat Greek yogurt with 1¼ cups Kashi GOLEAN cereal and 3 tablespoons of raw almonds) at breakfast experienced fewer junk-food cravings throughout the day than those who ate 13 grams of protein or no protein at all in a University of Missouri study published in the *American Journal of Clinical Nutrition*.[63] Protein also stimulates the release of leptin.

Always include produce, whole grains, and good fats. Healthy carbs and fats are tops at prompting your body to release lesser-known but important satiety hormones such as GIP (glucose-dependent insulinotropic polypeptide) and GLP-1 into your bloodstream.[64] Be sure to include healthy polyunsaturated fats such as sunflower oil, nuts, and fish oils; PUFAs (polyunsaturated fatty acids) were better than saturated fat at squashing ghrelin and boosting levels of the satisfaction hormone peptide YY in a Texas Tech University study published in the journal *Obesity*.[65] Omega-3 fatty acids, found in fatty fish such as salmon and sardines as well as in walnuts and flaxseeds, are also great at improving insulin sensitivity and also supporting an increase in leptin levels related to meal fullness.[66]

Choosing foods like lentils, black beans, kidney beans, green peas, barley, and oats also gives you a hefty dose of resistant starch. This starch digests slowly, increased fat-burning by 20 percent in one study, and prompted the release of fullness-signaling hormones that resulted in study volunteers consuming 320 fewer calories a day—without actually *trying* to eat less.[67] Thankfully, resistant starch is easy to get when you're eating clean. You can even swap some resistant-starch–rich flours, like potato, whole grain, bean, and green banana flour and some high-fiber, non-GMO corn flours, for some of the refined white flour in baked goods. And you can increase the amount of resistant starch in some carbs—like pasta and potatoes—by letting them cool after you cook them. (Reheat before you eat them, of course!)

High-fiber foods may help with hormones in a surprising way, too: Because they require more chewing, they force you to eat more slowly, and slower eating has big metabolic benefits. In one study from Athens University Medical School, people who took 30 minutes to eat a snack saw levels of appetite-controlling hormones GLP-1 and peptide YY rise 20 to 30 percent higher than they did for people who wolfed down the same snack in 5 minutes.[68] And in a 2015 study from Texas Christian University, people who ate breakfast slowly (taking 30 minutes) were less interested in eating more an hour later than those who rushed through their morning meal.[69]

#4: Retrain your cravings. Cravings are super common—97 percent of women and 68 percent of men experience them every week.[70, 71] But wouldn't it be great to crave mangoes and asparagus instead of corn chips and cupcakes? With clean foods, you can. In a fascinating Tufts University study, 13 overweight people had brain scans before and after a 6-month period of a weight loss program or no intervention and eating their usual way. The scans showed brain activity when the volunteers saw photos of high-calorie junk foods and low-calorie nutritious foods. The reward center in participants' brains lit up at the sight of the high-cal food on the first scan. But afterward, the dieters' brains were more stimulated by the healthy foods,[72] showing evidence for the brain to change around the food reward system.

#5: Slower digestion. It stands to reason that when food moves through your digestive system more slowly, you feel full for longer. And that's exactly what happens when you fill your plate with produce, whole grains, and lean protein. In fact, having these foods on board even slows digestion of less-healthy stuff you might be eating at the same time. Now that's teamwork!

NURTURE YOUR "GOOD BUGS"

You're not alone! Right now, you've got 100 trillion bacteria living in your digestive system. Most of us are familiar only with these tiny critters' embarrassing habit of releasing smelly gas at the wrong moments, but the truth is, your gut bugs are intimately involved with your weight.[73] There's growing evidence that the right mix of bacteria in your intestines can help you make healthier food choices and stay slim, while the wrong mix encourages weight gain and a taste for junky processed foods.[74]

When researchers from the Washington University School of Medicine carefully checked the types of bacteria found from the digestive systems of 154 people, they found that those who were obese had the smallest variety of gut bacteria.[75] A lab study with mice from the same team found that having more of a type of bacteria called Firmicutes may be related to weight gain. These bugs are great at sucking more calories out of food—digesting complex sugars that other bacteria can't and converting them into simple sugars and fatty acids that get absorbed from your intestines into your bloodstream.[76] In contrast, having more of a type of bacteria called Bacteroidetes has been associated with a slimmer physique.

Gut bugs help control your weight in several ways, research suggests. Some send more calories into your body, where they're likely to be stored as fat. But that's not all. Scientists from New York University Langone Medical Center have found that the bacteria *Helicobacter pylori* is involved in the regulation of certain hormones, including the hunger hormone ghrelin. While nobody wants an overabundance of *H. pylori* (it can cause painful stomach ulcers), the researchers note that the widespread use of antibiotics has reduced levels of *H. pylori* and could be making weight loss more difficult. In a 2011 study of 92 people published in the journal *BMC Gastroenterology,* those who were prescribed antibiotics to knock out *H. pylori* (due to digestive-system problems) also saw ghrelin levels rise sixfold after the bacteria were completely eliminated.[77] And in a recent Yale University lab study in mice, researchers found that a fatty acid called acetate, which is pumped out by gut bacteria, increased eating behaviors. The elevated release of acetate also increased production of ghrelin and of insulin, a key blood sugar control hormone that also promotes the storage of body fat.[78]

FEED THE SLIM BUGS

The big news about the microbiome (the catchall name for your personal bacterial "zoo") is that what you eat can help determine which bacteria gain the upper hand in your digestive system. Change happens quickly when you change your diet—and can go either way depending on what you eat. For example, when 21 people increased their daily intake of fiber by 21 grams, they had more Bacteroidetes and fewer Firmicutes in their systems after 3 weeks, according to a University of Illinois at Urbana-Champaign study published in the *American Journal of Clinical Nutrition.*[79] Bacteria, especially the good guys, love munching on the fiber found in abundance in clean foods like fruits, vegetables, and whole grains.

But loading up on processed junk food takes things in the other direction in a hurry. In a headline-grabbing study, a British genetics professor asked his college-student son to munch nothing but fast food for 10 days. The son's microbiome was checked at Cornell University and the British Gut Project, using stool samples, before and after. In just 10 days, his microbiome was "devastated" by the steady diet of burgers, chicken nuggets, fries, and soda, according to an informal report from his father published on the British science Web site TheConversation.com. Forty percent of the bacterial species in his gut were wiped out—a loss of 1,400 types. "I felt good for 3 days, then slowly went downhill, I became more lethargic, and by a week my friends thought I had gone a strange grey color," the son noted.[80] When the study ended, he rushed to the supermarket for fruit and salad.[81]

While the young man didn't gain much weight during the 10-day study, his

(continued on page 28)

STEVE B. *and* JENNY S.

TOTAL POUNDS LOST IN 6 WEEKS

STEVE:

22 lbs

JENNY:

7 lbs

TOTAL INCHES LOST

STEVE:

13"

JENNY:

5"

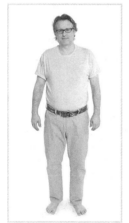 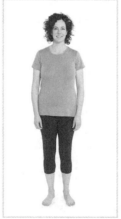

BEFORE

Steve and Jenny were already familiar with eating clean, and they ate that way some of the time. Jenny says, "I didn't have a terrific amount of weight to lose. But I was at my highest weight, and even the fat pants weren't fitting. So it was really more of a shift of focus."

Before they started on the program, the couple would sometimes have nutritious foods like beans or kale. But living in New York City, they also tended to dine out a lot with friends—which meant that their meals were often heavy on the bread, pasta, and wine. Portion control was another big issue. Steve used to eat spoonfuls of peanut butter, treating it like ice cream, without thinking twice. And he'd help himself to some chocolate almost every day.

After committing to eating clean, the couple quickly learned what counted as a reasonable serving size. Now Steve serves himself a tablespoon of peanut butter and pairs it with an apple. And they figured out how to make the plan work with their social life. Now Jenny orders salmon and lentils with a side of Brussels sprouts for dinner and skips the extras that she realized were making her bloated and puffy. When Steve goes to his friend's house for dinner, he brings ingredients to make a salad that the group can enjoy alongside their spaghetti and meatballs.

It's that kind of flexibility that makes the couple feel like they could eat this way for life. "I don't think I could fall out of this, because I know I can even go to a diner and get two poached eggs, some whole wheat toast, and berries. I don't have to do anything special," Steve says. "You should just call this the Easy Diet."

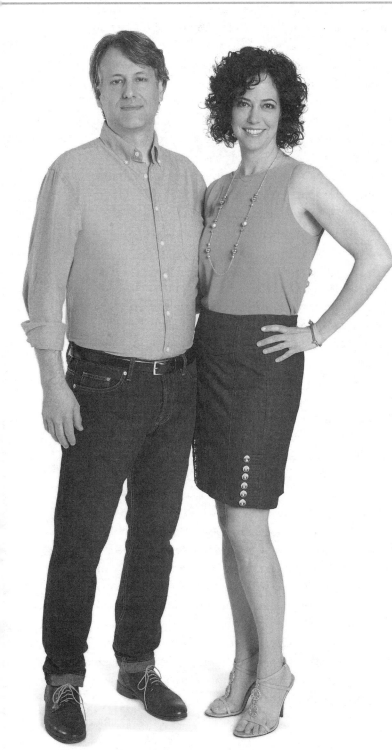

Dr. Wendy Observes:

People often tell me that an active social life makes it harder to make healthy choices, and at times, that can certainly be true. But as Steve and Jenny discovered, having a plan, a partner, and some know-how makes it easier—especially with a bit of practice. Plus, the fact that Steve's itchy skin and chronic heartburn were completely gone within days of starting the program is tremendously motivating and helps him continue to make healthy choices. And the plan's flexibility with guidelines helped both of them succeed individually, as well as together.

father commented that the shift in gut bacteria could lead to that over time. "Loss of diversity is a universal signal of ill health in the guts of obese and diabetic people," he noted.

There are clear-cut differences in the ways clean foods and processed foods affect your microbiome—and by extension, may affect your weight. Here are a few examples, all backed by science.

Fiber feeds the good guys. One science magazine calls it the "workhorse" that feeds "a healthy gut microbiome."[82] Your good bacteria love all sorts of fiber, but two especially beneficial types—*Bifidobacteria* and *Lactobacilli*—love fibers called fructans, especially a type called inulin.[83] You'll find inulin in plant foods including bananas, onions, garlic, leeks, asparagus, Jerusalem artichokes, chickory root, soybeans, and whole grain foods like rye and barley. In other research, people who ate whole grains such as whole wheat bread saw an increase in beneficial *Bifodobacteria*, while those munching refined wheat products saw levels decline.[84] You'll get plenty of good-for-you natural fiber from food when you eat clean. In fact, experts call fiber a "prebiotic"—a compound that primes your digestive system for optimal good-bug health.

Probiotic-rich foods invite more good bacteria in. Yogurt, kefir (a fermented milk drink), and fermented foods such as sauerkraut, kimchi, and tempeh (a soy-based meat alternative) all contain beneficial bacteria. Case in point: Yogurts that contain "live, active cultures" contain good bacteria including *Lactobacillus gasseri*, shown in at least two recent studies in animals to discourage weight gain and even help with weight loss.[85] That's why you should only buy yogurt that says right on the label that it contains live, active cultures. And yes, these bacteria can survive your digestive system and thrive. Evidence of this comes from research on people who've taken antibiotics, which can wipe out some good bacteria. Those who had yogurt daily cut their risk for antibiotic-related diarrhea by two-thirds.[86]

Good fats favor good bugs, too. A diet rich in omega-3 fatty acids—found in fatty fish like salmon and trout, as well as in walnuts and flaxseeds—fostered a mix of gut bacteria that kept mice slim in a recent University of Gothenburg study.[87] In contrast, a diet packed with saturated fat in the form of lard encouraged bacteria that caused weight gain. That's a great reason to grill salmon instead of a fatty steak for dinner tonight! While this was a lab study on mice, results like these can spark or stem important lessons for humans, too.

Artificial sweeteners feed obesity bugs. In a 2014 lab study from Israel's Weizmann Institute of Science, mice fed aspartame, sucralose, or saccharin developed a microbiome strikingly similar to that of obese mice.[88]

The researchers note that in some studies, people who used artificial sweeteners were more likely to be overweight and have impaired glucose tolerance than those who didn't—and differences in their microbiome may explain this difference.[89]

GET ENERGIZED!

Giving your body the nutrients it needs, stopping the exhausting cycle of blood sugar peaks and valleys that comes with eating processed foods, and sweeping chemical additives out of your system—that's a fatigue-fighting, metabolism-boosting recipe for renewed physical and mental energy! And the more energy you have, the easier it is to make healthy, clean food choices and to be more active all day, whether that means taking a morning Zumba class, getting outside for a lunchtime stroll, or jumping on your exercise bike while you watch television at home tonight.

Feeling tired is a top reason Americans skip exercise and make less-than-stellar food choices, surveys reveal.[90] And too often, processed food bears some of the blame. As you'll read later in this book, highly-processed, low-nutrient food makes it more difficult to fall asleep, stay asleep, and wake up refreshed—a huge energy drain. Unhealthy, high-fat stuff can also make you more tired in a matter of minutes after a meal. In a 2013 Pennsylvania State University study, participants who ate the most fat at lunch felt the sleepiest afterward.[91] According to another study published in the *British Journal of Nutrition*, a high-fat meal significantly reduced mental energy (alertness and sustained attention), compared to a lower-fat meal.[92] It turns out that eating fat triggers the release of a digestive hormone called cholecystokinin that lulls your brain into a foggy slump that scientists call "postprandial somnolence." (That kind of sleepiness can quickly lead to a midafternoon trip to the vending machine for a cola and a candy bar!)

In contrast, clean foods support high energy. Start with breakfast. In one study, people who ate a whole grain cereal felt 10 percent less fatigued than usual.[93] In another, people who ate protein in the morning felt 12 percent more alert at midmorning and 18 percent more alert by lunchtime than people who skimped on this important metabolism-boosting nutrient.[94]

MAKE OVER FOR GREAT HEALTH

HERE'S A SCARY STATISTIC: More than half of the calories in the typical American diet come from "ultraprocessed" foods—stuff like baked goods, chicken nuggets, fish sticks, hot dogs, instant noodles, energy bars, and many canned and packaged soups.[1] As you've read, it's bad news for your waistline—and even worse news for your health. There's no doubt about it: Research demonstrates that processed foods and the typical American diet are closely linked with a higher risk for diabetes, high blood pressure, heart disease, and high cholesterol—and even with cancer, depression, and chronic pain.

The antidote? Clean food, of course. A cornucopia of scientific research shines a spotlight on the body-wide benefits of reaching for fiber-rich produce, whole grains, lean meats, good fats, healthy dairy products, and even dark chocolate every day!

Clean eating can help you prevent or control some of the most disabling and deadly health problems confronting America in the 21st century. At the same time, it can help you sleep better, help you feel more energetic, and boost your mood.

Let's take a minute to check in and see how you're feeling while you read this. Are you wide awake or kind of tired? Relaxed or tense? Content or cranky? No matter your answers, chances are they have a lot to do with whatever you've eaten today. Enjoyed a bowl of oatmeal with chopped nuts and fresh fruit? You might be bright-eyed, bushy-tailed, and ready to tackle whatever comes your way. Went for the giant cinnamon bun, instead? Exhausted and frazzled may be your mood du jour.

You know that old phrase "You are what you eat"? It's usually used to make the point that you'll have a healthy, lean body if you eat mostly healthy foods and a not-so-healthy, not-so-lean body if you eat mostly unhealthy ones. But the foods that make up the majority of your diet can also help determine your mood, stress level, and overall sense of well-being. In other words, your food affects your external, internal, and emotional health.

Physically, you are what you eat. But in a way, you also feel what you eat. And when you feel good, you're more motivated to make smart choices that support your health and weight loss, such as taking the time to cook a clean meal instead of ordering pizza, or heading outside for a walk instead of watching your favorite TV shows all night. Sure, those might sound like small choices that don't matter much in the grand scheme of things. But it's the little decisions like these that, over time, form the healthy (or not-so-healthy) habits that end up determining your weight.

Of course, no one's saying you have to be perfect. We all have those days where there's zero time to cook dinner and the mere thought of doing yoga is too exhausting to contemplate. As long as those days are the exception instead of the rule, you don't need to worry. Your goal is to focus on making choices that foster wellness—and healthy weight loss—most of the time. One of the most effective ways to do that? You guessed it. It's by eating clean.

Eat to Your Heart's Content

Heart disease. It's the leading killer of women and men in America, taking 610,000 lives each year. Behind that scary statistic, tens of millions more of us are at risk. According to the Centers for Disease Control and Prevention, half of all Americans have at least one major risk factor for heart disease, such as high blood pressure or high cholesterol levels.[2] That sounds formidable, but did you know that clean food can help reduce your heart disease risk by a whopping 80 percent if you also exercise regularly, don't smoke, and lose a few pounds?[3]

That's right—and that's the power of prevention. The same clean food that helps raise your metabolism, trim your waistline, and take off pounds can also tackle America's leading killer and all of the nasty risk factors behind it.

Perhaps no study highlights the real-world benefits of choosing clean foods more than a recent look at 30 years of diet and heart-health data for 84,628 women and 42,908 men. The study, conducted by researchers from the Harvard T. H. Chan School of Public Health and published in the *Journal of the American College of Cardiology,* found that people who swapped just 5 percent of the calories they'd been getting from saturated fat (found in butter, fatty meats and dairy products, and plenty of processed foods) with the same amount of a healthier fat (such as the kind found in nuts, olive oil, and fatty fish) or from whole grains saw their heart disease risk fall by as much as 25 percent.[4]

But people who swapped saturated fat for refined carbs (by reaching for an extra cookie because they skipped the cheese on their sandwich at lunch, for example), had the same heart disease risk as people who kept on eating saturated fat. "People who choose refined carbs and sugars instead of saturated fat, thinking they're making a healthier choice, are not doing themselves any favors in terms of heart health," one study author noted in a Harvard news story with the headline "Butter is Not Back."[5]

The exciting news is that every element of clean eating works together to pamper your heart and your arteries by doing the following:

Lowering LDL cholesterol. LDLs are the "lousy" cholesterol that contributes to the fatty, foamy, nasty plaque that can narrow your arteries or cause an aneurysm. Soluble fiber in whole grains, fruits, veggies, and legumes grabs extra *LDLs* from your digestive system and whisks *them* out of your body when you have a bowel movement. This is a great reason to enjoy soluble fiber all-stars such as oats, barley, and every type of bean (red, white, black, navy, pinto . . . you get the idea), as well as sweet, juicy pears and plums and satisfying winter squash and parsnips.

Boosting HDL cholesterol. Helpful *HDLs* act like garbage trucks, picking up extra *LDLs* and hauling *them* away. The good fat in walnuts is especially adept at supporting healthy HDL levels.

Soothing your blood pressure. Your body needs plenty of the minerals calcium, potassium, and magnesium to regulate blood pressure. Skimping can make pressure levels climb—especially if you're eating too much sodium-packed processed food. In the landmark Dietary Approaches to Stop Hypertension (DASH) study, 70 percent of people with high blood pressure who ate lots of produce and got calcium from their diets saw their blood pressure fall to healthier levels.[6]

Clean food also helps soothe blood pressure by making weight loss easy. According to experts, our systolic blood pressure may fall by as much as 1 or 2 points for every 2.2 pounds you lose.[7] In one small study, women who lost just 5 percent of their weight (that's 8 pounds, if you weigh 160) saw blood pressure fall 7 points. Blood tests show that levels of hormones that drive up blood pressure fell from 30 to 40 percent.[8]

Pampering your arteries. Clean food can help keep artery walls flexible and healthy, making them less likely to pick up plaque or to constrict, raising blood pressure. Bright orange winter squash, as well as leafy greens like spinach, for example, provide lutein. This natural plant compound helps reduce chronic inflammation and keeps arteries supple.[9]

Cooling off body-wide inflammation. Processed foods and deep belly fat can increase levels of inflammation in your body. Inflammatory compounds increase the amount of plaque in artery walls and can also make plaque burst, causing heart attacks and strokes. A recent study of more than 2,500 people from Greece's Harokopio University of Athens revealed that adults who followed a Mediterranean-style diet filled with (you guessed it!) produce, whole grains, good fats, and lean protein were 47 percent less likely to develop heart disease over a 10-year period. Why? This way of eating cools inflammation and also helps control high blood pressure and diabetes.[11]

THE POWER OF ONE

Eating one small apple or another small serving of fresh fruit every day can reduce risk for a deadly heart attack by one-third, according to an Oxford University study of a half-million people.[10]

Walnuts, flaxseed, canola oil, and fatty fish like wild sardines, wild salmon, and trout are terrific sources of inflammation-cooling omega-3 fatty acids.[12]

This natural way of eating may help you out even if you take medications to protect your heart. In a European study of 197 people, male participants taking cholesterol-lowering statins and other medications for heart disease, a healthy diet (along with regular exercise and quitting smoking) reduced their 5-year risk for a heart attack by an additional 22 percent.[13] And in a different study, when people whose blood pressure wasn't responding to medication reduced their sodium intake by cutting out salty processed foods and eating foods like fruits, veggies, whole grains, and lean protein, their systolic and diastolic blood pressures dropped an average of 22 and 9 points, respectively, without adding more drugs or increasing doses.[14]

Defeat Diabetes

If you're among the nearly 28 million Americans with type 2 diabetes or the 86 million with prediabetes, keeping tabs on balancing blood sugar control is a top priority.[15] Diabetes and prediabetes don't just mess with blood glucose levels. They also raise your risk for heart disease and complications like vision loss, kidney damage, and circulation problems.

The typical American diet—full of white bread and sweets made with refined grains, burgers, fried potatoes, and soda—could boost your odds for a prediabetic condition called metabolic syndrome by at least 18 percent, according to a shocking University of Minnesota study published in the journal *Circulation*.[16] It followed more than 9,000 people for nearly a decade and found that munching two or more daily servings of meat, especially processed stuff like bacon and hot dogs, boosted risk by 26 percent. A fried food habit raised it by 25 percent.

Metabolic syndrome is an important but all-too-often overlooked marker for future diabetes—it quadruples your risk![17] Consult your doctor about the possibility of metabolic syndrome if you have at least three of these warning signs.

1. A wide waistline—more than 35 inches for women or 40 inches for men.
2. High triglyceride levels—over 150 mg/dl. These blood fats can be a heart disease risk factor, but high levels can also be a sign of metabolism changes that raise risk for type 2 diabetes.
3. Low levels of HDL cholesterol—under 40 mg/dl for men or under 50 mg/dl for women.

4. High blood pressure—130/85 or higher or taking blood pressure medications.
5. High fasting blood sugar—100 mg/dl or higher.

Prediabetes is another serious risk factor for diabetes. It increases your odds for developing full-blown diabetes by 5 to 10 percent every year.[18]

Here's where clean food comes to the rescue! The proof? Look no further than the headline-grabbing Diabetes Prevention Program (DPP), a government-backed study of people with prediabetes. The program's healthy diet, which focused on fiber-rich fruits, vegetables, and whole grains and limited amounts of saturated fat from fatty meats and other sources, slashed risk for diabetes by 58 percent.[19] One key: People on this plan, who also exercised, lost 5 to 7 percent of their body weight and thereby improved insulin sensitivity. Their bodies responded better to insulin, the hormone that tells cells to take in blood sugar. Weight loss—easier than ever when you reset your metabolism with clean foods—made a big difference. For every 2.2 pounds lost on the program, people lowered their risk for developing diabetes by 16 percent.[20]

Clean foods work hard to improve insulin sensitivity for easier blood sugar control whether you're trying to prevent or manage diabetes. Some exciting examples of clean foods that improve insulin sensitivity include:

- **Leafy greens.** Adding an extra 1½ servings of green leafy vegetables to your diet each day—that's just a small side salad with your lunch or a big helping of sautéed kale or spinach at dinner—could cut your diabetes risk by 14 percent, according to a British study from the University of Leicester.[21] The fiber in greens may help your body absorb food carbohydrates and sugar more slowly and help with weight loss. But researchers also suspect that magnesium and small amounts of alpha-linolenic acid (ALA) in greens may help with healthy blood sugar processing, too.
- **Whole grains.** Harvard T. H. Chan School of Public Health researchers who tracked the diets and health of more than 161,000 women for up to 18 years found that those who munched just two servings of whole grains a day (like a bowl of steel-cut oats for breakfast and some brown rice with dinner) were 21 percent less likely to develop diabetes compared to those who ate fewer daily servings of whole grains.[22]
- **Good fats.** From avocados and nuts to olive oil and dark chocolate, foods that contain monounsaturated fats have been shown to improve insulin

sensitivity.[23] In a recent Tufts University analysis of 102 studies involving 4,220 people, researchers found that replacing one daily serving of saturated fat (like a slice of cheese or a fatty hamburger) or of refined carbohydrates (like a slice of bread) with a small amount of good fats—for example, one-quarter of an avocado, a small handful of nuts, or a tablespoon of peanut butter—could reduce diabetes risk by an impressive estimate of 22 percent.[24]

We hear a lot about processed foods, but what about processed *drinks*? Loaded with sugars or artificial sweeteners, beverages like soda, store-bought tea, fruit punch, sports drinks, and even specialty coffee drinks could increase your risk for diabetes. Sweetened drinks send blood sugar soaring. All those extra calories can pack on pounds that tax your body's ability to process blood sugar. Meanwhile, the fructose found in high-fructose corn syrup and in other sweeteners may interfere with insulin sensitivity.[25]

But switching to zero-calorie and low-calorie artificial sweeteners could backfire, more and more research shows. In that University of Minnesota study, people who sipped one can of diet soda each day were 34 percent more likely to develop metabolic syndrome compared to those who avoided diet soda. Why? A lab study from Israel's Weizmann Institute of Science suggests a connection: These chemicals may change the balance of digestive-system bacteria in ways that lead to glucose intolerance (difficulty processing blood sugar).[26]

Healthy sips do make a difference. In one study from the United Kingdom's University of Cambridge, researchers kept tabs on 25,639 people for 10 years.[27] They concluded that swapping one sugar-sweetened drink a day for water or unsweetened tea or coffee could lower risk for type 2 diabetes by 14 percent. Skipping artificially sweetened drinks could lower your odds by as much as 11 percent.

Ease Pain

Let's be honest. Food, on its own, does not cause or cure chronic pain. But compelling research suggests that what you eat could play a role in helping to control a wide variety of chronic pain conditions that 114 million Americans cope with every day.

CLEAN FOOD TO THE RESCUE

Talk about the power of fruits, vegetables, and other whole, unprocessed plant foods! Thirty-seven people with osteoarthritis of the knee followed their regular diets or switched to a plant-based diet in a recent Michigan State University study published in the journal *Arthritis.* The plant diet featured plenty of produce, whole grains, and protein-rich beans (legumes like navy and pinto beans), no animal products, and almost no refined or processed foods. After 6 weeks, the plant-based group reported more energy and easier day-to-day functioning.[28]

One big component of the diet/pain connection is weight. For people with painful osteoarthritis of the knee, gaining just 10 pounds puts an extra 30 to 60 pounds of added force on already-achy knee joints with every step they take. Carrying extra weight also raises your risk for lower-back pain, tension and migraine headaches, fibromyalgia, abdominal pain, and chronic widespread pain.[29] So it's no surprise that losing weight eased aches significantly in one University of Cincinnati study of people with back pain, elbow pain, hip pain, and all-over pain.[30]

When British and Canadian researchers surveyed 8,572 people about their lifestyle habits and pain levels for a study published in the journal *Pain Research and Management,* diet emerged as a factor.[31] Women who said they were eating fewer fruits and vegetables than they used to were more likely to have chronic, widespread pain. Being overweight or obese increased the odds for pain that lasted 1 day or longer by 50 to 80 percent, too.

Reduce Cancer Risk

It's America's leading health fear. Cancer ranked ahead of Alzheimer's disease, heart disease, diabetes, and stroke as the disease people worried about most in one nationwide survey conducted by the polling group Harris Interactive.[32] With good reason: One in eight women will develop breast cancer, one in seven men will develop prostate cancer, and about one in 20 adults will receive a diagnosis of colorectal cancer.[33]

Science continues to debate the importance of diet in cancer prevention, but this much is clear: For many cancers—including the ones that strike most often—what you eat makes a difference. And once again, clean eating rises to the top of the list of preventive measures you can take.

In 2013, researchers from the United Kingdom's University College London published the results of a study that tracked the eating habits and health of 65,226 people for 7½ years. The result? Eating five or more daily servings of fruits and vegetables was associated with 25 percent lower cancer mortality.[34] Why? It could be that plants contain a rainbow of protective compounds that discourage cancer from forming, growing, and spreading, or it could be the way produce helps you reach and maintain a healthy weight.

According to the renowned American Institute for Cancer Research, no single food can fight cancer. It takes a team. But when you put together a great plate, meal after meal, the nutrients in produce, good fats, beans, whole grains, and lean protein work together. But that's not all: Clean foods also aid in the battle against cancer by helping keep you leaner. Research shows that extra body fat can boost the risk for 11 types of cancer—including those of the breast (for postmenopausal women), colon, kidney, liver, pancreas, and prostate.[35] In fact, obesity may be responsible for 130,600 cancer cases every year.

Cancer is a complex disease. A growing stack of research reveals the many ways that clean foods rise to the occasion when it comes to cancer protection, fighting this killer disease on all fronts.

Broccoli, cabbage, kale, and other cruciferous vegetables. These veggies contain compounds called isothiocyanates that may protect against cancer by slowing down cell growth and reducing cancer-fueling inflammation.[36]

Whole grains. Undigestible fibers in whole grains seem to protect against colon cancer by feeding the good bacteria in your digestive system, which in turn produce compounds called short-chain fatty acids that prompt potentially cancerous cells to self-destruct.[37]

Coffee. Java has both chlorogenic and caffeic acid, which may activate the body's antioxidant defenses to protect cells from DNA damage that could trigger cancer. Coffee also contains compounds called kahweol and cafestol, which seem to neutralize some cancer-causing substances. One to two cups a day cut the risk for colorectal cancer by 25 percent in one University of Southern California (USC) Norris Comprehensive Cancer Center study published in the journal *Cancer Epidemiology Biomarkers & Prevention*.[38]

* * *

"I have more energy, less stress, and I'm happy that I'm doing something for *myself.* I'm definitely going to continue eating clean because now I know I can do this."

—MARYANN L.

Blueberries, blackberries, raspberries, and strawberries. Sweet, luscious berries like these contain compounds called phenols that lead cancer cells, in lab studies, to self-destruct.[39] Ellagic acid in berries may also protect the DNA in healthy cells from damage that can lead to cancer.

Cooked tomatoes (such as in a sauce, soup, or quick sauté). Cooked tomatoes provide plenty of lycopene, a carotenoid that one recent Harvard Medical School study found that higher consumption was linked with a 9 percent lower odds of developing prostate cancer and with a 28 percent reduced risk of fatal prostate cancer.[40] Lycopene seems to help by inhibiting the growth of blood vessels that deliver oxygen and fuel to tumors, slowing down cancer growth.

Fish. Good-for-you omega-3 fatty acids found in fish cool inflammation, which can fuel cancer growth if left to flourish. Men with the highest blood levels of omega-3s were linked to a 25 percent lower risk for prostate cancer than those with the lowest levels.[41] In women, those who ate the most fish high in omega-3s were associated with 14 percent lower risk for breast cancer than those who had the least in an analysis of 21 studies involving 883,585 people, published in the *British Medical Journal.*[42]

Eat for Energy

Once you have the right tools (like this book!), you'll find that the principles behind making over your metabolism, losing weight, and keeping it off are pretty simple. But putting them into practice *does* take more effort than you'd expend hanging out on the couch and ordering takeout. You don't have to spend hours in the kitchen, but you do need to devote some time to thinking about what you'll eat, shopping for your ingredients, and prepping clean meals and healthy snacks. You don't have to train to become a marathon runner, but you do need to find ways to move more.

All of that stuff requires energy, and if you're used to eating the standard

American diet, you might not feel like you have all that much of it to spare. When it comes to the nutrients that keep your body fueled and your mind focused, processed foods are a veritable wasteland. To make matters worse, they're brimming with the sugar and refined carbs that practically guarantee exhaustion and brain drain. Skeptical? Try subsisting on sugary granola bars for a day or two and see how you feel. Or take science's word for it: Sugar actually inhibits neurons in your brain that promote feelings of wakefulness, according to British findings published in the journal *Neuron*.[43] No wonder that afternoon candy bar always ends up leaving you feeling even fuzzier than you did before you peeled back the wrapper.

With clean foods, it's just the opposite. Fiber-rich complex carbohydrates and lean proteins get digested more slowly than their processed, refined counterparts, so you stay revved for longer and don't end up crashing. And whole foods are rich in important nutrients, including magnesium, iron, and vitamin B$_{12}$, all of which are essential for helping you feel energized. The bottom line? When you eat clean, you have more oomph to tackle your day—and to put in the work needed to meet your weight-loss goals. Certain nutrients play particularly important roles in staving off sluggishness. Pay attention to these three biggies to increase your focus and fight fatigue.

IRON

Why it matters: Your red blood cells need this mineral to transport oxygen throughout your body, and when you don't get enough, you can end up feeling foggy, weak, and even out of breath.

Aim to get: 18 mg daily for women under age 50, 8 g daily for men and women over age 50

Find it in: Oysters, lean beef, sardines, non-GMO soybeans and tofu, lentils, beans (kidney, lima, black, and pinto), clams, and spinach

MAGNESIUM

Why it matters: Your body relies on magnesium to convert food into energy, as well as for proper muscle function. Fall short, and even basic activities like carrying a bag of groceries can feel harder.

Aim to get: 320 mg daily for women, 420 mg daily for men

Find it in: Halibut; almonds, cashews, and other nuts; peanuts; black beans; spinach; avocado; milk; whole grains; and dark chocolate

VITAMIN B$_{12}$

Why it matters: Vitamin B$_{12}$ plays a role in building the red blood cells that transport oxygen throughout your body, and too little will leave you weak and foggy-headed. Since the vast majority of plant foods don't naturally contain B$_{12}$, vegetarians and vegans should take extra care to meet their needs. Look for fortified foods or consider taking a supplement.

Aim to get: 2.4 mcg daily for women and men

Find it in: Clams, fatty fish, canned light tuna, lean beef, dairy foods, eggs, nutritional yeast, fortified nondairy milks, and fortified cereals

Beat the Blues

There's no doubt that an ice cream cone or a plate of freshly baked chocolate chip cookies will put a smile on your face. But that kind of happiness, while worthwhile, is only temporary. If you were in a crummy mood before you treated yourself to a scoop of rocky road, chances are you'll go back to feeling rocky yourself after the last lick. But sometimes, that can be tough to remember—since in the moment that you're eating it, junk food can make you feel terrific. That's because loading up on sugar or refined carbs activates the reward system in your brain, prompting it to pump out megadoses of the pleasure hormone dopamine.[44]

Of course, all good things have to end sooner or later. The problem with pounding back the junk food is that once you stop, the dopamine release shuts down. You're left wondering why the party ended—and craving more junk to get the good times going again. It might've taken a brain scientist to understand exactly how the process works, but it doesn't take one to figure out that that sort of habit could end up leaving you pretty moody—not to mention on a constant hunt for your next sugar fix.

Clean foods are free of the added sugars and refined carbs that send your dopamine levels into overdrive. But that doesn't mean that they can't make you happy, too! By delivering a steady source of energy and keeping

My Metabolism Makeover

* * *

"Before I would get my period, I'd have bad PMS. I don't have that now. No mood swings, nothing. I'm going to keep eating clean. It's a no-brainer."

—GIGI D.

you off the emotional roller coaster, clean foods work to keep your mood nice and steady. Sure, the highs might not be as extreme as the highs that come from eating sugary, processed foods, but the lows won't be as low, either. What's more, research suggests that eating clean can actually lead to greater happiness overall. One Australian study of nearly 14,000 people found that those who ate nine or more daily servings (about 6 cups or more) of fruits and vegetables reported feeling more satisfied with their lives compared to those who consumed less.[45] People also report feeling calmer, happier, and more energetic on days when they eat fruits and vegetables, according to findings published in the *British Journal of Health Psychology*.[46] It all sounds pretty nice, right?

Do This Now!

Why not start harnessing the feel-good powers of fruits and vegetables right now? Think about how you can amp up the produce power of each of your meals and snacks for the rest of the day—and reap the benefits of happier, more even moods. (Or do it tomorrow, if you're reading this before bed.) How about two kiwifruit instead of a brownie with lunch? The carbohydrates will boost your brain's production of the feel-good hormone serotonin while the fiber promotes a steady, even mood. What about some nuts at snack time, or sprinkled on top of a salad? Almonds, cashews, and peanuts are top sources of magnesium, which promotes feelings of calm. Can you do a juicy orange or some crunchy broccoli florets with your dinner? Both are rich in folate, a vitamin that's linked to lower rates of depression.

Bust Stress, Big-Time

You know that tense, frazzled feeling that makes you want to run straight for something comforting, like a frosted doughnut or a gooey, melty bowl of mac and cheese? Of course you do. Scarfing down junk is a pretty normal response to feeling anxious or stressed—and at some point or another, we've all done it. But it won't help you relax for long, and it definitely won't help you lose weight!

Eating clean can actually help keep stress—and the snack-crazy urges that often come with it—at bay. When you eat foods that aren't packed with refined sugars and carbs, you avoid the extreme blood sugar spikes and dips that can leave you feeling moody, irritable, and ready to reach for the cookie jar. In fact, research shows that eating a diet based on whole, unprocessed foods is associated with lower risks for both anxiety and depression, while sticking to a Western-style diet of processed or fried foods, refined grains, and excess sugar is linked to risks for both conditions.[47]

That's important, because once you get tangled up in the vicious cycle of sugar and stress, it can be tough to find your way out. Say you're at the corner deli, planning to get a turkey-and-veggie sandwich on whole wheat with a side salad for lunch. As you're waiting in line, you get an e-mail from your boss asking if you can send over that report by the end of the day instead of by the end of the week. You immediately feel frenzied and start eyeing the bologna sandwich on white bread and side of creamy macaroni salad that the guy in front of you just ordered. Because stress makes it harder to exert self-control—even when you *want* to make healthy choices—you cave and copy his order. You'll get that more nutritious combo you had actually planned on tomorrow.

As you're inhaling your meal, your boss sends *another* e-mail asking you for a status update, ASAP. Now you're in full-on anxiety overload. Your body's levels of the stress hormone cortisol start surging, which sends your body right toward storing fat. If that's not bad enough, all of that unspent cortisol leaves you feeling ravenous and desperate for anything made with sugar and white flour. So you grab a giant chocolate chip cookie before running back to the office, thinking it will calm your nerves and help you plow through the crazy amount of work you now have to take care of.

At the end of what turns out to be a very long day, you finally hand in the finished report. Exhausted, you pick up a container of greasy stir-fry for din-

DR. WENDY SAYS . . .

If losing weight feels like one *more* thing to worry about, try shifting your perspective a little bit: While stress is inevitable, you have in your possession one simple tool that's proven to help you feel less frazzled—and that's eating clean. Eating real, balanced meals on a regular schedule keeps your blood sugar steady so you stay focused and energized. Plus, planning clean meals and snacks in advance saves you time—not to mention the anxiety of scrambling to figure out what's for dinner every night. So close your eyes and take a few deep breaths. (Really—try it now!) Don't you feel better already?

ner. Thanks to who-knows-how-much sugar in the stir-fry sauce and a mountain of white rice, your energy crashes half an hour after dinner and you fall asleep without even putting on your pj's. In the morning, you wake up totally frazzled, so you grab a sugary blueberry muffin at the coffee shop. So starts another day.

For many of us, these sorts of scenarios happen all the time. And of course, no one's saying that eating quinoa and salmon can stop stressful situations from happening. But picking clean foods over processed ones *can* help your moods stay more even. That way, when life throws you the inevitable curveball, you can remain (somewhat) calmer—instead of flying off the handle and reaching for the candy bowl.

Feel a case of the crazies coming on? Resist the urge to nix those nerves with an empty-calorie snack, and try one of these clean, calming picks, instead.

SWAP: A CANDY BAR FOR 1 OUNCE OF DARK CHOCOLATE.
Findings suggest that the flavonoids in dark chocolate could keep levels of the stress hormone cortisol from spiking during tense times, while cocoa may help lower your blood pressure.[48] For the most phytonutrients and the least amount of added sugar, stick with dark chocolate that's at least 80 percent cacao.

SWAP: POTATO CHIPS FOR 1/4 CUP OF ROASTED, SALTED CASHEWS.
Both are rich, salty snacks. But cashews pack the mineral selenium and the amino acid tryptophan, both of which can elevate your mood. (As for potato chips, we don't need to remind you that they're practically devoid of nutrition, right?)

SWAP: COOKIES FOR A MEDIUM BANANA.
An all-carbohydrate snack ramps up your brain's production of the feel-good hormone serotonin within minutes of consumption, so you start to feel calmer—stat. And sure, cookies are loaded with carbs, but they don't offer

(continued on page 48)

RICHARD *and* SUZANNE M.

TOTAL POUNDS LOST IN 6 WEEKS

RICHARD:

21 lbs

SUZANNE:

4.5 lbs

TOTAL INCHES LOST

RICHARD:

8.75"

SUZANNE:

4.25"

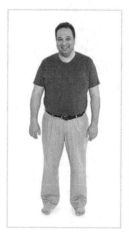
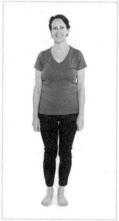

BEFORE

Travel and weight loss aren't exactly known for going hand in hand. And traveling to a place that's renown for some of the most delicious food in the world? Impossible.

But that wasn't the case for Richard and Suzanne, who already had a vacation in Italy planned before they decided to start eating clean. Instead of just taking time off from their weight-loss goals, they decided that they'd enjoy themselves without letting their trip turn into a week-long pizza-and-pasta binge. And the proof is in the results they reaped by sticking with the program.

For breakfast, they'd usually stop at a local grocery store for fresh fruit. "We never once missed having a big breakfast, and it allowed more time to get out and tour," says Suzanne. For lunches or dinners, they'd order what they wanted—but in a way that made it easy to keep their portions in check. "We didn't binge on pasta or bread. We tried to balance our meals," she says. Instead of ordering two appetizers and two pasta dishes, Suzanne would get a grilled vegetable dish and Richard would get pasta. Then they'd split the two plates.

The couple also made trade-offs by skipping the stuff they didn't care about that much; that way, they had room for the foods they really loved. For instance, they'd always pass on the bread basket at mealtimes. And since Richard and Suzanne aren't big drinkers, they didn't bother with wine or cocktails. But Suzanne, who's always loved sweets, *did* treat herself to delicious gelato made from high-quality ingredients.

In fact, after realizing how delicious simple meals made with fresh, quality ingredients could be, Suzanne was inspired to re-create at home many of the produce-centric dishes she and Richard enjoyed in Italy. These days, they're eating tasty foods sparked by their travel memories, like cabbage and bean soup, minestrone soup, and even homemade pasta with fresh sauces. "Now, eating clean just seems like common sense," Richard says.

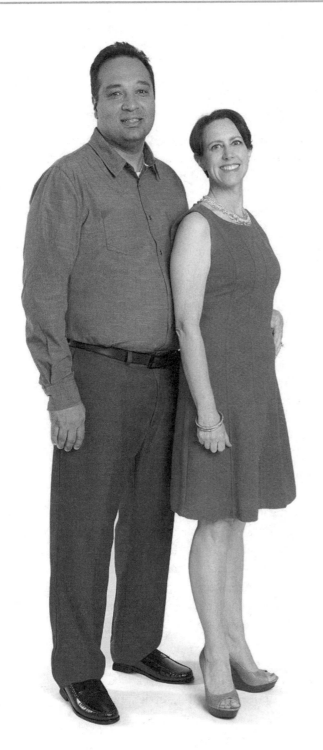

RICHARD: His systolic blood pressure (the top number) dropped by 24 points and his diastolic blood pressure (the bottom number) dropped by 11 points, bringing both out of the high blood pressure range. His LDL ("bad") cholesterol dropped by 17 points, bringing him from borderline high to just 4 points outside of the desirable range.

SUZANNE: She used to crave sugar on a daily basis, but now her taste for sweets has started to disappear.

Dr. Wendy Observes:

Richard and Suzanne are a testament to the fact that travel can be exciting, delicious, and still supportive of your health. They turned what had been a potential obstacle to their weight-loss progress into a major success, complete with great food, memories, and even new recipe inspirations for their clean-eating lifestyle. It's proof of how much you can achieve in virtually any life situation—without deprivation!

much else. Eat a medium banana, instead, and you'll get the same chill-out benefits, plus fiber (to slow digestion and keep you happy longer) and loads of potassium.

Sleep Soundly

Nearly half of all Americans say that they regularly struggle to get enough quality sleep.[49] If you're one of them, listen up: You might not realize it, but the way you eat has a major impact on how much—and how well—you snooze. And the better rested you are, the easier it is to reach or maintain a healthy weight. Want proof? When Harvard researchers followed some 60,000 women for nearly 2 decades, those who regularly slept for fewer than 5 hours per night were 32 percent more likely to gain 30 or more pounds compared to those who regularly slept for 7 or more hours.[50] When it comes to getting lean, sleep is *that* important.

Even so, the relationship between sleep and weight is complicated, and experts still have a lot to learn about how the two are connected. What does seem to be clear, though, is that a steady stream of highly processed, inferior food can make it harder to get the quality sleep you need. Research published in the *Journal of Clinical Sleep Medicine* found that people who eat diets high in sugar and refined carbs tend to take longer to fall asleep and wake up more frequently during the night.[51] Meanwhile, unhealthy fats could negatively affect your body's normal sleep–wake cycle, making it harder to doze off at night and wake up refreshed in the morning.

In part, that's because staying up later can seriously impact your ability to make choices that can help you get leaner. When you're zonked, you simply have less energy for things like shopping for fresh food, preparing clean meals, or even exercising. To make matters worse, running short on shut-eye makes it harder to resist junky snacks. In fact, one *SLEEP* study found that sleep deprivation cranks up the pleasurable effects of salty, sugary, and fatty foods.[52] And to top it all off, when you don't get enough sleep, your body prompts you to eat *more* calories and burn *fewer* of them. If that's not an ugly recipe for spending countless unproductive hours watching TV and eating sugary snacks, nothing is.

There's more to it, though. Eating clean doesn't just pull you out of the cycle of eating junk food, sleeping poorly, and then eating more junk food because you're sleep-deprived. Clean foods actually deliver the nutrients your body needs to sleep *better*. Research shows that people with adequate levels of vitamin D—found in foods like eggs, mushrooms, fortified milk, and fatty fish—are 33 percent less likely to experience insomnia than those with insufficient levels of this nutrient.[53] And speaking of fatty fish, some findings suggest that the omega-3 fatty acids found in fish like tuna and salmon can contribute to a better night's rest.[54] (So far, the research has been conducted on kids, but it's likely that adults would reap similar benefits.[55]) Your body relies on potassium (found in foods like sweet potatoes and bananas) and magnesium (found in foods like avocados, nuts, and seeds) to help your muscles relax so you can drift off to dreamland sooner. And it needs the calcium in foods like plain yogurt and leafy greens in order to produce the hormone melatonin, which tells your body when it's time to feel sleepy. (A few foods, including tart cherries and walnuts, actually *contain* melatonin.) With all of that in mind, it might not come as much of a surprise to learn that people who eat diets high in fiber-rich foods, like many of those just mentioned, report getting deeper, more restful sleep than their processed-food-eating counterparts.[56]

Ready to stop counting sheep? Pick an evening snack that helps you drift off to dreamland sooner, like one of these. Enjoy it 2 to 3 hours before going to sleep, since eating too close to bedtime can disrupt your sleep.

- **4 whole grain crackers topped with ¼ cup of cottage cheese.** Cottage cheese is rich in protein, which your body needs to make the sleep-promoting amino acid tryptophan. And crackers have carbohydrates, which boost tryptophan's availability to your brain.

SLEEP YOUR WAY SLIM

Getting enough sleep doesn't just promote the kind of clearheaded thinking that helps you pick salmon over a bacon double cheeseburger or a handful of nuts instead of a handful of candy. Adequate sleep appears to play a role in keeping your metabolism humming along at a healthy rate, so you burn more calories. When University of Pennsylvania researchers tracked the metabolic rates of unlucky subjects who were limited to just 4 hours of sleep for 5 nights, they found that the subjects burned about 42 fewer calories per day than they did when they weren't sleep-deprived.[57] At that rate, a week of poor sleep could cause you to burn nearly 300 fewer calories—the equivalent of a breakfast of a creamy bowl of oatmeal with nuts and fruit. That's right! You can actually earn more calories just by making it a point to get more snooze time. Next time you're tempted to stay up and watch another hour of TV, remember your metabolism makeover goal—and hit the hay.

- **8 ounces of tart cherry juice.** Tart cherries are a top source of melatonin, the hormone responsible for regulating your sleep–wake cycle. Plus, research shows that tart Montmorency cherries can help people with insomnia sleep longer—and better.[58]

- **10 walnut halves.** Like tart cherries, walnuts contain melatonin—and eating them has been shown to increase levels of the hormone in your blood, according to a study in *Nutrition*.[59]

- **Half a slice of whole grain toast with 1 tablespoon of almond butter.** Both deliver magnesium, which can offer protection against insomnia and sleep-disrupting leg cramps.

- **8 ounces of low-fat milk.** Many of us struggle with getting enough calcium and vitamin D, but these nutrients can reduce your odds of having trouble falling asleep and staying asleep. Milk is one of the few foods that serves up *both*.

- **A cup of chamomile tea.** This naturally sweet herbal sipper has long been used to promote feelings of calm and relaxation. Plus, it's calorie-free, so it can help you doze off even if you've already reached your snack limit for the day.

Reap Big Beauty Benefits

You know those days when you wake up and something just feels off? Maybe your skin is starting to break out, or your hair seems dull and lifeless. Or you feel weirdly bloated, and the jeans that always look good suddenly *don't*. Deep down, you know this kind of stuff is small and short-lived and that you shouldn't let it bother you. But often, it still does. So you head out the door feeling sort of down about yourself—and those negative feelings start to affect the decisions you make throughout the day. You're already feeling a little yucky, so why bother taking a walk or making healthy food choices?

When you make clean foods the mainstays of your diet, you're getting more of the important nutrients that can help you look your best—think clearer, more radiant skin; bouncier, shinier hair; and even a flatter, bloat-free belly. The sugar, refined carbs, and sodium abundant in highly processed foods can actually ramp up sebum production and promote breakouts, not to mention that it can cause water retention that can leave you feeling puffy. Overdoing it on the sweet stuff could be particularly bad because too much sugar can make your skin duller and more wrinkled. That's thanks to a process called glycation, where the sugar in your bloodstream attaches to proteins to form harmful new products called advanced glycation end products (or—appropriately—AGEs, for short). AGEs do damage

to collagen and elastin, the protein fibers that keep skin firm and elastic. And the more sugar you eat, the more AGEs develop.

Eating clean can help fight *all* of this stuff. Fruits and vegetables pack powerful phytonutrients that keep sugar from attaching to proteins, helping your skin stay smooth and supple instead of turning tired or lifeless. Whole foods boost your beauty in other big ways, too. Fresh produce, whole grains, and nuts are all brimming with beta-carotene, iron, zinc, vitamin C, and B vitamins that can strengthen your hair follicles. Yogurt, raw sauerkraut, artichokes, and onions deliver probiotics and prebiotics that help promote good digestion and keep uncomfortable bloating at bay. And animal findings suggest that the good bacteria play a role in protecting skin against the sun's harmful UV rays and even stimulate the growth of healthier, shinier hair. [61]

In other words, clean foods are beautifying foods that can help jump-start a sort of feel-good feedback loop. When you're already happy with what you see when you look in the mirror, you're more likely to feel motivated to do *more* of the good-for-you things that can help you lose weight.

For a radiant, more healthful complexion, make an effort to work more of these foods into your meals and snacks.

For a Radiant Glow: Carrots, Sweet Potatoes, Pumpkin, and Butternut Squash. Orange fruits and vegetables get their bright hue from the antioxidant beta-carotene. And when you eat these foods, findings show that they can quite literally give dull, sallow complexions a brighter, sun-kissed appearance—minus the UV-ray exposure.[62]

For Younger-Looking Skin: Avocados, Walnuts, Flaxseeds, and Chia Seeds. The monounsaturated fats in avocados and omega-3 fatty acids in walnuts, flaxseeds, and chia seeds play an important role in helping your

(continued on page 54)

GIGI D.

TOTAL POUNDS LOST IN 6 WEEKS

7.5 lbs

TOTAL INCHES LOST

6.5"

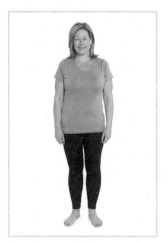

BEFORE

Want proof that eating clean can lead to amazing changes? Just look at Gigi. After several weeks of eating clean, a friend called her up at 6:30 in the morning to invite her on a 17-mile bike ride. Feeling energetic, Gigi decided to go. "Before that, the last time I [rode a bike], I was 10 years old! And it was *not* for 17 miles. So that was huge," she beams.

Huge, indeed. Gigi had been taking steps to eat better for about 9 months before fully committing to eating clean. She started getting serious about eating as much organic food as possible. She had wine or sugar only once in a while. She even made sure to bring clean food to social events like holidays and birthday parties so she always had something delicious to eat.

"I really was very careful with what I ate," she says. But for Gigi, going from pretty clean to squeaky clean was exactly what she needed. The sugar cravings that used to plague her at night disappeared. Her mind felt clearer. And her moods were consistently positive instead of up and down, as they had often been before.

What's more, she's sticking with her new habits. "If you want to be healthy, this is how you should be eating," she says. "It's really not a program, it's not a diet. It's a way of life."

MOST NOTABLE IMPROVEMENTS

Eating clean gave Gigi a major energy boost. Her moods were more even-keeled, too, even before her period, when she would usually deal with mood swings.

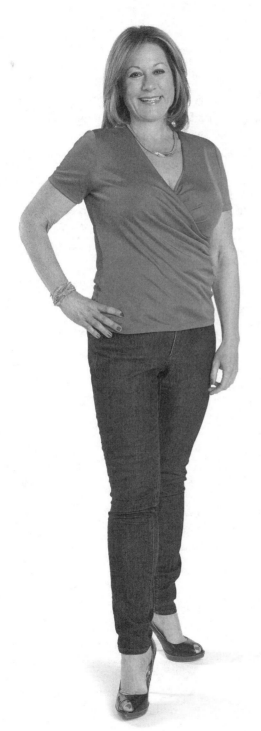

Dr. Wendy Observes:
Surprising things can happen when you start eating clean! Your mood shifts and you just might turn back the hands of time to tap some youthful energy you didn't realize you had. Small shifts paid off for Gigi in ways that she didn't expect. Sure, she lost weight and inches, which was great. But to engage life with a more positive, vibrant outlook? That's a reward worth seeking!

skin stay hydrated. As a result, skin looks smoother and more supple, and it shows fewer fine lines. Monounsaturated fats, too, are essential for the creation of healthy skin cells.

For Extra Sun Protection: Coffee, Green Tea, Grapes, Tomatoes, and Ginger. At first glance, these foods and drinks might not seem to have much in common. But *all* of them deliver dermis-friendly phytonutrients that can both help protect against future and fight existing damage and inflammation caused by the sun's UV rays. (They won't replace your sunscreen, though, so keep applying it daily!)

For Healthy, Nourished Skin Overall: Kiwifruit, Strawberries, Blueberries, and Oranges. All of these are rich in vitamin C, an essential nutrient that speeds wound healing, prevents easy bruising, and staves off dryness. It also aids in the production of the protein collagen, which helps skin stay firm and elastic.

MAKE OVER YOUR WEIGHT LOSS

EATING CLEAN IS ALL ABOUT giving your body the nourishment it needs to thrive, boost your metabolism, and shed excess weight. And in order for your body to work optimally, you have to listen closely to what it's telling you. That's where mindfulness comes in. By tuning in to your hunger, your emotional state, and even your cravings, you can learn how to make clean choices that are right for you. And that can play an important role in helping you get the maximum enjoyment from your food, feel great about what you eat, lose weight, and keep that weight off—for life.

What Is Mindful Eating?

Mindfulness is a bit of a buzzword these days, so you may have heard of it. But what exactly does it mean? In short, being mindful means paying attention. You can walk mindfully by focusing on your surroundings—the sound of birds chirping or the people around you—instead of staring at your phone. You can have a mindful conversation by listening closely to what the other person is saying instead of only thinking about what you'll say next. You can even fold the laundry mindfully by homing in on the fresh scent and soft feel of your freshly dried towels.

In short, you can perform practically any activity with mindfulness—including eating. When you eat mindfully, you pay closer attention to your food. How does it look on your plate? How does it taste and smell? How does it feel in your mouth? More importantly, you zero in on how your food makes you *feel*. Are you physically hungry, or do you just feel like eating because you're bored or stressed? Are you eating until you feel satisfied, or are you polishing off everything on your plate just because it's there? Do you feel content and energized after you eat, or do you feel sluggish or guilty?

Mindful eating is the part of losing weight—and keeping it off—that takes *you* into account. At this point, you're likely convinced that the best way to lose weight is by following the principles of clean eating. But mindfulness is the awareness that helps you figure out *how* to make those things work for you. Do you stay fuller after eating a breakfast of cornflakes and fruit or after a vegetable omelet? Do you really need a handful of almonds to satisfy your hunger in the afternoon, or do you just reach for them out of habit? Does splurging on two cookies leave you feeling crabby and stuffed, and if so, can you enjoy that same treat more fully by having only one cookie? When you're mindful of the way you eat, you uncover the answers to these questions. In turn, you get the maximum amount of enjoyment out of your food—and you learn how to approach food in a more balanced way. That can add up to more pounds lost—and kept off for the long term.

How Mindful Are You?

As you work to make more conscious food choices, it can be helpful to know where you're starting from. To find out, read each one of these statements and check off how many of them apply to you. After completing the *Your Metabolism Makeover* plan, you can revisit this list to see just how much progress you've made.

☐ When I'm stressed out or overwhelmed, I basically eat whatever I want.

☐ Once I start eating junk, I keep eating because I've "already blown it."

☐ I tend to give up on healthy-eating goals when I'm busy or have a lot going on in my life, waiting until sometime I think will feel right to start.

☐ Sometimes I have a plan in place to eat well, but other times, I have no strategy at all.

☐ What people might think or say about me sways my food choices.

☐ I keep myself busy with food when I'm bored.

☐ Sometimes I eat when I'm putting off doing something else.

☐ Eating helps distract me from how I'm feeling. It calms me and comforts me when I'm stressed, sad, or anxious.

☐ When I celebrate something, I usually eat larger amounts and more indulgently.

☐ I make better food choices in the morning and worse choices at night.

☐ I spend a decent amount of time worrying about my weight, appearance, and eating habits.

☐ I often eat while I'm checking e-mail, watching TV, or doing work.

☐ I typically finish everything on my plate.

☐ I often have intense cravings for unhealthy foods, to the point where I think about those foods continuously.

☐ I often eat most of my food for the day in one sitting or over the course of a few hours.

☐ I couldn't tell you what I ate for breakfast 2 days ago.

☐ I regularly binge eat, or consume too much food in one sitting, to the point where I feel uncomfortable or ill.

Getting Rid of Good and Bad

Many of us tend to think of food in black-and-white terms. If you eat a salad or a bowl of oatmeal, you're being good. If you eat a slice of pepperoni pizza or a cinnamon roll, you're being bad. And though you might think that that kind of mind-set would help you make better choices, it can often do the exact opposite. When you eat something that you think is "bad," you likely end up feeling shameful and guilty. As a result, you throw in the towel and start making rationalizations. Since you already blew your diet, you figure that you might as well keep on overeating for the rest of the day. Or, just as unproductive, that you need to make up for it tomorrow by being extra good—which is often code for eating the foods that are lowest in calories, not necessarily the ones that are the most nutritious. It's this cycle of guilt that tends to be the downfall of most diets.

When you practice mindfulness, though, you learn to enjoy your food without feeling guilty, so you're less susceptible to the cravings and binges that can throw you off the clean-eating wagon. Foods are no longer good or bad, and they aren't grounds for reward or punishment. Instead, *all* foods sit on a spectrum of more nutritious to less nutritious and more clean to less clean to highly processed—and there's no judgment over what's on your plate. Sure, you can still have a slice of pie for dessert sometimes. But since it's on the less healthful side of the spectrum, it's better to have something more nutritious, like fruit, *most of the time*. And when you *do* have your pie, you take the time to really enjoy the way it tastes and smells, and even how it feels in your mouth. Mindfulness lets you walk away from the table feeling content instead of guilty, and satisfied instead of stuffed.

DR. WENDY SAYS . . .

What is it about mindfulness that seems to help the pounds melt off? Let us count the ways!

I. It helps you take in fewer calories. When you start paying closer attention to your hunger and fullness signals, you'll probably start to eat less. Plus, when you start paying attention to how different foods make you feel, you'll start to naturally gravitate toward cleaner, leaner options rather than their processed counterparts.

2. It improves your relationship with food. By becoming aware of the nonhunger feelings that trigger you to eat, you can take steps to change how you respond to those situations. And that can make eating a less emotionally charged event.

3. It makes you feel good about your food choices. When you eat according to your true hunger and stop when you're full, you'll probably feel less deprived and learn how to enjoy the foods you love without feeling bad about eating them. By taking the guilt and anxiety out of eating, you'll be able to satisfy your hunger, enjoy your meal, and move on.

What You Want versus *Whatever* You Want

When you decide to eat mindfully, you're making choices about what and how to eat based on what your body wants. At first, mindfulness might sound like a woo-woo name for chowing down on chips and ice cream whenever the mood strikes. But eating what you want and eating *whatever* you want, *whenever* you want it, are not the same thing. And as you start to make mindfulness the name of your clean-eating game, you'll learn to tell the two apart.

Practicing mindfulness is about learning to tune in to your feelings—both physical and emotional—to figure out what it is that you really need and how to meet that need in a healthy way. Sometimes, that might mean treating yourself. But most of the time, it means eating the clean, wholesome foods that help fuel you. And when you pay attention, you'll become familiar with the difference.

For example, if you're hankering for a candy bar at 3:00 p.m., being mindful means that before you hit the vending machine you pause to ask yourself, *Am I actually hungry for chocolate right now, or am I really just running low on energy?* Chances are, the real answer is that you're in the middle of an afternoon slump and you can get the boost you need from drinking some water, eating a piece of fruit or a handful of nuts, or taking a quick stretch break. Or perhaps you just heard some good news and want to celebrate with a cupcake. Being mindful means realizing that you're still full from lunch or have some delicious apples in the refrigerator. This momentary pause can help you clarify that in the long run, you'll feel much better if you celebrate with a manicure than with a short-lived infusion of sugar.

Here are some ways to focus on what we eat and why to help you change your habits and patterns.

> **Your Metabolism Makeover**
>
> ∗ ∗ ∗
>
> **"As we age, our bodies don't need all the food we've been programmed to eat. When I get the urge to eat [for reasons other than hunger], I remind myself that it's not necessary. This program is rewiring my thoughts about food."**
>
> **—GEORGE S.**

ASK, AM I *REALLY* HUNGRY?

Do you sometimes find yourself eating out of stress, boredom, or loneliness? Or, on the flip side, because you're happy or downright giddy? Don't worry, you're not the only one. At some point, most people have been driven to eat for emotional reasons that had absolutely nothing to do with how empty—or full—their stomachs were. But learning to listen to your appetite—and in particular learning (or *re*learning) your true hunger cues—is the cornerstone of eating clean to boost your metabolism and lose weight.

Hunger is your body's way of saying that you're running low on energy and need to start thinking about fueling up. Unlike the other feelings that can drive you to eat, hunger comes with some distinct physical sensations that are pretty obvious. When you're hungry, your stomach feels empty and hollow. The hungrier you get, the stronger that feeling becomes. And when you get *really* hungry, you might also start to feel light-headed or shaky, or you might have trouble concentrating.

Your goal is to eat when you're hungry, not starving. Not only does getting *too* hungry feel terrible, but it also increases the risk that you'll eat too much food and sometimes even make unhealthy choices. So when's the right time to eat? The next time you think about wanting to have a certain food, ask yourself if you'd also be up for eating fruits or veggies. If the answer is yes, then you're genuinely hungry, and you should eat. If the answer is no, you probably aren't physically hungry, and you should hold off on eating. Instead, reach for a cup of hot tea, which can quell your urge to nibble on something.

FOCUS ON YOUR FOOD

You know how food always seems to taste more delicious when you're hungry? Well, it's true: Eating after you've worked up an appetite will go a long way toward helping you get the maximum amount of pleasure out of your food— whether it's your regular lunchtime Creamy Chicken, Green Grape, and Farro Salad (page 137) or a decadent slice of devil's food cake. But paying more attention to what you're eating also goes a long way toward helping you feel more satisfied, so it takes less food to fill you up and you're less tempted to scrounge around for more after getting up from the table.

Of course, paying attention to your food doesn't mean doing something crazy like talking to your chicken breast. It just means making your meal or snack the main focus—and taking the time to *really* enjoy it. Here are three simple ways to do just that.

- **Eat sitting down.** You might tell yourself that the calories in that bite of pasta or handful of crackers don't count if you're standing up, but they do. Plopping yourself at the kitchen table, the counter of your local sandwich shop, or even on a bench in the park can help you acknowledge that you're eating an actual meal or snack. And that in and of itself can make you less inclined to start noshing again in an hour or two.

- **Ditch the distractions.** TVs, phones, computers, and books (even this one!) all count as distractions. Make eating the main event instead of eating while you do something else—and home in on the flavor, texture, aroma, and appearance of your food. Chances are, you'll feel satisfied sooner than if you ate with your eyes glued to a screen or a page.

- **Slow down.** This isn't a race! Eating at a more relaxed pace gives your body time to release fullness-signaling hormones that tell you when you've had enough, and those hormones are key to weight loss. Research shows that when people at a healthy weight eat their meals slowly, they take in fewer calories and feel fuller for longer, compared to when they eat their meals quickly.[1] Sure, it's tough to always make eating a leisurely event—but try to devote *at least* 20 minutes to meals as often as you can.

ZERO IN ON YOUR TRIGGERS

A lot of us have foods that we can't stop eating once we start. Typically, these foods tend to be high in sugar, fat, or salt—or, very often, a combination of all three. Throughout most

WHAT'S *YOUR* TRIGGER?

Keeping a food journal is one of the most effective ways to become more aware of your triggers. If you're consistent, journaling can help you pinpoint the emotions that trigger you to eat and the specific foods that you like to reach for. That can help you figure out what tends to prompt you to eat mindlessly—and to avoid those triggers in the future.

Every night or after every meal, write down what you ate along with at least three adjectives to describe how you felt at the time. Try to be as descriptive as possible. For instance, instead of just writing *angry,* maybe you write *frustrated, sad,* or *overwhelmed.* Digging deeper helps you learn more about how you're feeling—and helps expose the triggers that cause you to overeat so you can start figuring out other ways of dealing with them.

Of course, remember to write about the good stuff, too! Jotting down the small victories or what you're doing well can encourage you to keep doing it.

(continued on page 64)

GEORGE S.

**TOTAL POUNDS LOST
IN 6 WEEKS**

11.5 lbs

TOTAL INCHES LOST

4"

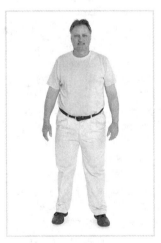

BEFORE

George had always been a self-described food addict who loved sugary treats and letting loose at happy hour on Friday night. But as he got older, he realized that his free-for-all eating style could be putting his health at risk. (Not to mention that many of his clothes no longer fit.) Having lived with type I diabetes for 40 years, the 58-year-old knew that he needed to start building better habits if he wanted to be around for his children as they began starting families of their own. "I'm in pretty good shape. But as I get older, I have to work harder and harder to stay there," he acknowledges.

Transitioning to cleaner meals and snacks wasn't always easy. A business owner, George had a tendency to get lost in his work and skip meals. When he finally remembered it was time to eat, he'd usually just order something from the deli for lunch or dinner. So he started packing clean lunches, dinners, and snacks to take to work, and he made an effort to eat every couple of hours to avoid getting too hungry. "I told myself, you have to focus on good meals. So I'm stopping [my old habits] and this is what I'm doing," he resolves.

Eating smaller portions came with a learning curve. George had long been used to eating or drinking what—and as much as—he wanted, whenever he wanted. But soon after starting on the plan, he realized that he didn't need as much food as he had thought. George also confessed that sometimes he'd eat out of habit, not because he was actually hungry. "I realized I actually don't need to eat as much as my 24-year-old son," he says. "I'd be watching golf on TV and think that I should be having chips. Then I'd think, no, I don't really need that. I'm good."

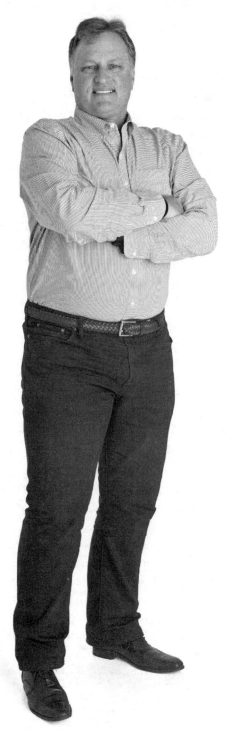

Dr. Wendy Observes:
Sometimes it's hard to break out of certain eating habits when you're successful and productive in other areas of your life, such as work. But George realized that something had to change. And once he gave clean eating with smaller portions and regular timing a real try, he discovered that he could have success in work and weight loss, too.

of human history, these kinds of calorie-dense foods were tough to come by, and we evolved to binge on them when we found them in order to avoid starvation. Unfortunately, our brains haven't caught up with the fact that we now live in an environment where binge-worthy fare is available 24/7. So it's no surprise that once you start munching on chips or cookies, it can be really hard to stop.

That doesn't mean we're completely powerless against the lure of sugary, fatty, high-calorie treats. Often, the compulsion to eat junky stuff is triggered by something completely unrelated to food, such as stress at work, a fight with your spouse, the loneliness of coming home to an empty house, boredom, or sheer exhaustion. Or it could just be a habit: Maybe you're used to eating a bowl of pretzels while you watch your favorite show. Or maybe you would eat ice cream for dessert growing up, so you get the urge to have a scoop whenever you visit your parents.

The point is, we each have our own triggers—and it doesn't really matter what your specific ones are. If they happen regularly and prompt you to eat for reasons other than hunger, they can lead to mindless overeating and weight gain. But simply becoming more aware of your triggers and the effect that they have on you can actually help you deal with them in a healthier way.

ORGANIZE YOUR KITCHEN

Have you heard people joke that they're on the *see-food* diet? You know, where they see food—and then they eat it? Turns out, there's some truth behind this funny play on words. Findings show that when food is in our visual path, we actually *are* more likely to eat it. Of course, that can spell bad news when you're trying to lose weight. (If the first thing you see when you open your pantry is a box of cookies, you'll be pretty tempted to eat it.)

However, the see-food thing can work to your advantage to help you make *cleaner* choices, too. All it takes is know-how in the kitchen. Here are five simple steps that can have a significant impact on what you do—and don't!—decide to eat.

Declutter those counters. On your countertop, swap sugary or processed snacks for a bowl or basket of fresh fruit. Women who keep things like potato chips, cereal, or soda on their counters tend to weigh more than women who don't, according to one study. And those who keep fruit on their counters tend to weigh *less*.[2] Opt for fruits like apples, oranges, bananas, pears, apricots, and peaches, which ripen best at room temperature. (They're also pretty, so they practically serve as a decoration for your kitchen.)

Reconfigure your fridge and pantry. Make fruits and vegetables more visible by moving them up to the shelves instead of storing them in the crisper, and store less-healthy items on the bottom shelves or toward the back of the fridge. In your pantry, put the healthy grains, dried fruits, and other clean staples front and center, and push sweets and treats toward the back. Better yet, if you have the space, store special-occasion treats in a less-visible space altogether, like another drawer or cabinet that you don't open often. When food is out of sight, it's more likely to be out of mind.

Designate a clean-eating snack drawer. Just like you have your own closet and drawer space for your clothes, it's perfectly reasonable to designate a drawer or two for yourself in the kitchen. Having your own space means that you'll only see *your* snacks when you open the drawer, not any of the more tempting stuff that might be stocked in the pantry for other members of your family.

Rethink your serving dishes. Consider rearranging your cupboards to put the smaller dishes, bowls, and cups right up front; that way, you'll get into the habit of reaching for them when it's time to eat. We serve ourselves more when we use bigger cups, plates, and utensils, and research shows that we eat 92 percent of what we serve ourselves—regardless of how hungry we are.[3]

Keep the kitchen for cooking and eating. Cook and prep in your kitchen, and eat sitting down at the kitchen table. (No spoonfuls over the sink or loitering in front of the fridge. Small bites add up!) Chat, play, or work in another part of your home. If your family tends to congregate at the kitchen table even when it isn't mealtime, consider setting up another gathering spot. A desk or a small table in your family room is a good spot to be together while going through the mail, doing homework, or flipping through magazines.

FIND NONFOOD REWARDS

Remember how foods that are high in sugar, salt, and fat activate the reward center in your brain? Negative trigger emotions cause you to seek out those highly processed foods—often without even thinking about it!—because they make you feel good. But eating a brownie won't actually solve whatever problem you're dealing with, and the happy feeling it gives you disappears as soon as you've polished off the last bite. And to make matters worse, it's usually replaced with guilt over eating something junky.

When you become aware of your triggers and the foods that they drive you to eat, look for ways to reward yourself without food. Think about the feeling you need to achieve to get past your trigger, then brainstorm ways to get that feeling without eating. Say your commitments have you booked all day and you're being asked to fit in one more thing. Notice if this stress makes you crave a sweet treat. You can't change the craving, but you *can* change how you react to it. Instead of reaching for that snack, start a new habit, like taking a 5-minute walk when you feel a craving. Not only will the walk boost your levels of feel-good hormones, it will also give you time to get some air, gather your thoughts, and come up with a game plan for fitting the new commitment in or finding someone to help you with it. Or skip the walk and get into the habit of reaching out to a friend for support when you feel stress-related cravings creeping up on you.

Of course, you can harness the power of nonfood rewards for smaller situations, too. If you're just feeling tired, do some jumping jacks to boost blood flow to your brain instead of popping a piece of chocolate into your mouth. When you want a quick mood boost, watch a video of a kitten doing something silly. Need a temporary escape when you just can't deal? Keep a novel in your bag and read a couple of pages rather than snacking.

COPE WITH CRAVINGS

If you've ever experienced the sudden, intense desire to devour a hot slice of pizza or indulge in a fudgy brownie, you know that cravings can be pretty tough to resist. You should definitely enjoy treats once in a while. But when you're plagued by overpowering urges to eat those kinds of foods every day, it can get in the way of your weight loss.

Clean foods can help keep cravings in check because they're free of the refined carbs and added sugars that send your blood sugar on a roller-coaster ride and drive you to eat more junk food. Still, even the cleanest eater isn't entirely immune to cravings. We're often surrounded by delicious, easy-to-access food—everything from the doughnuts in the office break room to the free chip-and-dip samples at the grocery store to the well-meaning neighbor who brings over a frozen dinner that was buy one, get one free. Sooner or later, temptation is bound to happen. And when it does, mindfulness can help you keep a clear head: Reminding yourself of the fact that you're in the throes of a craving and aren't actually *hungry* can often be enough to snap you back to reality.

(continued on page 70)

YOUR CRAVINGS Rx

Got chocolate and curly fries on the brain? That could be a sign that you're among the 90 percent of Americans missing out on at least one important vitamin or mineral. While a blood test is the only sure way to diagnose a nutrient deficiency, cravings can sometimes be a red flag. Here's a list of six common nutrients that are tough to get enough of and some tips on how to eat to beat the cravings they cause.

CALCIUM AND MAGNESIUM

Craving: Sweet or salty
Food fix: Make it a point to get more calcium from plain Greek yogurt, milk, or leafy greens. Get more magnesium from almonds, spinach, edamame, or avocado.

B VITAMINS

Craving: Sweet or salty
Food fix: B vitamins are found in many foods, but in varying quantities and combinations. Eating the following would give you a good mix: animal protein (such as poultry, lean beef, or salmon), yogurt, green veggies, beans, lentils, sweet potatoes, winter squash, sunflower seeds, avocado, and bananas.

ZINC

Craving: Sweet or salty
Food fix: Only certain proteins, such as oysters, crab, liver, and dark chicken meat, are high in this mineral. It's found to a lesser extent in eggs, black beans, cashews, and oatmeal.

IRON

Craving: Fatty meat
Food fix: Beef, poultry, and fish have the most absorbable iron, but you can also increase your levels by eating dried fruits, cashews, pumpkin seeds, legumes (such as soybeans, lentils, and garbanzo beans), leafy greens, and iron-enriched pastas and grains. Boost your absorption of plant-based iron sources by eating them with vitamin C–rich foods such as citrus fruits, kiwifruit, berries, broccoli, or bell peppers.

OMEGA-3S

Craving: Cheese
Food fix: Focus on fatty fish, such as salmon, sardines, and canned tuna, as well as plant sources, such as walnuts, flaxseeds, and chia seeds.

MARY PAT S.

**TOTAL POUNDS LOST
IN 6 WEEKS**

9 lbs

TOTAL INCHES LOST

7.5"

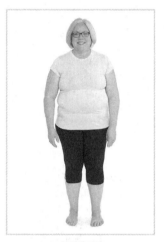

BEFORE

As a self-described emotional eater, Mary Pat was quite literally used to eating whenever the mood struck her. Eating clean not only helped her learn to tell the difference between her hunger and her cravings, but it also helped her find a daily rhythm for her meals and snacks that kept her from ever getting overly hungry.

"I felt like I had a lot of knowledge in my head about nutrition and what's healthy for you. But I wasn't able to sync it up with my actions," she says. Since she woke up to see her teenage daughter off to school, Mary Pat was used to eating breakfast early. She'd usually start to feel hungry by midmorning, but she'd try to hold off on eating. As a result, she'd be ravenous by lunchtime and would often end up overeating. "When I started following a schedule and having my morning snack, I noticed that what I ate for lunch satisfied me," she says.

Mary Pat reinforced the regular eating schedule by taking time to pause and fully enjoy her snacks. "I'd have a pumpkin ball [see page 114] or some walnuts and tart cherries with a cup of herbal tea, and it was very satisfying," she says. Often, she'd even picture the hot water from the tea causing the nuts, seeds, or whole grains to expand in her stomach, which helped her feel fuller.

And when the urge to nosh off-schedule did strike? She'd try to respond with her head instead of her heart. "In the evening, when I'd be most likely to want to snack, I'd tell myself, *You know you just ate dinner. Those growls from your stomach are just digestion, not hunger*," she says. "It worked like a stop-pause for me."

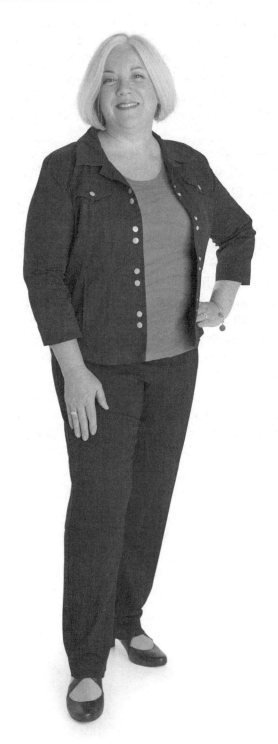

Dr. Wendy Observes:
Learning to differentiate between hunger and cravings can seem overwhelming, especially when you're prone to energy ups and downs that come from eating on an irregular schedule. I like to remind clients like Mary Pat to use their intellect as well as their emotions (*both* matter) and remember that often, we really do confuse healthy digestive sounds and rumblings with hunger. It's important to simply pause to consider that possibility before choosing to eat. Learning about balanced timing and snacks helped Mary Pat have foods ready to go and stable energy to make smart decisions about eating.

Try some of these ways to curb a craving.

Take a walk. A quick bit of exercise can help slash stress, reducing your urge to eat. And it doesn't take much: Walking for just 15 minutes can curb cravings for sugary snacks, according to one Austrian study.[4] Before you give in, take a brief stroll around your neighborhood and see how you feel.

Get distracted. Call a friend. Check your e-mail. Grab a magazine or book. Your brain can only juggle so much stuff before it forgets about that cupcake, so take advantage.

Use your nose. Keep a vanilla or green apple candle around and give it a sniff when a craving strikes. Smells that are sweet but that don't remind you of specific junky foods are thought to help curb appetite.

Imagine yourself indulging—a lot. Thinking repeatedly about eating the thing that you're craving might be enough to make you want it less, according to research published in the journal *Science*.[5] Visualize yourself enjoying the experience, and then move on.

Just have a small taste. You might find that it's all you really wanted, anyway. Eating less than half an ounce of chocolate or potato chips satisfied subjects' cravings just as well as eating a portion as much as 10 times bigger, according to one Cornell University study.[6] (Unless the food you're craving is a trigger for you. If it is, it's probably better to have it as a planned snack, rather than eating it on impulse.)

Have a zero-calorie beverage. Sip some water, sparkling water, or green tea. (Add a squeeze of fresh lemon or lime, if you like a little extra flavor.) Drinking can satisfy the urge to have something in your mouth, plus you might find that your hunger was really just thirst in disguise.

MAKE OVER YOUR MEALS

NOW THAT YOU UNDERSTAND THE importance of clean eating to boost your metabolism, here you'll learn how to do it simply and easily. You'll discover what is a clean food and what isn't. You'll learn how to find these foods among the many sneaky imposters lining the supermarket shelves. Daily, we are bombarded by a dazzling array of foods that tout themselves as healthy, natural, or even able to help you lose weight. But what *actually* counts as a clean food, and which ones will work hardest to boost your metabolism and help you slim down? Thankfully, the answer is much more straightforward than you might think. Use these tips, and you'll be jump-starting your metabolism while eating a truly clean diet—and getting leaner—in no time.

The Importance of Eating at Home: Your Metabolism Makeover Headquarters

Plenty of research supports a simple clean-foods truth: Eating at home is a powerful and affordable way to serve yourself and your family the clean foods that feed a strong, healthy metabolism. "Eating in" lets you sidestep the processed and additive-packed stuff that messes up your metabolism, too.

Throughout this chapter, you'll discover fast and simple ways to stock your pantry, refrigerator, and freezer with clean foods so that you can put a delicious, metabolism-friendly meal on the table in minutes. Yes, you can also eat clean away from home when it's necessary. (Don't worry!) Whether you're on vacation or out for a special dinner, or you simply must grab something fast on a busy day, it's easier than ever to find cleaner foods on menus. However, many studies have shown that homemade meals automatically help you eat cleaner, making it easier to achieve a healthier weight and a healthier body.

- **Homemade meals help you control calories without counting.** In a recent study of more than 18,000 people, University of Illinois researchers reported that when dining out, people ate 190 more calories per meal than they did at home.[1] They also took in more saturated fat and sodium—both shown in other studies to torpedo your metabolism and promote weight gain. The shocker: Restaurant meals had almost as much fat and even more sodium than fast-food meals.

- **You eat more metabolism-boosting clean foods at home.** People who make food at home eat more fruits, vegetables, and whole grains than those who rely on processed, packaged, or away-from-home meals, according to University of Minnesota

EATING OUT? SIT HERE

When you're eating out, sit at a high table close to a window—doing both can help you eat less and eat healthier, according to research done by Brian Wansink, PhD, director of Cornell University's Food and Brand Lab. In Dr. Wansink's experiments, people sitting by windows or at high tables ordered healthier food and tended to skip dessert and alcohol compared to people sitting in dimly lit booths. Why? Being more visible and sitting in a more upright, alert position may make you more tuned in to your hunger and food choices, making you less likely to indulge in something you know you should probably skip.[2]

researchers who checked up on the eating habits of 1,710 people for a study published in the *Journal of the American Dietetic Association*.[3] Lack of time was the main reason people in this study didn't make meals at home more often, but as you'll discover throughout this book, it's actually easy to put together a clean-foods meal in a matter of minutes.

- **You stay automatically slimmer when you eat at home.** In one revealing University of Minnesota study that tracked the eating habits and health of 3,031 people for 15 years, those who had fast food two or more times per week gained 10 pounds more than those who rarely ate this way.[4] In another study from the same university, women who went out for fast food one extra time per week during a 3-year study gained an extra 1.6 pounds.[5]

Load Up on Fresh Produce

This likely isn't the first time you've been told that it's important to eat plenty of fruits and vegetables. But it's worth repeating, because fresh produce is the foundation of a clean diet. From apples to zucchini (and everything in between), fruits and vegetables are loaded with the vitamins, minerals, and phytonutrients that your body needs to function at full capacity and help you feel your best. And because produce tends to be low in calories and high in fiber, it plays an essential role in boosting your metabolism while still making you feel satisfied.

Eating more of practically *all* types of fruits and vegetables can help rev your metabolism. But according to a recent *PLoS One* study that followed some 130,000 men and women for more than 2 decades, the following 12 fruits and vegetables seem to pack the biggest metabolism-boosting punch.[6]

Apples	Kale
Berries	Mustard greens
Broccoli	Pears
Brussels sprouts	Romaine lettuce
Cabbage	Spinach
Cauliflower	Swiss chard

What makes these guys so great? According to researchers, they tend to be especially high in belly-filling fiber—and that means you stay fuller, longer. They also have a low glycemic load, which can help prevent blood sugar spikes that can cause cravings for sugary fare.

Organic produce, by definition, is grown without synthetic, industrial fertilizers or pesticides. That's a big deal, since billions of pounds of agricultural chemicals are sprayed on our crops each year. And believe it or not, most of these chemicals haven't gone through extensive testing to ensure that they're safe.

When you choose organic, you know that the fruits and vegetables you're getting are truly clean. That's because organic produce:

- Can only be grown on land that has been free of fertilizers and pesticides for at least 3 years.
- Can't be fertilized with sewage sludge (in other words, treated human waste).
- Can't be irradiated to kill bacteria.
- Can't be grown from genetically modified seeds.

Since many of the chemicals used to produce conventional food haven't been thoroughly vetted, it's tough to know for sure just how harmful they really are. But why take a chance? Research has already linked synthetic pesticides and fertilizers to annoying side effects, such as headaches and nausea, as well as more serious issues, including cancer and reproductive problems. And some findings suggest that they could even be messing with the number you see on the scale.

But opting for organic isn't just about avoiding the bad stuff—it's also about getting more of the good stuff. For a while, experts believed that organic produce packed the same nutritional punch as conventional. But more recently, a review of 343 studies published in the *British Journal of Nutrition* found that organically grown fruits and vegetables contain an average of 17 percent more polyphenolic antioxidants than their conventionally grown counterparts.[7] Organic crops, experts think, probably get a boost from being grown in nutrient-rich soil that hasn't been sucked dry by years of exposure to chemical pesticides and fertilizers.

Even after you've washed them, different fruits and vegetables contain different levels of pesticide residues, so it makes sense to go organic when you're buying the worst offenders. The Environmental Working Group's "Dirty Dozen" list reveals which types of produce have the highest pesticide residues and are therefore the most important to buy organic whenever possible. Their "Clean Fifteen" list shows the types of produce with the lowest pesticide residues, which are therefore okay to buy conventional.

THE DIRTY DOZEN PLUS

1. Apples
2. Peaches
3. Nectarines
4. Strawberries
5. Grapes
6. Celery
7. Spinach
8. Sweet bell peppers
9. Cucumbers
10. Cherry tomatoes
11. Snap peas (imported)
12. Potatoes
13. Hot peppers
14. Kale/collard greens

THE CLEAN FIFTEEN

1. Avocados
2. Sweet corn
3. Pineapple
4. Cabbage
5. Sweet peas (frozen)
6. Onions
7. Asparagus
8. Mangoes
9. Papaya
10. Kiwifruit
11. Eggplant
12. Grapefruit
13. Cantaloupe
14. Cauliflower
15. Sweet potatoes

Basically, choosing organic can help you fuel your body with more of the nutrients it needs—which is key to boosting metabolism, losing weight, and feeling your best. (We'll get to that in much more detail later.) Still, that doesn't necessarily mean that you need to go organic 100 percent of the time. Eating fruits and vegetables in abundance—even conventionally grown ones—is seriously beneficial to your health and your waistline. So go organic when you can, but when you can't, don't let that stop you from enjoying as much fresh produce as possible.

DR. WENDY SAYS . . .

Remember: A produce-rich diet is essential for losing weight and optimizing your health—whether that produce is organic or not. It's great to choose organic when you can. But when organic isn't an option, never let that stop you from eating an abundance of fruits and vegetables.

Pick Clean and Lean Proteins

When it comes to losing weight and making over your metabolism, protein is pretty darn important. First, it forces your body to work harder and burn more calories during digestion, since high-protein foods are tougher to digest than ones that are mostly carbohydrates or fat. That means that protein-packed meals can help you stay satisfied for longer. Second, and most importantly, protein-rich fare supports healthy muscle tissue, which burns more calories than fat does. Add it all up, and it's easy to see why lean sources of protein—such as poultry, fish, eggs, dairy, beans, and moderate amounts of lean red meats—are essential for getting lean.

Choosing organic meat, poultry, eggs, and dairy might be even more important than choosing organic fruits and vegetables. Of course, conventionally raised cows and chickens aren't getting sprayed with chemical-laden pesticides or fertilizers. But their food—which consists mostly of corn, soybeans, and grains—is. So when you have a drumstick, a glass of milk, or a steak, *you* end up being subjected to the impact of that feed. Many conventional farmers also pump their cattle full of sex and growth hormones to increase meat and milk production, and some of these hormones are passed on to you. That's scary stuff, since the growth hormones rBGH and rBST are linked to an increased risk for breast and prostate cancers.

Evidence also suggests that all that added substances could affect your weight. One animal study from New York University found that mice who were given high doses of antibiotics had lower numbers of T cells, which is associated with obesity.[8] And some experts suspect that the steroid hormones given to meat and dairy cattle could also be contributing to the obesity epidemic. While the FDA maintains that these hormones don't pose a threat to human health, it's worth thinking about: If steroids can make cows and steers get bigger, why wouldn't they have the same effect on the people who eat the meat and dairy products of those animals?

Once upon a time, *all* of the seafood people ate was, of course, wild-caught. Over time, concerns about the harmful effects of heavy metals (such as mercury) and pollutants in our waters, combined with a higher demand for seafood, led to the rise of aquaculture, or fish farming. But fish farms—especially those located outside of the United States, which often lack strict regulations—are far from perfect: Like conventional livestock, the fish raised in these reservoirs are usually fed low-quality fish meal made from soy, wheat, and corn instead of the algae, krill, or smaller fish they'd eat in the wild. As a result, farmed fish can contain lower levels of beneficial omega-3 fatty acids than their wild counterparts. It's also common for farmed fish to be given a steady supply of antibiotics to help them avoid getting sick due to being crammed into small enclosures with too many other fish. Farmed fish can be exposed to harmful chemicals, too. For instance, farmed salmon grown on large-scale fish farms can contain up to 10 times more organic pollutants—including probable carcinogens such as polychlorinated biphenyls (PCBs), pesticides like DDT, and even flame retardants—than their wild counterparts, according to tests conducted by the Environmental Working Group.[9]

Still, cutting farmed fish out of your diet completely can really limit your seafood options. Wild-caught seafood can be expensive—and it's getting tougher to track down. Roughly half of our seafood is currently farmed, and according to World Bank estimates, that number could climb to two-thirds by 2030.[10] Fortunately, some types of seafood are being farmed in a cleaner, more responsible way. Many fish farms are growing their own algae to ensure that their fish eat a more natural diet, which helps them contain higher levels of omega-3s. And some high-end supermarkets have established standards for farmed seafood.

Since organic standards don't apply to fish and seafood, finding clean options might not be as straightforward as just looking for the USDA organic seal. But with a little know-how, you can shop for wild or sustainably farmed seafood with confidence.

SOMETHING FISHY'S GOING ON

Buyer beware! As demand for clean, wild seafood has skyrocketed, fish fraud has become a legitimate concern. There are two things to watch for.

✓ **"Organic" seafood.** Though the USDA has yet to establish guidelines for organic seafood, you might come across imported farmed options that call themselves organic. These "organic" offerings aren't subject to regulation, and the producers who farm them may still add contaminants to their fish feed or employ chemicals to fight parasites in fish, according to experts at the Environmental Defense Fund.[11] Steer clear!

✓ **Mislabeled wild salmon.** A recent report[12] by the environmental nonprofit organization Oceana found that out of 82 samples of "wild" salmon sold at grocery stores and restaurants, nearly half were actually farmed. Often, retailers will purposely mislabel farmed salmon as wild—especially during winter, when wild salmon isn't in season.

1. **Look for specifics.** The more information that's available, the less chance that your wild seafood is fake. For instance, salmon labeled Chinook, sockeye, or king is more likely to be the real deal than anything just labeled "salmon" or "wild salmon." But if the label doesn't specify . . .

2. **Ask questions.** Specifically, "Where was this fish caught?" Your fishmonger or restaurant server should be able to tell you the country (domestic is more likely to be clean than imported) and name a specific body of water (such as the Pacific Ocean). He should also be able to tell you whether farmed fish was raised in a clean environment and whether it was given antibiotics. If he can't tell you, or if it just doesn't seem to add up, pick something else. And if all else fails . . .

3. **Consider the cost.** Wild-caught and sustainably farmed fish usually isn't cheap (although prices do drop in late summer, when more fish is available). If the price simply seems too good to be true, it probably is.

4. **Or check with the pros.** The Monterey Bay Aquarium Seafood Watch is considered the top sustainable seafood shopping resource. Go to seafoodwatch.org to find their clean picks or download the app.

Remember Plant Proteins

Protein doesn't have to come from meat, dairy, and eggs. In fact, plant-based sources, such as beans and legumes, nuts and seeds, whole soy foods, and more, deliver plenty of the muscle builder, too—along with a side of belly-filling fiber and powerful antioxidants. Plus, people who eat a plant-heavy diet tend to weigh less than major meat eaters. Some important things to keep in mind:

- **Pick whole or minimally processed soy.** Edamame, tempeh, miso, and tofu are delicious, inexpensive sources of clean protein. Stuff like veggie "meats" and soy protein isolate are highly processed, so steer clear.

- **Don't worry about making "complete" proteins at a single meal.** You might have heard that you have to combine different plant foods to form a complete protein, such as beans and rice or whole grain bread and peanut butter. But as long as you're eating a variety of plant foods throughout the day, you don't need to worry about pairing different protein sources at the same meal. So much simpler, right?

- **Remember whole grains.** Yes, they're carbohydrates. But whole grains such as spelt, kamut, teff, amaranth, sorghum, and quinoa also pack more than 8 grams of protein per cup.

Refer to the following list to learn the best sources of plant protein to help boost metabolism and aid weight loss.

PLANT-BASED PROTEIN	AMOUNT OF PROTEIN PER COOKED SERVING
Organic, non-GMO edamame	17 g per 1 cup
Organic, non-GMO tempeh	15 g per 3 ounces
Lentils	9 g per ½ cup
Organic, non-GMO tofu	8 g per 3 ounces
Black beans	8 g per ½ cup
Amaranth	8 g per 1 cup
Kamut	8 g per 1 cup
Quinoa	8 g per 1 cup
Sorghum	8 g per 1 cup
Spelt	8 g per 1 cup
Teff	8 g per 1 cup
Almonds or almond butter	7 g per ¼ cup almonds or 2 tablespoons almond butter
Peanuts or peanut butter	7 g per ¼ cup peanuts or 2 tablespoons peanut butter
Wild rice	7 g per 1 cup
Chickpeas	6 g per ½ cup
Lima beans	6 g per ½ cup
Pistachios	6 g per ½ cup
Chia seeds	5 g per 2 tablespoons
Walnuts	5 g per ½ cup

Get Friendly with Healthy Fat

Let's get one thing straight: That whole thing about fat making you fat? It couldn't be further from the truth. True, fat *does* have more calories per gram than carbohydrates or protein do, which means keeping your portions in check is important, especially if you're trying to lose weight. But a few slices of creamy avocado, a spoonful of nut butter, or a drizzle of fruity olive oil can

Make the effort to seek out cleanly produced oils, like those labeled "cold-pressed" or "expeller-pressed." Cold-pressed oils are pressed at low temperatures, so they retain all of the flavors, aromas, and nutrients that can get destroyed by heat. "Expeller-pressed" means that the oil was extracted mechanically (through good old-fashioned squeezing!) instead of with chemicals.

leave you feeling fuller for longer and can even help your body burn more fat. Plus, let's be honest—fat makes food taste better.

The key is picking healthy types of fat, since not all fats are created equal. So how can you tell which is which? It's easiest to think about different types of fat like lights on a traffic light: Some are green lights (great anytime in moderate portions, of course), some are yellow (best once in a while, so be cautious), and some are red (stop and try to avoid these completely).

GREEN LIGHT FATS

Unsaturated fats such as monounsaturated (MUFA), polyunsaturated (PUFA), and omega-3 fats can help lower your risk for heart disease. They also play an important role in keeping your blood sugar levels stable, which could help stave off cravings for sugary junk. You can find them in lots of whole, unprocessed foods.

- **MUFAs.** Olive oil, olives, avocados, nuts, and nut butters
- **PUFAs.** Safflower oil and sunflower seeds
- **Omega-3s.** Fatty fish, such as salmon, trout, sardines, herring, and anchovies; walnuts; chia seeds, hemp seeds, flaxseeds; and flaxseed oil

YELLOW LIGHT FATS

In large quantities, the saturated fats found in meat and poultry, full-fat dairy (whole milk, full-fat yogurt, butter, and cheese), eggs, and tropical oils (such as coconut oil) can raise your risk for heart disease. But in moderation, they can be perfectly fine. If you're having an egg or two (with yolks) for breakfast, some diced chicken in your salad, or a stir-fry with vegetables and lean beef, you probably don't have to worry.

But if you're eating more than that on a regular basis, it's worth trying to cut back for the sake of your heart. Just make sure you swap your saturated fat with a healthier pick. Slashing saturated fat won't reduce your risk of heart disease unless you replace that fat with healthier foods, such as unsaturated fats or whole grains, according to findings published in the *Journal of the American College of Cardiology*.[13]

RED LIGHT FATS

Trans fats are artificial fats that are made by adding hydrogen to liquid vegetable oils, which makes them solid. And they're straight-up bad for you: Aside from the fact that they have zero nutritional value, trans fats have also been shown to raise your "bad" LDL cholesterol, lower your "good" HDL cholesterol, and increase your risk for heart disease and diabetes. Trans fats tend to show up in packaged items like cookies, crackers, and margarine—and if you spot them on an ingredients list (usually under the name "partially hydrogenated oils"), it's a surefire sign that the food is *not* clean. Don't eat these fats!

CAN COCONUT OIL MAKE ME THIN?

Coconut oil is often touted as a weight-loss wonder food, and there is some evidence to suggest that the medium-chain triglycerides (MCTs) in coconut oil could help you fit into your skinny jeans. One small study published in the journal *Lipids* found that women who consumed roughly 2 tablespoons of coconut oil daily for 12 weeks lost more belly fat than women who downed the same amount of soybean oil.[14] There's also some evidence suggesting that coconut oil's MCTs can rev your metabolism and boost satiety to help you eat less throughout the day.

So should you down it by the spoonful? All oils contain about 120 calories per tablespoon, so simply *adding* coconut oil to whatever you're already eating won't help with weight loss. But replacing other less nutritious things in your diet with coconut oil—using it instead of conventional canola oil in a stir-fry, for example—might help you lose weight faster. Just stick to less than 2 tablespoons of coconut oil per day as you're working to shed some pounds.

Go with the (Whole) Grain

You don't need to cut out carbs to boost your metabolism. You just need to choose complex, fiber-rich carbohydrates instead of their refined counterparts. Quinoa, barley, millet, oats, and brown rice are tasty and filling. And they can have *big* benefits for your weight: In a *Nutrition Journal* study of more than 45,000 adults and children, those who ate the most whole grains had lower body mass indexes and smaller waist circumferences and were more likely to be at a healthy weight compared to those who ate the least.[15]

But you don't have to limit yourself to individual grains. Pastas made from whole wheat, quinoa, and non-GMO corn are all great choices, too. Clean eating can even include bread—as long as it's made from whole grains. But be careful: Plenty of manufacturers add a touch of whole grain flour (or even just caramel coloring) to make their bread seem more wholesome than it is. The only way to tell for sure whether a bread is truly whole grain is to check the ingredient list. First up should always be something with the word "whole" in the name, like "whole wheat" or "whole oats." If you don't see the word "whole," that's a sign that the grains in your bread are likely refined.

Watch for Hidden Sugars

As mentioned earlier, the average American eats nearly 23 teaspoons of sugar every single day. Most of that comes from packaged foods—and not just desserts. Everything from jarred pasta sauce to microwave oatmeal packets to whole wheat bread can be loaded with added sugar. This is bad news if you're trying to boost your metabolism, since loading up on sugar zaps your energy, ramps up your cravings, and sends your body toward fat storage—all of which make it nearly impossible to lose weight. But manufacturers are crafty. They know that sugary foods are addictive, so they add the sweet stuff to virtually all of their products, including many that might surprise you, such as bread, barbecue sauce, crackers, salad dressings, and frozen dinners. To make matters worse, you won't always spot "sugar" on the ingredients list. The sweet stuff goes by many different names, including some that sound pretty wholesome, such as agave syrup, honey, or maple syrup. But to your body, it's all sugar. What follows is a surprisingly large list of different names for sugar that you might find on packages.

- Agave syrup
- Barley malt
- Beet sugar
- Brown rice syrup
- Brown sugar
- Buttered syrup
- Cane sugar
- Caramel
- Carob syrup
- Coconut sugar
- Corn syrup
- Date sugar
- Dextran
- Dextrose
- Evaporated cane juice
- Fructose
- Fruit juice
- Fruit juice concentrate
- Glucose
- Glucose solids
- Golden syrup
- Grape sugar
- High-fructose corn syrup
- Honey

- Invert sugar
- Lactose
- Maltodextrin
- Maltose
- Malt syrup
- Mannitol
- Maple syrup
- Molasses
- Raisin juice concentrate
- Raw sugar
- Refiner's syrup
- Rice/rice bran sugar
- Sorbitol
- Sorghum syrup
- Sucrose
- Sugar
- Turbinado sugar

Sugars aren't the only things to be aware of. Packaged foods can be full of certain additives that should be avoided. Here's something that might blow your mind: Some of the additives in packaged foods haven't actually been tested by the FDA because they're considered by certain experts to be "generally recognized as safe" (GRAS). This makes sense for basic ingredients, such as salt or pepper. (Do we really need to test those things to know that they're a-okay?) But the GRAS program has effectively created a loophole that lets some potentially harmful ingredients end up in our foods without adequate testing. Seems like a pretty terrible idea, right?

Unless you're growing and preparing all of your own food, it can be tough to avoid food additives completely. But eating clean isn't about being perfect—it's about doing your best to pick the best option that you can with the resources that you have at the time. For those times when you have to choose a packaged food, it's a good idea to try to avoid these potentially sketchy additives as much as possible.

- **Artificial sweeteners, including aspartame, sucralose, and acesulfame K.** These fake sweeteners often pop up in "diet" or "sugar-free" items such as diet soda, sugar-free gum or desserts, chewable vitamins, cough syrup, toothpaste, and cereal. And as you've read, they have the potential to wreak havoc with your metabolism. In part, that could be because the sweet flavor of aspartame and other artificial sweeteners appears to stimulate taste receptors in your taste buds and digestive tract in the same way that sugar does. That can trick your brain into thinking you're getting calories from real sugar when you're not, which can promote cravings for *more* sweet foods, as well as cause other ill effects. But there's an even more serious problem: Some studies have shown that artificial sweeteners could also have a negative impact on the bacteria in your gut, which play a role in metabolism. It's no wonder that groups like the Center for Science in the Public Interest recommend avoiding artificial sweeteners altogether—and we agree.[16] Bottom line: They're not natural and they're not clean.

- **High-fructose corn syrup (HFCS).** This highly processed version of fructose (the sugar that occurs naturally in fruit) is added to bread, candy, yogurt, salad dressing, canned vegetables, cereal, and more. Too much HFCS can increase insulin resistance, which can raise your risk for diabetes and heart disease. If you spot it in an ingredients list, it's a dead giveaway that what you're looking at is not a clean food.

- **Monosodium glutamate (MSG).** This flavor enhancer is found in potato chips and snacks, cookies, seasonings, canned soups, frozen meals, lunch meats, and some Chinese food. It's known to trigger migraines in some people, and it has a crazy addictive flavor that makes you want to eat, and eat, and eat.

- **Added trans fats.** This lab-produced fat is used to extend the shelf life and improve the flavor of things like margarine, chips, crackers, baked goods, and fast foods. It's strongly linked to heart disease and diabetes, which is why the FDA ruled that added trans fats must be phased out of most packaged and restaurant foods by 2018. (Meat and dairy contain small amounts of naturally occurring trans fats, but if you're eating these foods in moderation, these trans fats aren't something to worry about.)

- **Food dyes: blue #1 and #2, red #3 and #40, and yellow #5 (tartrazine) and #6.** Found in fruit cocktail, maraschino cherries, ice cream, candy, baked goods, American cheese, mac and cheese, and many other foods, these colors might *look* pretty, but they're petroleum-based, and several have been linked to hyperactivity in kids and cancer in lab animals. Now that you know the risks, you don't *really* need pink yogurt, do you?

- **Caramel color.** This common food coloring is used in soda, beer, brown bread, chocolate, cookies, doughnuts, ice cream, and even pickles. It can be processed with ammonia, which leads to the creation of the potentially carcinogenic compound 4-methylimidazole.

- **Sulfites.** These preservatives and flavor enhancers are found naturally in wine and beer, and they're added to soda, juice, dried fruit, condiments, and potato products. In some people, they can cause allergy-like symptoms ranging from hay fever to anaphylaxis.

- **Sodium nitrite and sodium nitrate.** A possible carcinogen, sodium nitrite is a synthetic preservative used in processed meats such as hot dogs, lunch meats, bacon, and smoked fish. Natural sodium nitrates, which are derived from celery, are often used in "uncured" meat products and may be safer, but foods containing them aren't clean eats.

Avoid sodium nitrites altogether, and limit your consumption of sodium nitrates as much as possible.

- **Butylated hydroxyanisole (BHA) and butylated hydroxytoluene (BHT).** These petroleum-based preservatives are found in potato chips, gum, cereal, frozen sausages, enriched rice, lard, shortening, and candy. BHA is a likely human carcinogen, and BHT has been linked to cancer to a lesser degree.

- **Potassium bromate.** This flour-bulking agent is often used in breads and rolls, bagel chips, wraps, and bread crumbs to strengthen dough and shorten baking time. It could cause kidney or nervous system disorders and gastrointestinal discomfort.

Deciphering Food Claims

Whole foods are real, simple, and straightforward—usually! Sometimes even things as basic as a carton of eggs, a jug of milk, or a package of chicken breasts can have an awful lot of *stuff* on the label. And while the terms can be a bit confusing, they're worth paying attention to if you're committed to eating clean. Here are the important ones to become familiar with.

- **Organic.** For produce, this means that the plants weren't grown from genetically modified seeds; were not grown with pesticides, herbicides, or sewage sludge; and were not irradiated. For meats and poultry, this means that the animals were fed organic feed containing no animal by-products, were not given antibiotics or hormones, and had some (but not necessarily much) access to the outdoors. For a packaged food to be labeled organic, it must be made up of at least 95 percent organic ingredients; a label stating "made with organic ingredients" means the product must be made up of at least 70 percent organic ingredients.

- **Cage-free.** For eggs, "cage-free" means that the hens were not confined to cages—but they didn't necessarily have access to an outdoor space. Unless they're organic, cage-free hens can still be fed grains made from genetically modified crops that have been heavily treated with chemical pesticides, which can then be passed on to you. Since there's no mandatory third-party auditing for the term "cage-free," look for a third-party verification seal such as "Certified Humane" or "Animal Welfare Approved."

- **Free-range.** Found on both poultry and egg packaging, free-range means that the hens had some access to the outdoors. Like cage-free hens, free-range hens that aren't certified organic can still be given feed that contains antibiotics and pesticides. Since there's no mandatory third-party auditing for the term, look for a third-party verification seal such as "Certified Humane" or "Animal Welfare Approved."

- **Pasture-raised.** This term can apply to meat, poultry, and eggs. Pasture-raised animals spend some time on grassland, where they're able to eat a more natural diet of grass and bugs. Because of this, their meat and milk often have richer flavors and higher levels of nutrients such as omega-3s. But since there's no mandatory third-party auditing, it can be tough to tell how much time an animal actually spent on the pasture. For that reason, it's best to buy pastured meat, poultry, and eggs with a third-party verification seal such as "Certified Humane" or "Animal Welfare Approved." Or buy these foods from a local producer who can offer details on how his animals are raised.

- **Grass-fed.** Due to recent changes to labeling standards, the USDA grass-fed label only means that beef, bison, lamb, goats, and dairy cattle were fed grass *at some point* in their lives. The label doesn't stop producers from feeding animals grain, giving them antibiotics or hormones, or keeping them in confined spaces. For true grass-fed products, look for those certified by the American Grassfed Association, or buy from a local producer who can offer details on how his animals are raised.

- **Natural.** "Natural" foods are those made without artificial flavors, colors, or other synthetic ingredients. But these foods can still contain high-fructose corn syrup, and many also contain genetically modified ingredients. In short, natural is a vague term, so don't rely on it exclusively when you're looking for clean products. Inspect the ingredients list, instead.

- **No hormones.** When you see this label on meat or dairy products, it means that hormones weren't given to the animals involved. The USDA

COMMON GMO CULPRITS

Good news! The majority of real, whole foods aren't genetically modified. That means that by eating clean, you'll automatically be avoiding most foods that contain GMOs. However, it's common for conventional packaged, processed foods to contain genetically modified ingredients such as soy, corn, rapeseed (used to make canola oil), and sugar beets (used to make white sugar). When buying packaged or processed foods, look for certified organic products because by law, organic foods cannot be grown using genetically engineered seeds. Another good option: Look for non-GMO labels from third-party certifiers, such as the Non-GMO Project.

already prohibits the use of hormones in poultry and pork, so you don't need to seek out this label for those products.

- **No antibiotics.** This phrase can be found on meat or dairy items, and it means that no antibiotics were given to the animals involved. That's a good thing, since antibiotic use in animals is linked to drug resistance, as well as obesity. But if you're going to pay more for antibiotic-free products, you might as well buy organic ones.

- **Certified humane.** This means that the animals had access to enough space to allow them freedom to move, which is good for your conscience. But it also means that the animals weren't treated with artificial growth hormones or antibiotics—which is good for your health.

- **Heart healthy.** The American Heart Association Heart-Check Food Certification Program's standard certification requires that a product have less than 6.5 grams of total fat, 1 gram or less of saturated fat (or less than 15 percent of total calories), less than 0.5 gram of trans fats, and 20 milligrams or less of cholesterol per serving. It also requires that a food contain less than a certain amount of sodium, depending on the food category. The food must contain 10 percent or more of the Daily Value of one of six beneficial nutrients (vitamin A, vitamin C, iron, calcium, protein, or dietary fiber). While nuts are higher in fat than many foods (such as fruits and vegetables), they can also get the Heart-Check mark, thanks to the enormous amount of evidence backing their benefits for heart health. Still, because of the label's emphasis on certifying lower-fat foods—even as mounting research shows that quality fats are good for you—take the label with a grain of salt, and read the ingredients list and nutrition panel before you make a decision.

- **High-fiber.** High-fiber foods must contain at least 5 grams of fiber per serving, according to the Whole Grains Council. Whole grains typically contain between 0.5 and 3 grams of fiber per serving, so you'll usually see the "high-fiber" label on processed foods that contain added fiber in the form of resistant starch, inulin, or cellulose. If you're already eating a whole foods diet that contains plenty of vegetables and grains, you don't need to bother looking for this label.

- **Raw.** This label typically shows up on juices, fermented drinks and vegetables, dairy, and some snack foods, and it means that the product was not cooked or heated to a temperature that destroys certain beneficial nutrients and enzymes. In the case of things like kombucha, sauerkraut, and kimchi, it means that the product has retained its good bacteria and still offers probiotic benefits. The jury's out on juices, since pasteurized juice still retains many vitamins and minerals. For milk, the benefits may not outweigh the risks of food-borne illnesses. For packaged snack foods, such as kale chips, look for more specific quality indicators in addition to raw, such as organic or non-GMO.

- **Non-GMO or GMO-free.** Both terms imply that a food is free of genetically modified organisms—but neither one is regulated. To be most certain that the food you're buying is free of GMOs, look for foods that are certified organic and have a Non-GMO Project Verified seal.

Buy Clean Packaged Foods

Eating clean doesn't mean cooking every single thing from scratch and swearing off all foods that come in a box, can, or bag. Instead, choose packaged items that help support your health and weight-loss goals. Look for packaged foods made with real ingredients, not overly processed, and free of artificial additives. Your body and waistline will benefit from a little label reading.

Start by reading a packaged food's ingredient list. Foods with fewer, more simple ingredients tend to be better for you than foods with lots of—or unrecognizable—ingredients. Think about, say, an energy bar. You might think that, in general, any energy bar is probably good for you because it contains foods like oats, dried fruit, and nuts. But let's take a look at the ingredient lists for two different types of bars.

Energy bar A: Dates, almonds, unsweetened apples, walnuts, raisins, cinnamon

Energy bar B: Granola (whole grain rolled oats, brown sugar, crisp rice [rice flour, sugar, salt, malted barley extract], whole grain rolled wheat, soybean oil, dried coconut, whole wheat flour, sodium bicarbonate, soy lecithin, caramel color, nonfat dry milk), semisweet chocolate chips (sugar, chocolate liquor, cocoa butter, soy lecithin, vanilla extract), corn syrup, brown rice crisp (whole grain brown rice, sugar, malted barley flour, salt), invert sugar, sugar, corn syrup solids, glycerin, soybean oil. Contains 2% or less of sorbitol, calcium carbonate, salt, water, soy lecithin, molasses, Natural and artificial flavor, BHT (preservative), citric acid.

Once you look at the ingredient list, it's easy to tell that energy bar A is the cleaner choice: There are only six ingredients, and none of them are processed. Energy bar B, on the other hand, is packed with processed ingredients (when was the last time you found freshly picked sodium bicarbonate at the farmers' market?), loads of sugar, and potentially carcinogenic colors and preservatives.

Everyday Essentials

Learning about all the weird stuff that goes into most conventional food might have you running to clean out your kitchen—stat. But once all the junk is out, what do you put back in? Don't worry about the goji berries and sprouted hemp seeds for now. The basic staples listed below are all you need in order to build a clean refrigerator, freezer, and pantry. Here's how to stock your kitchen so eating clean is quick, easy, and delicious.

VEGETABLES AND FRUITS

- Leafy greens, like kale, spinach, or romaine lettuce
- Cruciferous vegetables, like broccoli, cauliflower, or Brussels sprouts
- Other vegetables, like bell peppers, mushrooms, or sweet potatoes
- Fresh fruits, like apples, oranges, bananas, or peaches
- Citrus fruits, like lemons or limes
- Frozen fruits, like berries, peaches, or mangoes
- Frozen vegetables, like broccoli, butternut squash, bell peppers, onion, or spinach
- Flavor-enhancing alliums, like leeks, scallions, onions, and garlic
- Avocados
- Olives
- Fresh herbs
- Dried fruits, like raisins or unsweetened dried cherries

PROTEINS

- Organic chicken, like boneless, skinless breasts or thighs or a whole roaster
- Organic turkey, like whole turkey breast or turkey cutlets
- Organic grass-fed beef, like London broil, flank steak, or cubed stew meat
- Organic ground meat, like ground chicken, ground turkey, or lean ground beef
- Organic pork, like a tenderloin, a roast, or chops
- Wild-caught fish, like Alaskan salmon or cod (fresh or frozen)
- Wild-caught shrimp (fresh or frozen)
- BPA-free canned tuna or wild-caught salmon

DAIRY

- Organic plain yogurt (Greek or regular)
- Organic dairy milk or organic unsweetened nondairy milk, like almond, soy, coconut, or hemp
- Organic butter
- Organic cheese, like Parmesan, ricotta, goat, feta, or mozzarella

GRAINS AND BEANS

- Whole grain or sprouted breads, tortillas, or pitas
- Whole grain or gluten-free pasta
- Whole grains, like quinoa and brown rice
- Whole wheat flour
- Rolled oats
- Legumes, like BPA-free canned, no-salt-added or low-sodium beans or lentils, or dried beans or lentils
- Organic, non-GMO edamame

NUTS, SEEDS, AND NUT BUTTERS

- Raw nuts, like almonds or walnuts
- Raw seeds, like pumpkin, chia, or flaxseeds
- Natural nut butters, like peanut, cashew, or almond

COOKING STAPLES AND FLAVOR ENHANCERS

- Anchovies
- Boxed lower-sodium chicken or vegetable stock
- BPA-free canned light coconut milk
- BPA-free canned or jarred tomatoes, like crushed, diced, or paste
- Capers
- Stone-ground mustard
- Dried herbs and spices and spice blends without added sugars or additives
- Low-sodium tamari
- Oils, like expeller- or cold-pressed olive oil, organic non-GMO canola oil, or coconut oil
- Unsweetened cocoa powder
- Vinegars, like balsamic, red wine, or apple cider
- White miso paste

Savvy Shopping for Clean Eaters

It's true that distinguishing clean foods from their not-so-healthy counterparts can sometimes be tricky. (Though it's nothing you can't handle and it gets easier with practice.) The good news is that more and more people are waking up to the fact that clean foods are key to losing weight and feeling great. This means that whole, unprocessed fare is more widely available than ever. Gone are the days when you had to drive 50 miles to reach a store that carried quinoa—only to find that it cost $20 a bag. We're living in a golden age of clean shopping, and there are more places than ever that offer fresh, clean foods at prices that won't break the bank. So grab your reusable bags and let's go!

The main thing to consider as you head into your supermarket is to look for whole foods and real ingredients at every turn. This will keep you focused on clean foods and prevent you from being distracted by the endless rows of chip bags and soda bottles. It's a grocery store's job to tempt you into filling your cart at every turn, but you don't have to cave to the pressure: Focus on the outer perimeter of the store, which is where whole foods like fresh produce, meat, poultry, seafood, and dairy are generally kept. As for the center aisles, that's where most of the processed stuff lives. Be on high alert when you walk through that zone, and check the ingredients list on any box or bag you pick up so that you can find your best clean options.

Where else can you find clean food? The question should really be, where *can't* you find it? All of these spots are stocked with the staples you need.

- **Megamarkets.** These days, even most megamart chains offer at least some organic produce, meat, dairy, and eggs. They also have a smattering of truly clean packaged goods. Just be sure to check those ingredients lists!

- **Natural food stores.** These stores tend to offer a bigger selection of clean produce, animal products, and more. Even better, they usually have large selections of bulk items—everything from whole grains and dried beans to nuts and seeds. And since you're avoiding all of the extra packaging, these bulk foods tend to be more affordable.

- **Farmers' markets.** More and more farmers' markets are popping up all across the country, which is good news for clean eaters. In addition to selling fresh, seasonal produce, most markets offer locally produced eggs, dairy products, meats, and breads. The best part? You can talk to the farmers and producers to find out *exactly* what goes into growing or making their food.

- **CSAs.** CSA stands for community supported agriculture. Buying a share of a CSA means that you're investing in a local farm and receiving a weekly box of produce in exchange. (Some CSAs also offer eggs, dairy, and meats.) Like shopping at the farmers' market, this gives you the opportunity to learn more about how your food is produced and to get to know what's truly local and seasonal in your area. Head to localharvest.org for everything from farmers' markets and CSAs to pick-your-own farms in your area.

Smart Ways to Save

At some point, you might've walked into a high-end grocery store and balked at a $4 bunch of broccoli or an $6 carton of eggs. It's easy to drop big bucks on clean fare, but fueling your body with the good stuff doesn't have to be expensive. In fact, when you start trading processed, packaged items for their whole-food counterparts, you might end up spending less! Consider these tips to save big.

- **Make a list—and stick to it.** It sounds obvious, but this is essential if you're going to stick to your budget and avoid the little impulse buys (fancy organic chocolate bar, anyone?) that can lead to sticker shock at the checkout counter. Make it a point to plan your meals and snacks ahead of time, and make a shopping list of all the ingredients that you'll need. (This will be a huge help with making clean choices and losing weight, too—but more on that later!) It's as simple as this: If you didn't write it down, it doesn't go in your cart.

- **Buy in season.** Produce grown out of season isn't just lacking in flavor, it's also usually flown in from far, far away—so it's often expensive. Stick to in-season fruits and vegetables that were grown nearby, and stock up on extras to freeze or even can so you can enjoy them all year long. Or look for produce that's available year-round, such as apples and broccoli.

- **Go veggie more often.** Plant-based proteins are considerably less expensive than their animal counterparts. Commit to eating vegetarian meals more often, or eat meat, poultry, or fish in small quantities instead of as the main event. Bonus: A largely plant-powered diet has been shown to help with losing weight—and keeping it off.
- **Join a co-op.** Co-ops are member-owned grocery stores that focus on whole foods, including organic produce, dairy products, and meats. Usually you pay a small membership fee up front to own a share of the co-op and then you reap the rewards in the form of significantly discounted fare.
- **Grow your own.** Whether it's a backyard raised bed brimming with vegetables or a pot of fresh herbs on the windowsill of your apartment kitchen, every bit of food you grow is food that you don't have to pay for out of your wallet. Plus, it's as fresh as you can get!

KELLEY S.

**TOTAL POUNDS LOST
IN 6 WEEKS**

11 lbs

TOTAL INCHES LOST

13.25"

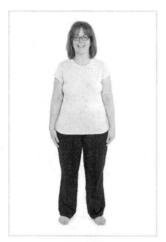

BEFORE

As a mom of three athletes, much of 50-year-old Kelley's free time is filled with cheering her kids on at games and shuttling them to tournaments. Her hectic schedule doesn't leave much time for cooking clean meals during the week, which meant that she had to get creative with prepping food for herself and her family.

"If I preplanned, I was successful. But if I didn't preplan, I wasn't successful," she says. Kelley got into the habit of shopping for groceries and cooking meals for the week on Sundays. But when one weekend got particularly busy, she didn't have time to do her usual prep work—and that threw her off. "So I felt like a failure. I was having cereal for dinner. I didn't go off the plan, I just didn't have great meals," she says.

That setback almost made her lose her resolve altogether. But then, someone noticed that she looked leaner. "When you work so hard and somebody notices, it's huge," Kelley says. Around the same time, *she* started picking up on the positive effects of eating clean, too. "The last 2 weeks, I could feel the weight loss," she remarks.

That's when she knew that she'd be able to stick with eating clean for the long haul. At the same time, she realized that always trying to aim for perfection might end up doing her more harm than good. For instance, when the teacher-appreciation luncheon was held at the school where she works, she knew that she wanted to indulge without feeling guilty. "Once a week, I might want to have a treat that isn't part of the plan," she admits. But even so, "I think that I'll be eating in more moderation than I would have normally."

MOST NOTABLE IMPROVEMENT

Kelley's cholesterol was high before she started eating clean. But afterward, it dropped into the healthy range.

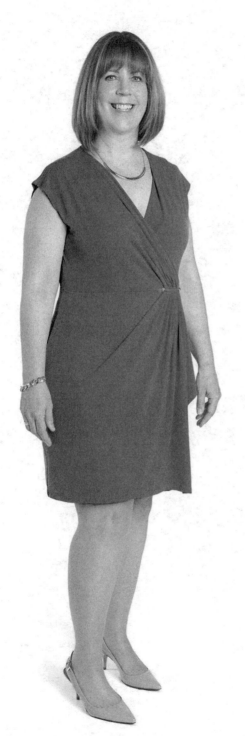

Dr. Wendy Observes:
It's easy to get sidelined when you hit a speed bump. But when Kelley ran into the all-too-common challenge of navigating a time-crunched schedule, she adapted instead of giving up. Sure, some of her meals during that challenging week may not have been as tasty or pretty, but they were still clean—and that's a success. It's about progress, not perfection.

PART

2

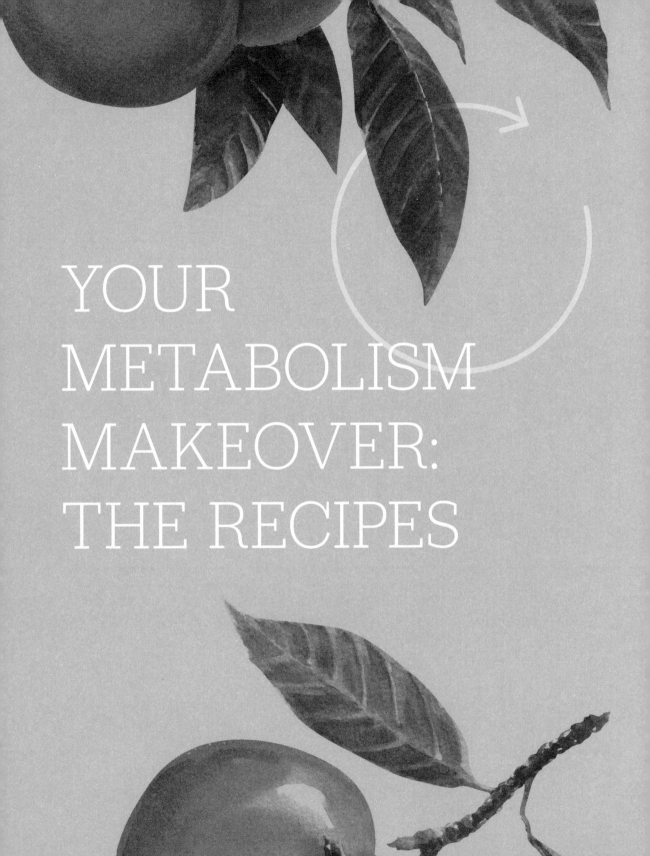

YOUR METABOLISM MAKEOVER: THE RECIPES

BREAKFASTS

SOUTHWEST SKILLET EGGS

PREP TIME: 5 MINUTES / TOTAL TIME: 55 MINUTES / **MAKES 2 SERVINGS**

Shown in photo insert pages.

I	tablespoon canola oil
½	large onion, diced
I	clove garlic, minced
I	can (I4.5 ounces) no-salt-added diced tomatoes
I	cup water
½	cup canned black beans
½	cup brown rice
I	tablespoon smoked paprika
I	teaspoon ground cumin
¼	teaspoon salt
	Ground red pepper
4	ounces baby spinach, roughly chopped
4	large eggs
½	cup chopped cilantro
½	cup 2% plain Greek yogurt
½	avocado, peeled, pitted, and sliced

1 In a large skillet over medium-high heat, heat the oil. Cook the onion and garlic until the onion is translucent, 2 to 3 minutes. Add the tomatoes (with juice), water, beans, rice, paprika, cumin, salt, and ground red pepper to taste. Reduce to a simmer, cover, and cook until the rice is tender, about 40 minutes. Add the spinach and cook until gently wilted, 3 minutes.

2 Form 4 indentations spaced evenly around the skillet. Place 1 egg in each indentation. Cover and cook until the eggs are opaque, 3 to 5 minutes. Uncover and garnish with the cilantro, yogurt, and avocado.

NUTRITION (PER SERVING): 528 calories, 27 g protein, 49 g carbohydrates, 13 g fiber, 11 g sugars, 26 g fat, 6 g saturated fat, 524 mg sodium

HEALTHY HINT

You can actually use eggs to increase the nutrient value of the other foods you eat. A recent study found that topping your salad with a hard-cooked egg can help you absorb a whopping 500 percent more beta-carotene from your veggies.[1] This antioxidant is essential for healthy eyes, skin, and immune function.

ZESTY BREAKFAST PIZZA

PREP TIME: 10 MINUTES / TOTAL TIME: 25 MINUTES / **MAKES 4 SERVINGS**

Shown in photo insert pages.

4   whole wheat flour tortillas (6" diameter)

2   tablespoons olive oil

I   small onion, thinly sliced

I   red bell pepper, cut into thin strips

½   jalapeño chile pepper, finely chopped (wear plastic gloves when handling)

8   eggs

2   teaspoons water

2   ounces pepper Jack cheese, shredded

4   tablespoons salsa

¼   cup chopped cilantro

1 Preheat the oven to 400°F. Coat both sides of each tortilla with cooking spray and place on a baking sheet. Bake until golden and crisp, 6 minutes.

2 In a large nonstick skillet over medium heat, heat the oil. Cook the onion, bell pepper, and jalapeño pepper until tender, about 5 minutes. Transfer to a plate.

3 In a medium bowl, beat the eggs and water. Pour the eggs into the same skillet and cook over medium heat, stirring to scramble until set, 2 minutes. Sprinkle the cheese over the eggs halfway through cooking.

4 Evenly divide two-thirds of the onion and peppers among the tortillas. Divide the cooked eggs, the remaining onion and peppers, and salsa among the tortillas. Sprinkle with the cilantro.

NUTRITION (PER SERVING): 360 calories, 19 g protein, 18 g carbohydrates, 9 g fiber, 3 g sugars, 23 g fat, 7 g saturated fat, 591 mg sodium

MINI SPINACH QUICHE

PREP TIME: 15 MINUTES / TOTAL TIME: 40 MINUTES / MAKES 4 SERVINGS

Shown in photo insert pages.

2	teaspoons extra-virgin olive oil
4	ounces lean ham, diced
2	cups diced mushrooms
½	onion, chopped
½	red bell pepper, chopped
2	cloves garlic, minced
½	teaspoon thyme
	Pinch of salt + ¼ teaspoon
4	cups baby spinach
8	large eggs
¼	cup 2% milk
1	cup shredded reduced-fat Jarlsburg cheese (4 ounces)

1 Preheat the oven to 375°F. Coat a 12-cup muffin pan with cooking spray.

2 In a medium nonstick skillet over medium heat, heat the oil. Cook the ham until lightly browned, 2 minutes. Add the mushrooms, onion, pepper, garlic, thyme, and a pinch of salt, and cook, stirring, until the vegetables have softened, 5 minutes. Stir in the spinach and cook until wilted, 3 minutes. Set aside to cool slightly.

3 In a medium bowl, whisk together the eggs, milk, and the remaining ¼ teaspoon salt. Divide the vegetables among the cups in the muffin pan. Pour the egg mixture over the vegetables until ¼" below the rim of each cup. Sprinkle with the cheese and bake until the quiches are puffed and set in the center, 25 minutes.

NUTRITION (PER 3 MINI-QUICHE SERVING): 314 calories, 29 g protein, 9 g carbohydrates, 2 g fiber, 4 g sugars, 18 g fat, 6 g saturated fat, 635 mg sodium

MAKE IT AHEAD! The quiches can be made and refrigerated for up to 4 days or frozen for up to 1 month. Reheat a serving in the microwave at 50% power for 2 minutes.

CHANGE IT UP! To make these vegetarian, leave out the ham and double the mushrooms.

SALMON BREAKFAST BURRITO

PREP TIME: 5 MINUTES / TOTAL TIME: 10 MINUTES / **MAKES 4 SERVINGS**

4   eggs

¼   cup low-fat milk

I   cup spinach leaves, chopped

4   scallions, sliced

4   fat-free whole wheat tortillas (8" diameter)

8   ounces wild salmon, cooked and flaked into pieces

4   tablespoons crumbled feta cheese

I   teaspoon chopped fresh dill or ⅓ teaspoon dried

1 In a large bowl, whisk together the eggs, milk, spinach, and scallions.

2 Heat a nonstick skillet coated with cooking spray over medium heat. Cook the egg mixture, stirring, until scrambled and set, 2 minutes.

3 Fill the tortillas with the eggs and salmon. Sprinkle with the cheese and dill. Fold in the outer edges and roll up the tortillas.

NUTRITION (PER SERVING): 265 calories, 23 g protein, 23 g carbohydrates, 3 g fiber, 2 g sugars, 11 g fat, 4 g saturated fat, 398 mg sodium

HASH BROWN FRITTATA

PREP TIME: 10 MINUTES / TOTAL TIME: 30 MINUTES / MAKES 2 SERVINGS

1   large russet (baking) potato

2   tablespoons extra-virgin olive oil, divided

1   small onion, chopped

1   red bell pepper, chopped

2   cups kale leaves (tough ribs removed)

4   large eggs

½   cup shredded part-skim mozzarella cheese (2 ounces)

½   cup 2% milk

½   teaspoon garlic powder

½   teaspoon onion powder

Pinch of salt

1 Position an oven rack 6" from the heating element, and preheat the broiler. Shred the unpeeled potato on the large holes of a box grater.

2 In a large ovenproof skillet over medium-high heat, heat 1 tablespoon of the oil. Cook the onion, bell pepper, and kale until lightly browned, 5 to 6 minutes. Remove to a medium bowl. Add the eggs, cheese, milk, garlic powder, and onion powder to the bowl with the vegetables; whisk to blend.

3 In the same skillet over medium-high heat, heat the remaining 1 tablespoon oil. Add the potato and salt and cook, stirring, until lightly browned, 5 minutes. Spread the potato evenly in the pan and gently press to form a base layer. Pour the egg mixture over the potatoes.

4 Return the skillet to medium heat. Cook until the eggs are set on the bottom, 2 to 3 minutes. Place the pan under the broiler until golden brown on top and cooked through in the middle (test with a knife), 8 to 10 minutes.

NUTRITION (PER SERVING): 536 calories, 30 g protein, 52 g carbohydrates, 7 g fiber, 9 g sugars, 24 g fat, 8 g saturated fat, 528 mg sodium

MUSHROOM OMELET

PREP TIME: 5 MINUTES / TOTAL TIME: 15 MINUTES / **MAKES 2 SERVINGS**

4   large eggs

2   tablespoons water

1½ tablespoons butter, divided

1½ cups thinly sliced mixed mushrooms

1   clove garlic, minced

¼   teaspoon dried ground sage

¼   teaspoon salt

2   tablespoons chopped fresh chives

1 In a medium bowl, whisk together the eggs and water.

2 In a medium skillet over medium heat, melt half of the butter. Cook the mushrooms until lightly browned, 8 minutes. Add the garlic, sage, and salt, and cook for 1 minute. Transfer to a plate.

3 In the same skillet, melt the remaining butter. Pour in the eggs and use a spatula to gently move the egg mixture from the sides to the center, allowing the liquid egg to fill in around the edges.

4 Flip the omelet over in the pan and top one half with the mushroom mixture and chives. Fold in half.

NUTRITION (PER SERVING): 235 calories, 14 g protein, 3 g carbohydrates, 1 g fiber, 1 g sugars, 18 g fat, 9 g saturated fat, 387 mg sodium

BLUEBERRY PROTEIN PANCAKES

PREP TIME: 5 MINUTES / TOTAL TIME: 15 MINUTES / **MAKES 2 SERVINGS**

½ cup rolled oats

2 scoops (¼ cup) vanilla-flavored, unsweetened egg, non-GMO soy, or plant whey protein powder

¼ teaspoon baking powder

¼ teaspoon salt

1 medium banana, mashed

1 large egg

¼ to ½ cup water

⅓ cup fresh or frozen and thawed blueberries

1 teaspoon coconut oil

1 In a blender or food processor, pulse the oats to a flour consistency. Transfer to a medium bowl. Stir in the protein powder, baking powder, and salt.

2 In another bowl, whisk together the banana, egg, and ¼ cup water until smooth.

3 Fold the oat mixture into the banana mixture until just smooth, adding more water if needed until pourable. Gently stir in the blueberries.

4 In a skillet over medium heat, heat the oil. Pour about ¼ cup of the batter onto the skillet for each pancake. Cook until small bubbles begin to appear on the surface of the pancakes, flip and cook until browned, about 3 minutes.

NUTRITION (PER SERVING): 255 calories, 17 g protein, 32 g carbohydrates, 4 g fiber, 10 g sugars, 7 g fat, 3 g saturated fat, 362 mg sodium

HEALTHY HINT

Don't just use protein powder for smoothies or shakes. Consider adding a scoop or two to your next batch of cookies, muffins, granola bars, or oatmeal to help thicken treats while infusing them with more stomach-filling, sugar-stabilizing protein.

PB AND J STUFFED FRENCH TOAST

PREP TIME: 10 MINUTES / TOTAL TIME: 20 MINUTES / **MAKES 4 SERVINGS**

Shown in photo insert pages.

4 tablespoons all-natural creamy peanut butter, divided

2 tablespoons all-fruit strawberry jam, divided

8 thin slices sprouted whole grain bread

1 cup sliced strawberries, divided

2 large eggs

½ cup unsweetened almond milk

1 teaspoon ground cinnamon

1 teaspoon pure vanilla extract

1 Spread 1 tablespoon of the peanut butter and ½ tablespoon of the jam on 4 slices of the bread. Evenly divide half of the strawberries in a single layer on the jam. Top with a second slice of bread and press lightly to form a sandwich.

2 In a shallow dish or pie plate, combine the eggs, milk, cinnamon, and vanilla. Dip the sandwiches, one at a time, into the egg mixture, turning to coat both sides.

3 Heat a large nonstick skillet coated with cooking spray over medium heat. Cook the sandwiches, turning once, until golden and cooked through, 8 minutes. Serve hot, topped with the remaining strawberries.

NUTRITION (PER SERVING): 331 calories, 15 g protein, 41 g carbohydrates, 9 g fiber, 6 g sugars, 12 g fat, 2 g saturated fat, 210 mg sodium

CHOCOLATE-BANANA STUFFED FRENCH TOAST

PREP TIME: 10 MINUTES / TOTAL TIME: 20 MINUTES / MAKES 4 SERVINGS

1 banana, thinly sliced

4 tablespoons almond butter

2 ounces bittersweet chocolate (70% cocoa), chopped

8 slices sprouted whole grain bread

2 cups milk

2 eggs

1 teaspoon ground cinnamon

½ teaspoon pure vanilla extract

½ teaspoon confectioners' sugar, divided (optional)

1 In a small bowl, mash about one-quarter of the banana slices with a fork. (You should have about 2 tablespoons.) Stir in the almond butter and chocolate until smooth.

2 Evenly divide the banana filling among 4 slices of the bread. Top with the remaining banana slices and bread slices to make 4 sandwiches.

3 In a shallow dish or pie plate, whisk together the milk, eggs, cinnamon, and vanilla until blended. Dip the sandwiches into the egg mixture, turning to coat both sides.

4 Heat a large nonstick skillet or griddle coated with cooking spray over medium-low heat. Cook the sandwiches until golden and cooked through, turning once, 8 minutes. Dust with confectioners' sugar, if using.

NUTRITION (PER SERVING): 352 calories, 15 g protein, 48 g carbohydrates, 9 g fiber, 11 g sugars, 12 g fat, 5 g saturated fat, 210 mg sodium

APPLE PIE PARFAIT

PREP TIME: 15 MINUTES / TOTAL TIME: 30 MINUTES / **MAKES 2 SERVINGS**

1⅓ cups plain low-fat yogurt

1 tablespoon pure maple syrup

1 teaspoon pure vanilla extract

⅓ cup rolled oats

2 tablespoons almond butter

¼ teaspoon ground nutmeg

¼ teaspoon ground ginger

1 teaspoon ground cinnamon, divided

2 teaspoons coconut oil

1 Pink Lady apple, diced

1 Preheat the oven to 350°F.

2 In a small bowl, stir together the yogurt, maple syrup, and vanilla. Cover and refrigerate until ready to serve.

3 In a small bowl, mix together the oats, almond butter, nutmeg, ginger, and ½ teaspoon of the cinnamon until well blended. Spread the mixture onto a baking sheet and bake until golden brown and fragrant, about 15 minutes. Remove from the oven and set aside.

4 In a medium skillet over medium heat, heat the oil. Add the apple and the remaining ½ teaspoon cinnamon, and cook until the apple is tender and golden, about 10 minutes.

5 Spoon ¼ cup of the yogurt mixture into the bottom of each of 2 parfait glasses. Top each with ¼ of the apple mixture and a heaping tablespoon of the oat crumble. Repeat the layers once more.

NUTRITION (PER SERVING): 375 calories, 14 g protein, 44 g carbohydrates, 6 g fiber, 1 g sugars, 17 g fat, 7 g saturated fat, 150 mg sodium

HEALTHY HINT

Calorie-packed pies, crisps, cobblers, and crumbles aren't the only option when you want an apple dessert. To get the taste of these treats without all of the calories, sauté organic apples in a skillet with a bit of coconut oil and finish with a sprinkle of cinnamon. The result is a delicious, healthy dessert that will help control blood sugar and satisfy cravings.

PB&J GRANOLA

PREP TIME: 5 MINUTES / TOTAL TIME: 30 MINUTES / MAKES 10 SERVINGS

1½ cups rolled oats

½ cup puffed brown rice cereal

2 tablespoons flaxseeds

¼ cup peanuts

Pinch of salt

2 tablespoons extra-virgin olive oil

2 tablespoons strawberry all-fruit spread

2 tablespoons all-natural creamy peanut butter

1 teaspoon pure vanilla extract

¼ cup dried tart cherries or raisins

1 Preheat the oven to 250°F.

2 In a large bowl, combine the oats, rice cereal, flaxseeds, peanuts, and salt. Set aside.

3 In a small saucepan over medium heat, heat the oil, fruit spread, peanut butter, and vanilla. Stir until combined and smooth. Pour over the oats mixture and toss together.

4 Spread evenly on a baking sheet, and bake, stirring every 10 minutes, until browned and crisp, 30 minutes. Let the granola cool to room temperature, and stir in the dried cherries or raisins. Store in an airtight container at room temperature for 1 week.

NUTRITION (PER SERVING): 295 calories, 11 g protein, 26 g carbohydrates, 5 g fiber, 5 g sugars, 18 g fat, 2 g saturated fat, 37 mg sodium

NOTE: This granola is very versatile. It can be enjoyed as a snack, sprinkled on yogurt for breakfast, or eaten on peanut butter toast.

HEALTHY HINT

Eat this granola with 1 cup of Greek yogurt to increase your protein intake by 19 grams and in turn boost your metabolism even more.

COCOA GRANOLA

PREP TIME: 15 MINUTES / TOTAL TIME: 55 MINUTES / **MAKES 8 SERVINGS**

⅔ **cup water**

½ **cup unsweetened cocoa powder**

2 **tablespoons pure maple syrup**

I **tablespoon pure vanilla extract**

½ **teaspoon ground cinnamon**

¼ **teaspoon salt**

½ **pound chopped, pitted Medjool dates, divided**

4 **cups rolled oats**

½ **cup whole raw almonds**

½ **cup raw pumpkin seeds (pepitas)**

1 Preheat the oven to 325°F. Line 2 baking sheets with parchment paper.

2 In a blender or food processor, combine the water, cocoa, maple syrup, vanilla, cinnamon, salt, and half of the dates. Process until smooth, 5 minutes. Scrape down the sides every few minutes. Pour the date mixture into a large bowl. Add the oats and toss to coat well.

3 Spread the mixture evenly on the prepared baking sheets. Bake until the granola is dry to the touch and somewhat crisp, 40 to 50 minutes, adding the almonds, pumpkin seeds, and remaining dates halfway through. Remove from the oven and place on a wire rack to cool. Store in an airtight container at room temperature for 1 week.

NUTRITION (PER SERVING): 385 calories, 13 g protein, 58 g carbohydrates, 10 g fiber, 23 g sugars, 13 g fat, 2 g saturated fat, 64 mg sodium

HEALTHY HINT

Eat this granola with I cup of Greek yogurt to increase the protein by I9 grams and in turn boost your metabolism even more.

SIMPLE OVERNIGHT STEEL-CUT OATS

PREP TIME: 5 MINUTES / TOTAL TIME: 5 MINUTES + OVERNIGHT SOAKING / MAKES 2 SERVINGS

1⅔ cups 1% milk or unsweetened milk alternative

⅔ cup steel-cut oats

2 Medjool dates, chopped

¼ teaspoon ground cinnamon

1 tablespoon almond butter

2 tablespoons chopped walnuts

1 In a blender, combine the milk, oats, dates, cinnamon, and almond butter and blend until the dates are nearly pureed. (Some small pieces might remain.)

2 Pour the mixture into a container with a lid, cover, and refrigerate overnight. In the morning, stir and top with the walnuts.

NUTRITION (PER SERVING): 435 calories, 18 g protein, 67 g carbohydrates, 8 g fiber, 27 g sugars, 14 g fat, 3 g saturated fat, 108 mg sodium

HEALTHY HINT

Eating oatmeal for breakfast can actually help you lose weight. In a recent study, when people breakfasted on oatmeal instead of consuming its caloric equivalent in sugared cornflakes or skipping the meal altogether, they took in 31% fewer calories at their next meal.

WARM BERRY BREAKFAST BARS

PREP TIME: 15 MINUTES / TOTAL TIME: 1 HOUR 10 MINUTES / **MAKES 8 SERVINGS**

¼ cup chia seeds

1 cup water

½ cup unsweetened coconut flakes

½ cup whole wheat flour

1 cup pitted dates

1 cup rolled oats, divided

¼ cup light brown sugar

2 tablespoons coconut oil

1 cup sliced almonds

3 tablespoons peanut butter

1 teaspoon pure vanilla extract

½ cup plain 2% Greek yogurt

1 tablespoon granulated sugar

½ cup blueberries

1 Preheat the oven to 350°F. Grease a 9" x 5" loaf pan.

2 In a small bowl, stir together the chia seeds and water. Let sit until a loose gel forms, 5 minutes.

3 In a food processor, combine the coconut flakes, flour, dates, and ½ cup of the oats. Pulse until the dates are broken into small, crumb-size pieces and are distributed evenly throughout the mixture. Pulse in the brown sugar and oil to combine. Transfer the flour mixture to a large bowl. Stir in the almonds, peanut butter, vanilla, soaked chia seeds, and the remaining ½ cup oats until thoroughly blended.

4 In a food processor, puree the yogurt, granulated sugar, and blueberries until smooth.

5 Press the oat mixture evenly into the prepared loaf pan. Pour the yogurt mixture on top. Bake until browned and set, 55 minutes. Cut into 8 bars.

NUTRITION (PER SERVING): 361 calories, 10 g protein, 43 g carbohydrates, 8 g fiber, 23 g sugars, 19 g fat, 8 g saturated fat, 37 mg sodium

HEALTHY HINT

Consider storing your whole grain flour in the fridge or freezer. Unlike all-purpose flour, whole grain still contains the bran and germ, which are high in nutrients and oils that make them more prone to spoilage. Chilling will extend your flour's shelf life and prevent off-flavors in your baked goods.

FRUITED BREAKFAST BALLS

PREP TIME: 20 MINUTES / TOTAL TIME: 35 MINUTES / MAKES 6 SERVINGS (2 BALLS EACH)

1¾ cups rolled oats

½ cup chopped almonds or pecans

¾ cup canned pure pumpkin puree (canned pure pumpkin)

⅓ cup unsweetened dried cranberries, dried tart cherries, or a mixture of both, chopped

⅓ cup toasted, salted pumpkin seeds (pepitas), roughly chopped

⅓ cup hemp seeds

¼ cup pure maple syrup

2 tablespoons grapeseed oil

½ teaspoon pumpkin pie spice

¼ teaspoon salt

1 Preheat the oven to 350°F.

2 Scatter the oats and almonds or pecans on a baking sheet. Bake until toasted and very fragrant, 10 minutes. Transfer to a large bowl.

3 Add the pumpkin, cranberries or cherries, pumpkin seeds, hemp seeds, maple syrup, oil, pie spice, and salt to the oats mixture. Stir until well blended.

4 Scoop the mixture into golf ball–size portions and roll firmly into balls. Set the balls on a tray or baking sheet and refrigerate until firm, about 15 minutes. Transfer to an airtight container and refrigerate for up to a week or freeze for as long as a month.

NUTRITION (PER SERVING): 377 calories, 13 g protein, 35 g carbohydrates, 7 g fiber, 12 g sugars, 22 g fat, 2 g saturated fat, 86 mg sodium

PEANUT BUTTER BALLS

¼ **pound (½ cup packed) pitted Medjool dates**

1 **cup rolled oats**

½ **cup unsalted dry-roasted peanuts**

¼ **cup + 1 tablespoon peanut butter**

1 **tablespoon pure vanilla extract**

1 **tablespoon honey**

1 In a food processor, combine the dates, oats, peanuts, peanut butter, vanilla, and honey. Process until crumbly, 3 minutes.

2 Use a 1½-tablespoon cookie scoop to make 12 balls. You may need to lightly squeeze or roll the balls between your hands to help stick together. Set the balls aside on a cutting board or piece of waxed paper until firm. Store in an airtight container.

NUTRITION (PER SERVING): 408 calories, 13 g protein, 47 g carbohydrates, 7 g fiber, 27 g sugars, 20 g fat, 3 g saturated fat, 94 mg sodium

ALMOND SPICE SCONES

PREP TIME: 20 MINUTES / TOTAL TIME: 40 MINUTES / **MAKES 6 SERVINGS**

Shown in photo insert pages.

- 2 cups whole wheat or white whole wheat flour, divided
- 1 cup almond meal/flour
- 2 teaspoons baking powder
- ¼ cup granulated sugar
- 1 teaspoon apple or pumpkin pie spice
  Pinch of salt
- 4 tablespoons coconut oil, solid
- ⅔ cup unsweetened vanilla almond milk
- 1 egg
- 1 teaspoon almond extract
- 2 tablespoons raw sugar

1 Preheat the oven to 350°F. Line a baking sheet with parchment paper.

2 In a food processor, combine 1½ cups of the whole wheat flour, almond meal, baking powder, granulated sugar, pie spice, and salt. Process until well blended.

3 Add the oil and pulse again until evenly distributed and the mixture forms fine crumbs. Add the milk, egg, and almond extract and pulse 8 to 10 times, until the dough is uniform and sticky.

4 Dust a clean, flat surface with the remaining ½ cup flour and scrape the dough onto the surface. Gently knead the dough to incorporate enough flour so the dough is no longer sticky. Pat into a round that is roughly 2" tall and 8" in diameter.

5 Cut into 6 wedges, and place each on the prepared baking sheet.

6 Evenly sprinkle the wedges with the raw sugar, and pat gently into the dough. Bake until golden with a light crust, about 20 minutes. Cool on a wire rack.

NUTRITION (PER SERVING): 376 calories, 10 g protein, 47 g carbohydrates, 7 g fiber, 13 g sugars, 19 g fat, 9 g saturated fat, 198 mg sodium

HEALTHY HINT

Breakfast can actually boost brainpower and help you fight disease all day long. Years of research shows that a morning meal—regardless of its effect on weight loss—hones cognitive performance, supplies extra energy for exercise (no matter what time of day you work out), and can help stave off type 2 diabetes, high cholesterol, and even heart disease.

MOCHA PEANUT BUTTER SMOOTHIE

PREP TIME: 5 MINUTES / TOTAL TIME: 10 MINUTES / **MAKES 2 SERVINGS**

1   scoop (33 grams) chocolate protein powder

½   cup brewed coffee

½   cup unsweetened almond milk

½   frozen banana

1   tablespoon almond butter

1   teaspoon pure vanilla extract

4   ice cubes

In a blender, combine the protein powder, coffee, milk, banana, almond butter, vanilla, and ice cubes. Blend until smooth.

NUTRITION (PER SERVING): 301 calories, 27 g protein, 23 g carbohydrates, 7 g fiber, 8 g sugars, 12 g fat, 1 g saturated fat, 490 mg sodium

HEALTHY HINT

Protein powders make getting a good meal a breeze on busy mornings. Whether you choose whey powder, pea protein, or egg whites, opt for an organic product that's high in protein (more than 15 grams per serving) and low in carbs (fewer than 5 grams).

PEACH SMOOTHIE

PREP TIME: 6 MINUTES / TOTAL TIME: 6 MINUTES / **MAKES 2 SERVINGS**

2   **scoops vanilla protein powder (25 to 35 grams)**

2   **cups frozen sliced peaches**

1½   **cups unsweetened plain almond milk**

½   **ripe avocado, peeled and pitted**

⅛   **teaspoon ground cardamom**

In a blender, combine the protein powder, peaches, milk, avocado, and cardamom. Blend until smooth.

NUTRITION (PER SERVING): 290 calories, 27 g protein, 21 g carbohydrates, 15 g fiber, 13 g sugars, 10 g fat, 1 g saturated fat, 139 mg sodium

GREEN GINGER SMOOTHIE

PREP TIME: 5 MINUTES / TOTAL TIME: 5 MINUTES / **MAKES 1 SERVING**

½ **cup chopped kale**

½ **cup water**

⅓ **cup plain, pineapple-flavored, or mango-flavored coconut water**

¼ **cup frozen pineapple chunks**

¼ **cup frozen mango chunks**

¼ **medium avocado**

1 **tablespoon chia seeds, unsweetened shredded coconut, hemp seeds, or ground flaxseeds**

½ **teaspoon grated fresh ginger**

In a blender, combine the kale, water, coconut water, pineapple, mango, avocado, seeds or coconut, and ginger. Blend until smooth.

NUTRITION (PER SERVING): 291 calories, 18 g protein, 29 g carbohydrates, 9 g fiber, 16 g sugars, 14 g fat, 4 g saturated fat, 112 mg sodium

YOUR VISUAL GUIDE TO CLEAN EATING

THERE ARE SOME CLEAN PACKAGED FOODS that can help you prepare healthy meals with minimal effort. This guide will give you confidence when reaching for packaged goods. In these pages, you'll find grocery items broken down into three categories: not clean, clean, and cleanest. You'll learn not only how to pick the best brand to purchase but also which ones to avoid. Can't find the "cleanest" version of the item you're looking for? Go for the "clean" version of that product and know that you're still getting metabolism-boosting benefits. The photos offer advice on the best brands to buy and countless tips on how to read a product's packaging. In no time, you'll become an expert at picking out the cleanest foods.

When reaching for something not shown on these pages, follow these rules to find a clean packaged food—*fast.*

1. Scan the ingredients. Do you recognize all (or most) of them? If you wanted to, could you buy the ingredients separately? If not, take a pass on that product.

2. Opt for organic. This guarantees that the food was produced without synthetic pesticides, is free of artificial additives, *and* is made without genetically modified ingredients. Check, check, check!

3. Scrutinize the sugar. Stick to products with fewer than 15 grams of sugar per serving and with most of that sweetness coming from real foods, like fruit—not from added sugars.

4. Watch the salt. A snack should have fewer than 250 milligrams of sodium per serving; a meal should have fewer than 600 milligrams.

PACKAGED FRUITS

LET'S START WITH OUR JUICY STAND-IN for all fruit—packaged peaches. As it turns out, frozen fruits without added sugar can actually have more nutritional value than their fresh counterparts. See, convenience doesn't always mean compromise.

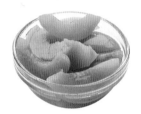

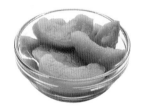

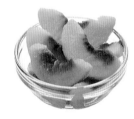

NOT CLEAN

Canned Peaches in Syrup

Peaches in syrup are basically low-nutrient sugar bombs. Thanks to the addition of corn syrup, they have more sugar than either frozen or canned-in-juice varieties. Another bummer: The high heat used in the canning process degrades those powerful antioxidants.

CLEAN

Canned or Jarred Peaches in 100% Juice

Peaches in 100% juice may contain some of the nutritional benefits of fresh and frozen, such as the antioxidants beta-carotene, vitamin C, and vitamin E, as well as B vitamins like folate. The big difference, though, is that they lack flavor.

CLEANEST

Organic Frozen Sliced Peaches

Frozen fruits are frozen just after they're harvested—at their nutritional peak—so their vitamins, minerals, and antioxidants are locked in and won't be depleted as they sit in the freezer. Bonus: They're insanely versatile. Blend them with yogurt for a protein-packed smoothie; bake them with oats, cinnamon, and a drizzle of olive oil for dessert; or simply use a few to top off your morning oatmeal.

PACKAGED VEGETABLES

POPEYE DIDN'T EAT IT FOR NOTHING. Spinach is our stand-in for veggies because it is one of the most nutrient-dense greens you can find—in addition to packing a healthy dose of vitamin C, it's loaded with vitamin K, which will help keep your bones healthy; lutein, which helps prevent cataracts and macular degeneration; and twice the iron of most other greens—but if you're not buying it fresh, you may not reap these benefits.

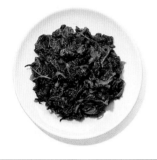 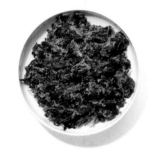 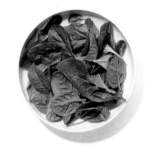

NOT CLEAN	CLEAN	CLEANEST
Canned Spinach	*Frozen Spinach*	*Organic Bagged Spinach*
Sure, a can of spinach is far from junk food and may still provide some health benefits, but by choosing canned you're going to lose out on taste and texture and add a bunch of unwanted sodium to your diet.	While some frozen fruits and veggies can actually have a higher nutritional value than their fresh counterparts, a study by the Frozen Food Foundation found that frozen spinach had less vitamin C than a fresh bunch.	A bag of washed and ready-to-eat fresh spinach retains far more nutrients and is far more versatile than other forms. Use it to quickly prepare salads and soups, sauté and use it as a base for your protein, or whip it into a smoothie.

LETTUCE

MOST GREENS LIVE UP TO THEIR superfood reputations, packing a good dose of potassium, vitamin K, and folate, as well as an array of antioxidants, and even calcium. But to be sure you're getting max nutrients per leaf—and avoiding pesticides in the process—opt for organic and locally grown whenever possible.

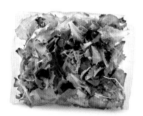 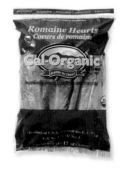 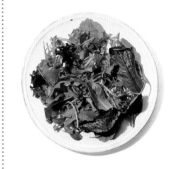

●	●●	●●●
NOT CLEAN	**CLEAN**	**CLEANEST**
Regular Bagged Greens	*Organic Bagged Greens*	*Organic Locally Grown Greens*

NOT CLEAN

Conventional bagged greens are often washed with a mix of chlorine and water—not exactly appetizing. And like organic bagged greens, they're likely to have fewer nutrients than fresh. But perhaps worst of all is that they're grown with, and contain residues of, pesticides and fertilizers that no amount of washing can completely remove.

CLEAN

Because they're free of pesticides and funky chemicals, bagged greens are a good backup plan. But greens of any kind—even organic—can be up to 2 weeks old by the time you get them home, meaning they contain fewer nutrients than they should. Even more important, a recent investigation of 16 brands of prewashed greens found that many contained coliforms and enterococci, bacteria linked to food-borne illnesses.

CLEANEST

To get the most nutritional bang for your leafy green buck, buy locally grown organic greens that aren't prebagged. These can pack four times as many antioxidants as precut, washed, and bagged varieties, which lose more nutrients the longer they're in transit. And the fact that they aren't bagged means they're less likely to encourage the growth of dangerous pathogens that can make you sick.

BEEF

GROUND BEEF AND STEAK ARE SOME of the most important foods to buy clean, given the dire state of factory farms and the overuse of antibiotics and hormones—but they also have some of the most confusing label terminology out there. Your safest and most nutritious bet will always be 100% grass-fed and organic. No question.

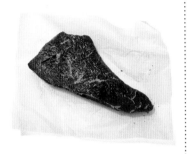
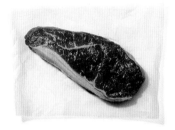
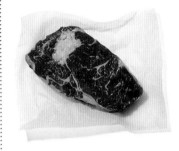

NOT CLEAN	CLEAN	CLEANEST
Conventional Beef	*Organic Beef*	*100% Grass-Fed Beef*

These animals spend much of their lives in cramped feedlots where they're fattened up on a diet of nonorganic grains and are often given growth hormones and antibiotics. Conventional beef contains far fewer omega-3s and more cholesterol and saturated fat than grass-fed and organic do.

Organically raised cattle start on pasture. Then, to increase their weight before slaughter, most cattle are fed a diet of organic grain, which diminishes the nutritional profile of their meat compared to that of 100% grass-fed cattle. On the plus side, they're never given hormones or antibiotics, and they have access to the outdoors throughout their lives.

Grass-fed cattle are never injected with hormones and antibiotics, and they graze on pasture their entire lives—no grains allowed. The meat from grass-fed animals contains more omega-3s, conjugated linoleic acid (CLA, a fat that may reduce risk of heart disease and cancer and even promote weight loss), and nutrients such as beta-carotene than conventional beef.

TURKEY

WHO DOESN'T LOVE TURKEY? IT'S LEAN, versatile, and just one serving delivers nearly half a day's worth of protein, plus a healthy dose of selenium and B vitamins. But to make sure you're getting all of the good stuff and none of the funky flavorings or antibiotics, opt for fresh and organic.

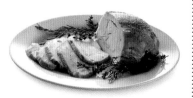 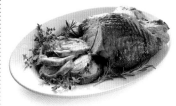 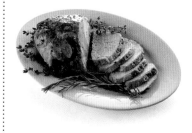

NOT CLEAN

Conventional Frozen Turkey Injected with Sodium or Flavor

Many store-bought frozen turkeys have been injected with a solution that contains preservatives, sodium, coloring ingredients, or artificial flavors. This solution can negatively impact your blood pressure.

CLEAN

Conventional Natural Turkey

No added sodium or flavorings here, but these birds were still most likely given antibiotics; fed a diet of nonorganic, potentially pesticide-riddled feed; and raised in cramped indoor cages.

CLEANEST

Organic Natural Turkey

Buying organic means avoiding antibiotics and pesticides (from the nonorganic feed the turkeys consumed), while natural, according to the USDA, means that your turkey hasn't been injected with sodium or flavorings. Pastured turkeys—ones that have been allowed to roam outdoors in their natural environment—are an added plus, but may be hard to find.

DELI MEATS

SURE, COLD CUTS ARE A QUICK and easy source of protein, but they're also a speedy delivery system for not-so-delicious synthetic nitrites, excess sodium, and fillers. To ensure that you're loading your organic whole grain bread or lettuce wrap with only the good stuff, go for organic and uncured.

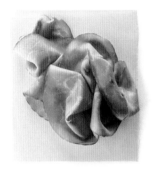
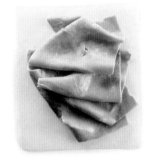
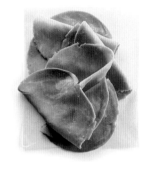

NOT CLEAN	CLEAN	CLEANEST
Traditional Cured Meats (with Synthetic Nitrites)	*Conventional Uncured Meats*	*Organic Uncured Meat*

NOT CLEAN

Traditional Cured Meats (with Synthetic Nitrites)

Traditionally cured deli meats are just kind of gross—they can contain synthetic nitrites, loads of fillers, and excessive sodium, which can lead to high blood pressure. Studies suggest that sodium may increase your risk of heart disease, diabetes, and cancer.

CLEAN

Conventional Uncured Meats

These won't deliver the same benefits as organic—the animals they're made from were likely given antibiotics and hormones—but they'll still be free of synthetic nitrites. To maintain freshness and kill pathogens, uncured meats do often contain celery powder or salt, a naturally occurring nitrate that's considered safer than its lab-produced counterpart. These might also contain fillers for texture, such as corn syrup and carrageenan—a seaweed extract that's been linked to gut inflammation.

CLEANEST

Organic Uncured Meat

The animals used to produce these meats were fed a cleaner diet of organic feed and not given antibiotics or hormones, and these meats weren't pumped full of synthetic sodium nitrite, either. All deli meats, however, can be high in sodium, so always be mindful of how much you eat. You can find presliced brands such as Applegate at most markets, and the deli counters at most natural food stores should have organic, uncured options.

SALMON

SALMON MAY BE EVERYONE'S FAVORITE SUPERFOOD of the sea—it has loads of heart-healthy omega-3s and lots of filling protein, and it pretty much tastes incredible however you prep it. But if you want to avoid seriously scary pollutants and antibiotics, go wild.

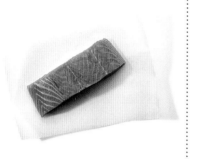 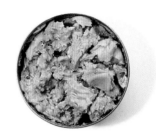 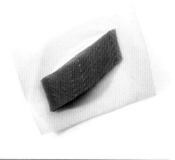

●	●●	●●●
NOT CLEAN	**CLEAN**	**CLEANEST**
Farm-Raised Salmon	*Canned Wild Salmon*	*Fresh Wild or Alaskan Salmon*

Farm-raised salmon are far more likely to be exposed to persistent organic pollutants (POPs) than fish that have lived their lives in a natural environment.

It seems strange, but if you can't get fresh wild salmon, go for canned instead of fresh farmed salmon. Canned salmon will still give you a helping of omega-3 fatty acids, essential nutrients that your body cannot produce on its own. These fats help promote healthy joints and skin, and they reduce your risk of heart disease.

Wild salmon is both more nutritious and safer than farmed salmon—it has fewer calories and a significantly lower fat content than farmed salmon, but it still packs a good dose of heart-healthy omega-3s. Eating wild also means you're avoiding POPs, which have been associated with obesity, diabetes, and cancer.

CANNED FISH

CANNED FISH IS AN EASY AND convenient way to get a dose of protein and omega-3s in your diet without doing all the prep work required with fresh fish. But fear about toxins is warranted when it comes to this convenience food, so minimize your exposure by choosing the safest seafood.

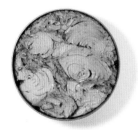
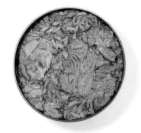
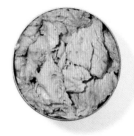

NOT CLEAN	CLEAN	CLEANEST
White or Albacore Tuna	*Light Tuna*	*Canned Wild Salmon*

Mercury levels in canned white or albacore tuna can be up to three times that of light tuna! Even worse, most conventionally processed brands on the market are lower in omega-3s than both light tuna and canned salmon.

If you can't give up your tuna salad, opt for light tuna over white or albacore. Light tuna, made from lower-mercury skipjack tuna, not only contains fewer calories than white or albacore but also has less sodium and more selenium, vitamin B_{12}, and iron.

Canned wild salmon provides more omega-3s in the form of DHA and EPA—two fatty acids that are essential for a healthy brain—than other canned fish (about 500 milligrams in an 8-ounce serving). Bonus: Because salmon is lower on the food chain (typically feeding on microscopic plankton), it's likely to contain fewer toxins (such as mercury) than tuna.

EGGS

SCRAMBLED EGGS—PACKED WITH NUTRIENTS LIKE CHOLINE, which is essential for healthy liver function—can be the perfect quick and clean breakfast. But all the different labels applied to eggs are enough to make your head spin. In reality, there's only one variety you can truly feel good about eating: organic and pasture-raised.

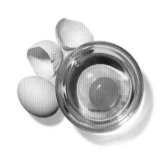 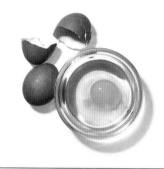 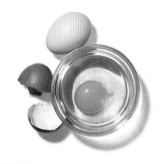

NOT CLEAN	CLEAN	CLEANEST
Conventional Eggs	*Cage-Free Eggs*	*Organic Pasture-Raised Eggs*

Conventional eggs are best avoided. Not only are they less nutritious than pasture-raised eggs, but studies show that they have higher levels of salmonella than eggs from organic and cage-free hens. This is in large part because the cramped quarters standard to conventional egg farming lead to a more concentrated amount of fecal matter in a small space, and this attracts more disease-carrying insects and rodents. Crowded cages are difficult to disinfect, and these conditions stress out hens, which may lower their natural immunity. Sounds pretty darn horrific, doesn't it?

Cage-free eggs come from hens that aren't confined to cages, but they could still be raised in close quarters. They can spread their wings and lay eggs in nest boxes. It's also easier to maintain sanitary conditions for cage-free hens. But unless they're raised organically, cage-free hens are fed grains made from crops heavily treated with chemical pesticides. There's no mandatory third-party auditing for the term "cage-free," so look for the term along with a seal such as "Certified Humane" or "Animal Welfare Approved."

Pasture-raised hens hunt and peck for grass and insects, and their diets may be supplemented with organic feed. These eggs can contain two and a half times the amount of omega-3s and twice as much vitamin E as conventional eggs. There's no mandatory third-party auditing for the term "pasture-raised," however, so seek these eggs out from a farmer you trust or from a brand that's been pasture-raised certified ("Certified Humane" or "American Humane Certified"), such as Vital Farms Alfresco Eggs.

BEANS

THINK OF BEANS AS A SUPERFOOD for your heart. Their high fiber, potassium, and magnesium contents work together to help keep blood pressure in check. Bonus: Just 1 cup of beans packs 15 grams of vegetarian-friendly protein. But packaging and added ingredients can make certain brands clean-diet killers.

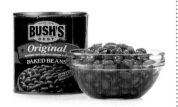
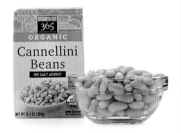
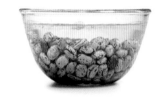

NOT CLEAN	CLEAN	CLEANEST
Baked Beans	*Unflavored Packaged Beans*	*Dried Beans*

Sure, they're delicious and may be okay for that once-in-a-while cookout, but in general, pass on the baked beans. They contain added sugar (some pack 12 grams in just ½ cup), salt, fat, and preservatives.

Regular packaged beans will still provide beneficial nutrients like protein and fiber, but you'll often end up consuming quite a bit of sodium, and, in the case of canned varieties, exposing yourself to dangerous BPA. Some canned beans—usually the organic brands, like Eden Foods—use BPA-free cans, so opt for those. Or choose beans that come in cardboard Tetra Pak packaging, such as Target's Simply Balanced organic brand beans, which are always BPA-free.

Buying dried beans, rather than beans in a can, will ensure that they're free of added salt and BPA—a chemical linked to a slew of health problems, including breast cancer. Recent research shows that avoiding BPA-containing packaging can immediately reduce BPA levels in your body. Soak dried beans overnight to cut down on cooking time the next day.

BREAD

DITCHING WHITE BREAD FOR WHOLE WHEAT is a no-brainer, but you shouldn't stop there. For maximum nutrition per slice, minimal additives, and fewer refined carb–induced cravings, your best bet is organic whole wheat bread.

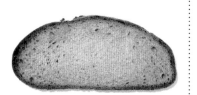 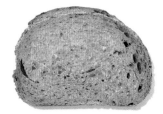 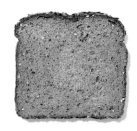

NOT CLEAN	CLEAN	CLEANEST
Wheat or White Bread	*Whole Wheat or Whole Grain Bread*	*Organic Whole Wheat or Whole Grain Bread*
Bread made with refined flour should be skipped altogether. Most of the naturally occurring nutrients from the wheat kernels have been stripped away, which means you're missing out on some of that blood sugar–stabilizing fiber and protein.	The grains used in nonorganic whole wheat or whole grain bread have likely been treated with pesticides called organophosphates—compounds linked to lower IQ and ADHD in children and which have unknown effects on adults. Nonorganic breads have also been found to have more preservatives, thickeners, and refined flours.	Whole wheat bread contains the original kernel (bran, germ, and endosperm), leaving fiber and protein intact. Bread made with other grains is also a good choice, as long as the word "whole" appears before them on the ingredient list. Studies have shown that consuming whole grains helps promote a healthy weight. Buy organic whenever possible to avoid pesticides.

RICE

DON'T KNOW ABOUT YOU, BUT THE last time we looked at the varieties of rice in the grocery store, we were a tad overwhelmed. It's not just a matter of white versus brown anymore—jasmine, basmati, arborio, black, red, and wild are all options. Next time you need a base for your stir-fry, pick the rice that packs the most nutrients: wild.

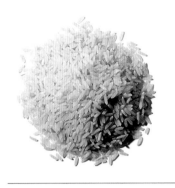
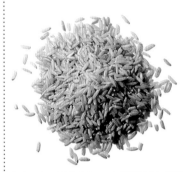
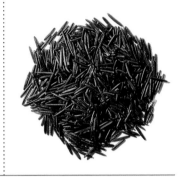

NOT CLEAN	CLEAN	CLEANEST
White Rice	*Brown Rice*	*Wild Rice*

Your typical white rice isn't necessarily unhealthy, but its nutritional value simply doesn't begin to measure up to wild or brown rice.

Mild and nutty brown rice beats white. It's considered a whole grain because, unlike white, it still contains the bran and the germ, which provide you with a dose of fiber. That fiber makes brown rice less likely to contribute to blood sugar spikes and drops.

Wild rice is actually the seed of a marsh grass found near the Great Lakes. It contains protein, fiber, folate, manganese, zinc, magnesium, phosphorus, niacin, and iron, making it more nutrient-dense (and lower in carbs!) than even our beloved brown rice.

CEREALS

THE PROBLEM WITH MOST CEREAL TODAY is that it's actually dessert in disguise. Let's be real—Reese's Puffs are anything but wholesome. Healthy options do exist, but you have to be a savvy shopper and keep the balance of sugar, fiber, and protein on top of your priority list.

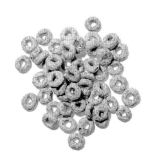 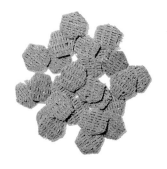 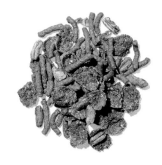

●	●●	●●●
### NOT CLEAN	### CLEAN	### CLEANEST
Most Store-Bought Cereal	*Whole Grain Cereal with Less Than 10 Grams Sugar*	*Organic Whole Grain Cereal Low in Sugar and High in Protein or Fiber*
Be careful with the majority of store-bought cereals—they're often made with refined grains, processed sugars, and a slew of preservatives. They also contain artificial colors that are derived from petroleum and which have been linked to behavior problems in children.	If you're having a hard time finding a cereal that meets all of our clean criteria, the most important factor to consider is sugar: Keep it under 10 grams per serving to avoid crazy spikes in blood sugar that put you at risk for overeating later.	To feel satisfied and energized, choose an organic whole grain cereal with fewer than 10 grams of sugar and at least 5 grams of fiber and/or protein per serving. And be wary of what that serving size is: You might find an option that fits the bill only to discover that the serving is a measly ¾ cup, putting you at risk of overdoing it on sugar if you pour a full bowl.

OATMEAL

WHOLESOME, FILLING, FIBER-PACKED OATMEAL: WELL, THAT'S what it should be, anyway. But not all oatmeal is created equal. Your best choice is the one that's least messed-around-with: steel-cut oats.

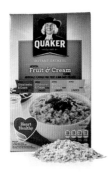

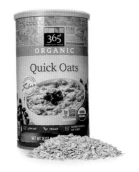

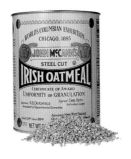

●	● ●	● ● ●
NOT CLEAN	**CLEAN**	**CLEANEST**
Flavored Instant Oatmeal	*Plain Rolled or Quick-Cooking Oats*	*Steel-Cut Oats*

Pass on packets of flavored instant oatmeal. The oats have been highly processed, and the packets contain artificial flavors, excessive sugar, and preservatives. If you want convenience, toss some quick-cooking oats in a plastic baggy to take to the office or to have on hand throughout the week.

While rolled oats also help lower cholesterol, the way they're processed—they're steamed, rolled, steamed again, and then toasted—gives them a higher glycemic index, meaning that your blood sugar will experience more of a spike. But these are still a great option for the time-strapped.

Steel-cut oats are simply whole oat groats that have been cut into neat little pieces on a mill. Because they're the least processed, they have the lowest glycemic index of all oat varieties, meaning it takes more time for your body to convert them into glucose for energy, keeping your blood sugar levels stable.

NUT BUTTERS

PEANUT, ALMOND, AND CASHEW BUTTERS (just to name a few) are perfect foods to eat when you want to add protein and healthy fats to your diet. Research even suggests that eating more nuts, in their various forms, can reduce your risk of heart disease and diabetes. That's good news, but you'll need to use some caution to make sure pesticides and nasty packaging don't counter these health benefits.

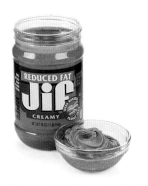

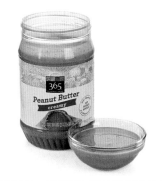

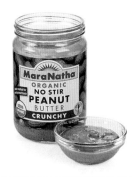

●	● ●	● ● ●
NOT CLEAN	**CLEAN**	**CLEANEST**
Reduced-Fat Nut Butters	*Conventional Nut Butters without Added Sweeteners*	*Organic Nut Butters without Added Sweeteners, in Glass Jars*

Don't buy into low-fat claims on nut butter jars: While there may be less fat, there's more sugar, and the healthy mono-unsaturated fats in nut butters are an important part of your diet that shouldn't be stripped away.

Nonorganic nut butters can contain pesticides and other synthetic ingredients. Plastic nut butter jars may also contain potentially dangerous chemicals that may leach into your food.

Whichever nut butter you prefer, select organic varieties sold in glass jars. They'll be free of pesticides and potentially carcinogenic chemicals found in plastic packaging. Also, since many manufacturers add sugar to peanut butter, check labels to be sure the product you pick doesn't include any sweeteners.

BUTTER

ONCE THOUGHT OF AS A COMPLETE "diet don't," real butter is finally making a comeback, and with good reason: High-quality varieties are thought to contain more beta-carotene and a healthier fatty acid profile than lab-made margarine, which is a sneaky source of dangerous trans fats.

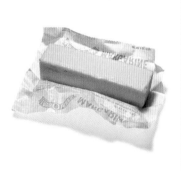

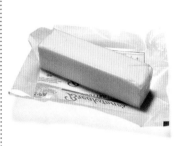

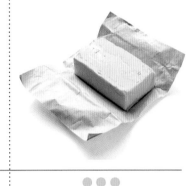

●	●●	●●●
NOT CLEAN	**CLEAN**	**CLEANEST**
Margarine	*Conventional Butter*	*Organic Grass-Fed Butter*

Margarine and other "buttery spreads" can contain trans fats—the fats that are most strongly associated with heart disease—as well as synthetic vitamins, soy protein isolate, and other additives and preservatives. Some studies have shown that people who eat margarine are twice as likely to suffer from cardiovascular disease.

Think twice about conventional butter, as it's likely the product of cows that have been given antibiotics and growth hormones. That being said, it's still more natural than margarine, and its fat will help boost your absorption of disease-fighting nutrients from the veggies you consume.

Butter from grass-fed cows has been shown to contain healthier fats than butter from grain-fed cattle. A grass-fed diet also contributes to larger amounts of beta-carotene, which your body converts to vitamin A.

SALAD DRESSINGS

TOPPING YOUR LOVINGLY PREPARED SALADS WITH a trans fat–loaded dressing (or even a fat-free one) should be a crime. Unfortunately, those dressings make up a lot of what's lining store shelves. Keep it simple and make your own—it literally takes 30 seconds! Try one of our three unique recipes in Chapter 11.

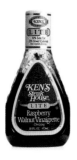

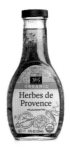

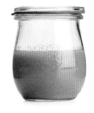

NOT CLEAN	CLEAN	CLEANEST
Conventional Store-Bought Dressings	*Organic or Non-GMO Store-Bought Dressings*	*Homemade Dressing*
Most of these are loaded with added sugar, sodium, artificial colorings, and preservatives. They may also contain trans fats in the form of partially hydrogenated vegetable oils, which are linked to heart disease.	If you buy bottled dressing, look for an organic or non-GMO dressing, nothing synthetic, few ingredients, and fewer than 5 grams of sugar per 2 tablespoons. Oh, and pick one that has some fat (at least 3 grams, although the more, the better) because it helps you absorb the nutrients in your veggies.	A homemade vinaigrette of olive oil and vinegar will make your salad even better for you. Olive oil contains anti-inflammatory monounsaturated fats, and apple cider vinegar consumed before a carb-heavy meal can slow the rise of blood sugar (reducing cravings) and improve insulin sensitivity.

PASTA SAUCES

WHOLE WHEAT PASTA, VEGGIES, AND A lean protein topped with a little marinara is an easy and nutritious meal. But don't ruin it all by choosing the wrong sauce. Pick something that will enhance your meal's nutrition, not detract from it.

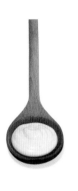

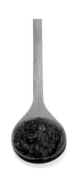

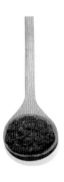

NOT CLEAN	CLEAN	CLEANEST
Store-Bought Cream Sauce	*Regular Tomato Sauce*	*Organic Tomato Sauce without Added Sugars*

Just say no to dairy-based cream sauces. They're full of unhealthy fats, sodium, and preservatives—and you definitely don't get the antioxidant benefits of tomatoes from these sauces. If you ever indulge in a cream sauce, make it yourself and use quality ingredients.

Standard store-bought tomato sauce can contain up to 12 grams of sugar per ½ cup, and this sugar may come in the form of high-fructose corn syrup. And don't forget about the excess sodium, preservatives, and traces of pesticides.

Low-sugar organic sauce is delicious and packs good doses of vitamin C and lycopene, an antioxidant that may help reduce your risk of heart disease, cancer, and macular degeneration. Want to make your own (and can't find grandma's recipe)? Try our homemade Tomato-Basil Marinara in Chapter 11.

MAYO

MAYO GETS A BAD REPUTATION, BUT this classic sandwich spread can actually be part of a clean diet if you know what to look for. The secret is finding a product that keeps its ingredients simple—just eggs, oil, vinegar, and a bit of salt—and uses high-quality oils. (If you can't find one at the supermarket, try our homemade version in Chapter 11.)

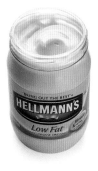 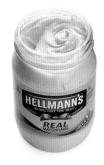 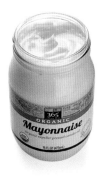

NOT CLEAN	CLEAN	CLEANEST
Reduced-Fat Mayo	*Regular Mayo*	*Organic Mayo Made with Non-GMO Expeller-Pressed Oil*
While it's tempting, resist the urge to cut calories by using low-fat mayo. These mayos generally include dangerous ingredients (such as high-fructose corn syrup) and fillers (like xanthan gum) to add texture in fat's absence, making them unwelcome additions to a clean diet.	Your typical supermarket mayonnaise is heavily processed and likely to contain genetically modified ingredients (thanks to the inclusion of genetically modified soy), as well as sugar or corn syrup, but it is generally free of funky fillers.	Unlike conventional and reduced-fat mayonnaise, organic and expeller-pressed mayonnaise is free of GMOs and uses oil that was extracted via pressure, as opposed to with potentially dangerous chemical solvents. Whole Foods 365 Everyday Value Organic brand and Spectrum Organic mayonnaise are both good choices.

YOGURT

BUYING YOGURT IS ALMOST AS CONFUSING as buying eggs. There are so many varieties and claims slapped on yogurts that it's hard to know what to focus on—Greek, probiotic, low-fat, plain, or fruit-filled. The solution happens to be refreshingly simple.

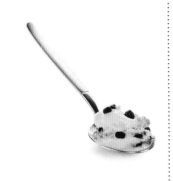

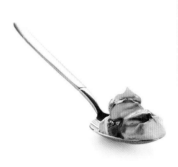

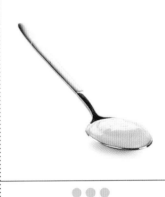

NOT CLEAN	CLEAN	CLEANEST
Sweetened Yogurt with Mix-Ins, or Artificially Sweetened Yogurt	*Naturally Sweetened Yogurt*	*Plain Yogurt*

Sweetened yogurts with mix-ins like granola or crushed cookies should be avoided at all costs. These yogurts are laden with added sugar and artificial ingredients—many contain more of the sweet stuff than a candy bar does. Also avoid yogurts that include artificial sweeteners like sucralose (Splenda) or aspartame.

If you want a yogurt with some flavor, look for "fruit" listed as an actual ingredient—otherwise you're just getting fruit flavoring. Or try a yogurt sweetened with honey or stevia, a natural no-calorie sweetener. But always avoid yogurts that list sugar as their first or second ingredient.

When choosing a yogurt, a plain and ideally organic yogurt (of any variety you like—Greek, Icelandic, whatever) is your most nutritious option. Plain will provide a healthy dose of protein and calcium without any added sugar, and organic will ensure that no hormones, antibiotics, or GMO ingredients are present. For some flavor, add your own clean ingredients, such as walnuts, blueberries, and a drizzle of honey.

VEGGIE CHIPS

VEGGIE CHIPS SOUND HEALTHY, RIGHT? WHILE they can be a good alternative to conventional greasy potato chips, it's important to choose varieties that are actually an improvement on the original, not just dressed-up corn and potato flour.

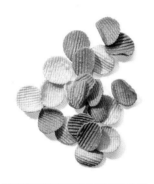 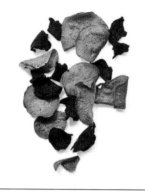 

●	● ●	● ● ●
NOT CLEAN	**CLEAN**	**CLEANEST**
Store-Bought Veggie Chips Made with Corn or Potato Flour	*Store-Bought Whole-Veggie Chips*	*Homemade Kale, Sweet Potato, or Beet Chips*
Veggie chips made with corn or potato flour are best left on the shelf. Many of these chips are high in fat, calories, and sodium, and they're actually more processed than conventional potato chips. Talk about deceptive.	If you buy premade kale or other veggie chips, an actual vegetable should be listed as the first ingredient, followed by ingredients like oil, salt, and spices. The shorter the list, the better.	DIY chips offer the most nutrients and fewest funky ingredients per crunch since you get to control how much oil, salt, and other seasonings you use. The easiest: kale chips. Just rinse, pat dry, coat in oil and spices, and bake. Kick the flavor up a notch by making one of the two delicious recipes in Chapter 10. Bonus: Kale is packed with vitamin K, which helps build strong bones and ensure that your blood clots normally.

POPCORN

EATING CLEAN DOESN'T MEAN YOU HAVE to forgo your "movie and popcorn" habit. Plain popcorn is actually a great whole grain snack that's loaded with fiber. Bonus: A cup of air-popped popcorn has only 30 calories. But most movie theater and microwavable stuff is another story. We've got seven exciting flavor combos for you to try in Chapter 10.

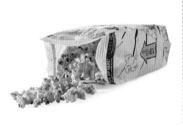

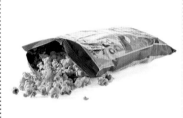

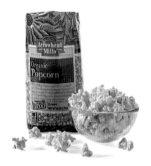

NOT CLEAN

Microwave Popcorn

Conventional microwave popcorn is actually pretty sketchy. That smell that hits you after you open the bag comes from a chemical called diacetyl, or synthetic butter flavoring. Even worse, the bag is typically lined with a chemical called perfluorooctanoic acid (PFOA)—the same chemical used on nonstick pots and pans. Research shows that PFOA in the blood is linked to health problems such as high cholesterol and various cancers. Steer clear.

CLEAN

Organic Bagged Popcorn

For convenience, organic bagged popcorn is a great alternative. It will be free of pesticides, genetically modified corn, and synthetic ingredients, but it may still contain salt and oils—not necessarily "unclean" ingredients, but you won't be able to control how much you're getting.

CLEANEST

Stove-Top, Non-GMO Popped Corn with Olive Oil and Sea Salt

Simply buy organic kernels and pop them in a saucepan with olive oil, then top with sea salt. You'll avoid pesticides, genetically modified corn, and funky chemicals.

CHOCOLATE

NUTELLA MAY NEVER MAKE IT ONTO our "clean" list (yeah, we're bummed, too), but there's definitely a whole bunch of chocolate out there that you can feel good about eating. Cocoa beans contain the antioxidants known as flavonols, which have been found to protect skin from sun damage, reduce blood pressure, and improve cardiovascular function.

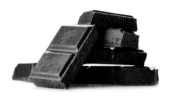 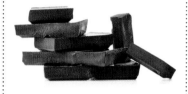 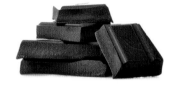

NOT CLEAN	CLEAN	CLEANEST
Milk Chocolate	*Regular Dark Chocolate*	*Organic 80% Cacao Dark Chocolate*

NOT CLEAN

Milk Chocolate

Since milk chocolate doesn't have the same cocoa content, it doesn't offer the cardiovascular benefits you'd get from dark chocolate. Milk chocolate is also full of added sugars, putting you at risk for weight gain and obesity.

CLEAN

Regular Dark Chocolate

Regular dark chocolate is certainly better than milk chocolate, but it may still contain pesticide residue, and you'll have to watch out for added sugars.

CLEANEST

Organic 80% Cacao Dark Chocolate

The next time you treat yourself with chocolate, make it organic dark chocolate with at least 80% cacao. You'll be avoiding lindane, a pesticide used in cocoa production that's been shown to cause reproductive and neurotoxic issues in animals. Plus, the darker the chocolate, the greater the health benefits.

MILK

MILK IS A CONVENIENT SOURCE OF protein and essential nutrients. One cup contains 8 grams of protein, 30% of your recommended Daily Value of bone-building calcium, and 40% of your vitamin B_{12}. But milk from conventionally raised cows may not be worth the perks.

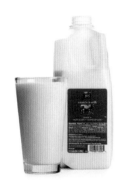

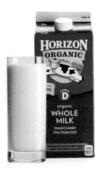

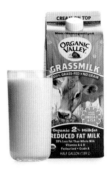

NOT CLEAN

Conventional Milk

Conventional milk comes from cows fed a processed diet containing genetically modified grain and will lack the omega-3 fatty acids you'll get from higher-quality milk. If you have to buy it, try to at least choose a brand that's rBGH- and rBST-free—cows given these growth hormones are more likely to require antibiotics.

CLEAN

Organic Milk

Non-grass-fed organic milk will still provide protein and be free of dangerous growth hormones such as rBGH or rBST, but you're not going to get the amazing benefits of fat- and inflammation-fighting fatty acids. Opt for 2% or whole, which have some fat to boost satiety and keep you full for longer than skim.

CLEANEST

Organic Grass-Fed Milk

Grass-fed cows graze in pastures and are not pumped full of growth hormones or fed a processed diet. This results in milk with more omega-3 fatty acids, vitamin E, beta-carotene, and conjugated linoleic acid (CLA), a fatty acid associated with reduced body fat and inflammation. To reap the benefits, choose a milk with adequate fat.

MILK ALTERNATIVES

IF YOU DON'T DRINK COW'S MILK, the bevy of nondairy options can be totally overwhelming. Most are at least fortified, so they've got you covered in terms of calcium and vitamin D, but you need to be careful about additives such as sugars, flavorings, and others.

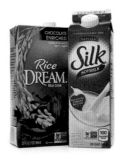

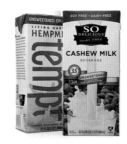

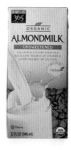

NOT CLEAN

Flavored and Sweetened Alternative Milks

Flavored nondairy milks tend to have an even higher sugar content than "original" varieties. One brand of chocolate almond milk has a whopping 17 grams per serving! That's more sugar than a chocolate frosted donut from Dunkin' Donuts (13 grams).

CLEAN

"Original" Alternative Milks, Preferably without Carrageenan

So-called "original" nondairy milks usually have around 7 grams of added sugar in the form of cane sugar. Not totally outrageous, but if you're drinking it frequently, those calories and sugar grams will add up fast. Carrageenan-free options exist even among nonorganic varieties, so opt for those.

CLEANEST

Organic Unsweetened Alternative Milks without Carrageenan

Nearly all "original" varieties of these nondairy milks contain added sugars, so ideally you should opt for "unsweetened." Choose organic varieties to avoid pesticide residue and, if possible, steer clear of brands with carrageenan—a controversial thickening agent that has been linked to GI inflammation in animals.

SUGAR

WE'LL BE HONEST: THERE'S NO MAGIC sweetener that you can eat with abandon. All should be consumed in moderation and in the context of a healthy diet that emphasizes whole foods. But certain options are less evil than others and even offer trace nutrients that plain old table sugar doesn't.

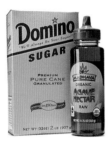 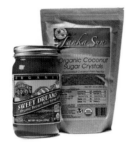 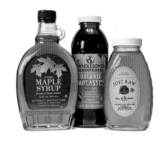

NOT CLEAN	CLEAN	CLEANEST
●	● ●	● ● ●
Table Sugar, Agave Nectar	*Coconut Sugar, Date Sugar, Brown Rice Syrup*	*Raw Local Honey, Pure Maple Syrup, Molasses*

NOT CLEAN

White table sugar consumption has been linked to obesity, type 2 diabetes, dementia, high blood pressure, and heart disease. And agave, once the go-to natural sweetener of the uber–health conscious, is likely even worse due to its extremely high fructose content. Too much fructose may contribute to unhealthy changes in liver function, triglyceride levels, and insulin sensitivity.

CLEAN

Coconut sugar, date sugar, and brown rice syrup are natural options that are less processed than table sugar, but in terms of added health benefits, they don't offer much. There's also some concern about high levels of arsenic in certain products that contain brown rice syrup.

CLEANEST

Raw local honey, pure maple syrup, and molasses are all clean options that offer trace minerals. Raw honey retains its natural enzymes, and research shows it has antimicrobial properties and may be effective at fighting cold symptoms. Maple syrup and molasses contain antioxidants and an array of minerals, including iron, potassium, magnesium, and calcium.

FLOUR

CHANCES ARE YOU'VE BEEN FLYING ON autopilot, reaching for the same type of flour for as long as you've been buying your own groceries. But switching from an ultraprocessed and bleached version of this staple to one that incorporates the whole grain can be a huge first step in cleaning up your diet.

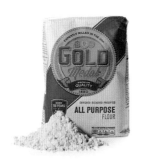
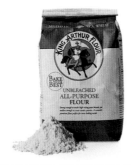
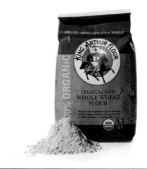

NOT CLEAN	CLEAN	CLEANEST
Regular All-Purpose Flour	*Unbleached All-Purpose Flour*	*Organic Whole-Grain Flour*

Regular all-purpose flour is best avoided, as it quickly spikes blood sugar and may contain alloxan, a chemical left over from the bleaching process. Alloxan has been shown to produce diabetes in animals, likely because it can destroy cells in the pancreas, but the effect of small quantities (like those found in flour) on humans is unknown.

These flours are missing the healthiest parts of the plant—the wheat bran and germ—and have little protein and fiber as a result. A diet full of refined flours puts you at greater risk for cardiovascular disease, type 2 diabetes, and obesity. But they are free of the chemicals used in the bleaching process, which makes them your second-best choice.

Swap out white flour for whole wheat flour. Not only will it add a more complex, nutty flavor to baked goods, but it's also nutrient-rich, featuring protein, fiber, B vitamins, antioxidants, and minerals. Bonus: A recent study showed that people who eat whole grains have less abdominal fat.

COOKING OIL

FROM OLIVE TO COCONUT TO FLAX, it's no secret that oils are having a major culinary moment. Good thing, too, since most of them are rich in healthy fats that'll help keep your heart in tip-top shape. But what's the smartest way to fit all of these different lipids into your kitchen repertoire?

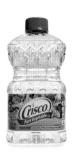 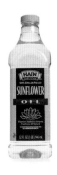 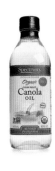

NOT CLEAN	CLEAN	CLEANEST
Conventional (Uses Hexane or Chemical Extraction)	*Expeller-Pressed*	*Organic Expeller-Pressed*

The chemicals used during the process of making conventional oils are toxic—hexane is classified as a neurotoxin by the Centers for Disease Control and Prevention, as it's destructive to nerve tissue when inhaled. (Little is known about the effects of consumption.) These toxins then need to be removed from the oil in a process called deodorization, which involves steaming oils at extremely high temperatures (often over 500°F). This can damage fatty acids and speed up oxidation, causing oils to go rancid. No thanks.	While organic is the safest choice because you're limiting your exposure to pesticides, at the very least, make sure your oil is expeller-pressed and not conventionally extracted with hexane, a toxic chemical, or deodorized at dangerously high temperatures that can damage the oil's fatty acids.	Olive oil, canola oil, coconut oil, sesame oil, and sunflower oil are all healthy options for clean eating. But while the type of oil you choose is important, so is the method that's used to make it. To keep the food you're cooking clean, buy organic expeller-pressed oils.

PROTEIN POWDER

PROTEIN POWDER CAN INSTANTLY MAKE A smoothie more satisfying and boost muscle-building potential after a workout. According to most experts, as long as you don't have an intolerance, your best bet is whey—a complete protein that enters your bloodstream quickly and contains a high amount of leucine, an amino acid that delivers energy to muscles. But still, choose your whey wisely.

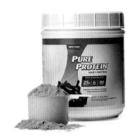 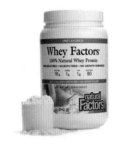 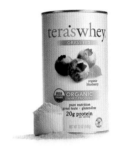

NOT CLEAN

Whey Protein with Added Sugar

Steer clear of flavored whey proteins and those that have been sweetened with sugar or artificial sweeteners to make them more palatable. These are often highly processed and contain corn- and soy-based ingredients.

CLEAN

Whey Protein Isolate or Hydrolysate with a Short Ingredient List

Whey protein isolate and hydrolysate are two other good options, delivering large amounts of protein, but you can't guarantee that they're made from high-quality, organic dairy. Plus, a recent study found that some whey protein isolates contained trace amounts of harmful metals, so be sure to buy yours from a reputable source.

CLEANEST

Concentrated Whey Protein from Organic Grass-Fed Dairy

Your cleanest whey protein powder will be a whey concentrate (80% protein) that's organic and made with milk from grass-fed cows. This means your powder contains no hormones, pesticides, or additives. No other variations of whey protein (e.g., isolate and hydrolysate) meet these specifications.

PACKAGED SOUPS/BROTHS

SOUP IS ONE OF THOSE COMFORTING, soothing meals that never gets old. But unfortunately, most store-bought soup is loaded with preservatives or packed in cans that contain toxic chemicals. Consider making your own to get only the perks.

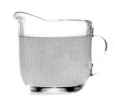 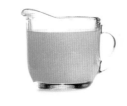 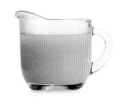

NOT CLEAN

Soup and Broth in Cans

Unless specified on the label, the epoxy linings of cans generally contain BPS and BPA, two chemicals that have been associated with hormone disruption, prostate cancer, diabetes, obesity, and aggressive behavior in children. A few brands, such as Eden, offer canned soups free of BPA and BPS. Canned soups also often contain excessive levels of sodium, sugar, artificial colors, and preservatives.

CLEAN

Soup and Broth in Tetra Pak

If you're buying soup or broth, know that it's safer to buy them in a Tetra Pak than in a can.

CLEANEST

Homemade Soups and Broths

After you've roasted a chicken, don't ditch that carcass—make a soup that's loaded with organic veggies, whole grains such as brown rice or whole wheat pasta, and beans. Start with our Homemade Bone Broth in Chapter 11. Not a meat eater? Try our hearty Homemade Vegetable Broth (also in Chapter 11) as a base for your favorite soups.

FLAVORINGS

TAKE ORGANIC VEGETABLES, WHOLE GRAINS, AND lean proteins to another level of flavor with the right herbs and spices. Just don't fall victim to the convenience of packaged spice blends and most conventional condiments.

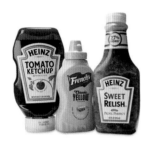 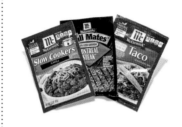 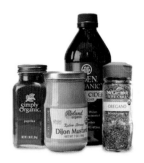

NOT CLEAN	CLEAN	CLEANEST
Store-Bought Condiments or Sauce Packets	*Store-Bought Spice Packets*	*Fresh Herbs, Organic Jarred Herbs and Spices, Vinegars, Salt, Mustards, and Other Low- or No-Sugar Condiments*
Store-bought sauce packets and condiments generally contain synthetic ingredients as well as added sugar and salt—and bring nothing to the table as far as health benefits go.	These typically contain a mix of herbs, spices, and salt. They're not likely to be organic, but they're generally not loaded with funky additives and preservatives, either.	Use organic spices and herbs, vinegars, salt, and mustards to enhance the flavors of the meals you're preparing. All are very minimally processed and even pack health benefits of their own—herbs and spices contain a variety of antioxidants and phytonutrients, and vinegars contain acids that help curb cravings.

SOUPS AND SALADS

BEEF BARLEY SOUP

I	tablespoon olive oil
I	pound well-trimmed lean boneless beef top sirloin, cut into ¾" cubes
2	onions, halved and thinly sliced
3	cloves garlic, minced
8	ounces cremini mushrooms, sliced
3	carrots, sliced
2	ribs celery, thinly sliced
I	parsnip, halved lengthwise and sliced
½	teaspoon dried thyme, crumbled
3½	cups low-sodium beef broth
3	cups water
¼	cup no-salt-added tomato puree
½	cup pearl barley

1 In a Dutch oven or a large saucepan over medium heat, heat the oil. Lightly brown the beef until the liquid evaporates, 3 minutes.

2 Cook the onions and garlic until the onions soften, 3 minutes. Add the mushrooms, carrots, celery, parsnip, and thyme, and cook until the vegetables begin to soften, about 6 minutes.

3 Reduce the heat to medium-low. Add the broth, water, and tomato puree. Bring to a boil over medium-high heat. Reduce the heat to low, cover, and simmer for 45 minutes.

4 Stir in the barley and simmer until the barley is tender, 45 minutes.

NUTRITION (PER SERVING): 263 calories, 24 g protein, 28 g carbohydrates, 6 g fiber, 7 g sugars, 7 g fat, 2 g saturated fat, 138 mg sodium

CHICKEN SOUP WITH ASIAN NOODLES

PREP TIME: 20 MINUTES / TOTAL TIME: 50 MINUTES / **MAKES 6 SERVINGS**

I	tablespoon olive oil
3	carrots, thinly sliced
2	red bell peppers, thinly sliced
2	ribs celery, thinly sliced
2	cloves garlic, thinly sliced
4	thin slices fresh ginger
4	cups low-sodium chicken broth
3	cups water
4	ounces buckwheat soba noodles (or whole wheat thin spaghetti), broken in half
3	cups shredded cooked chicken
2	scallions, sliced
¼	cup small fresh basil leaves

1 In a large pot over medium heat, heat the oil. Cook the carrots, bell peppers, celery, garlic, and ginger, stirring, until the vegetables have softened, 6 minutes.

2 Stir in the broth and water. Over medium-high heat, bring to a boil. Add the noodles, reduce the heat to medium-low, and simmer until just tender, 5 minutes. Stir in the chicken and simmer until heated through, 3 minutes. Remove the ginger with a slotted spoon and discard. Season to taste with salt and black pepper. Ladle into bowls and top with the scallions and basil.

NUTRITION (PER SERVING): 247 calories, 22 g protein, 20 g carbohydrates, 3 g fiber, 3 g sugars, 7 g fat, 1 g saturated fat, 385 mg sodium

MINESTRONE

PREP TIME: 10 MINUTES / TOTAL TIME: 45 MINUTES / MAKES 6 SERVINGS

2¼ cups water

¾ cup wild rice

1 tablespoon olive oil

4 ounces Italian chicken or turkey sausage, thinly sliced

5 cups shredded green cabbage

2 cloves garlic, minced

1 medium zucchini, thinly sliced

1 rib celery, chopped

8 cups (2 quarts) low-sodium chicken broth

1 can (14.5 ounces) no-salt-added diced tomatoes

1 can (15 ounces) no-salt-added chickpeas, rinsed and drained

2 sprigs parsley, finely chopped

1 In a microwaveable glass bowl, combine the water and the rice and microwave on high for 5 minutes. Set aside.

2 In a large soup pot over medium-high heat, heat the oil. Cook the sausage, stirring, until no longer pink, 4 minutes. Add the cabbage, garlic, zucchini, and celery. Cook until just tender, 4 minutes. Add the broth, tomatoes (with juice), and chickpeas. Bring to a boil over high heat, reduce the heat to medium-low, and simmer for 10 minutes. Stir in the rice and parsley, reduce the heat to low, and simmer to blend the flavors, 10 minutes.

NUTRITION (PER SERVING): 228 calories, 13 g protein, 33 g carbohydrates, 5 g fiber, 4 g sugars, 5 g fat, 0 g saturated fat, 257 mg sodium

CAJUN SHRIMP SOUP

PREP TIME: 10 MINUTES / TOTAL TIME: 1 HOUR 15 MINUTES / **MAKES 4 SERVINGS**

1   bulb garlic

1   tablespoon olive oil

3   ribs celery, chopped

2   green and/or red bell peppers, chopped

1   onion, chopped

3   cups low-sodium chicken broth

2   cans (14.5 ounces each) no-salt-added diced
     tomatoes

1   teaspoon oregano

1   teaspoon chili powder

⅛   teaspoon ground red pepper

1   pound medium shrimp, peeled and deveined

1   cup frozen corn kernels, thawed

1 Preheat the oven to 350°F. Place the garlic bulb on a piece of foil, moisten with water, and wrap to seal. Bake for 45 minutes. When cool enough to handle, squeeze the garlic from the bulb into a small bowl.

2 In a large saucepot over medium-high heat, heat the oil. Cook the garlic, celery, bell peppers, and onion until soft, 10 minutes. Add the broth, tomatoes (with juice), oregano, chili powder, and ground red pepper. Bring just to a boil. Stir in the shrimp and corn and cook until the shrimp are opaque, 5 minutes.

NUTRITION (PER SERVING): 219 calories, 17 g protein, 27 g carbohydrates, 4 g fiber, 10 g sugars, 5 g fat, 1 g saturated fat, 589 mg sodium

HEARTY LENTIL MUSHROOM SOUP

PREP TIME: 25 MINUTES / TOTAL TIME: 1 HOUR / **MAKES 4 SERVINGS**

½ ounce dried porcini mushrooms

I cup hot water

8 ounces fresh shiitake mushrooms, stems removed

I tablespoon olive oil, divided

I medium yellow onion, diced

2 cloves garlic, minced

2 medium carrots, peeled and diced

½ teaspoon dried thyme

½ teaspoon salt

½ teaspoon black pepper

4 cups low-sodium vegetable broth

I cup French lentils

I teaspoon red wine vinegar

4 teaspoons shaved Parmesan cheese

1 In a small bowl, soak the porcini mushrooms in the water until soft, 15 minutes. Drain, reserving the soaking liquid, and coarsely chop the mushrooms.

2 Preheat the oven to 400°F. Coarsely chop half of the shiitake mushrooms and set aside. Slice the remaining shiitake mushrooms into ¼" pieces and place on a baking sheet. Toss with 2 teaspoons of the oil. Spread the mushroom slices in one layer and roast until browned and crisp, turning once, 10 minutes. Set aside.

3 In a medium saucepan over medium heat, heat the remaining 1 teaspoon oil. Cook the onion and garlic until soft, 2 minutes. Add the chopped porcini and shiitake mushrooms, carrots, thyme, salt, and pepper, and cook for 2 minutes. Add the broth, lentils, and mushroom-soaking liquid, and bring to a boil over medium-high heat. Reduce the heat to low, cover, and simmer until the lentils are soft, about 25 minutes. Stir in the vinegar.

4 Serve topped with the cheese and the roasted mushrooms.

NUTRITION (PER SERVING): 268 calories, 14 g protein, 42 g carbohydrates, 11 g fiber, 7 g sugars, 6 g fat, 1 g saturated fat, 433 mg sodium

CREAMY POTATO, LENTIL, AND HAM CHOWDER

PREP TIME: 10 MINUTES / TOTAL TIME: 45 MINUTES / **MAKES 8 SERVINGS**

I tablespoon olive oil

2 onions, chopped

2 tablespoons whole wheat flour

3 cups low-sodium chicken broth

2 cups water

4 red potatoes, cut into ¾" cubes

I rib celery, chopped

½ cup green lentils, rinsed

I teaspoon mustard powder

1⅔ cups 1% milk

½ pound fully cooked lean, low-sodium ham, cut into ¾" pieces

1 In a large saucepan over medium-high heat, heat the oil. Cook the onions, stirring occasionally, until translucent, 5 minutes. Stir in the flour and cook for 1 minute. Gradually stir in the broth until well blended.

2 Add the water, potatoes, celery, lentils, and mustard powder. Bring to a boil. Reduce the heat to low, cover, and simmer until the potatoes are tender, 20 minutes.

3 In a blender or food processor, working in batches, puree the soup until smooth. Return the soup to the saucepan. Stir in the milk and ham. Gently simmer until heated through, 5 minutes.

NUTRITION (PER SERVING): 224 calories, 15 g protein, 32 g carbohydrates, 4 g fiber, 6 g sugars, 5 g fat, 1 g saturated fat, 352 mg sodium

HEALTHY HINT

Did you buy more kale and carrots than you could eat in a week? To avoid waste and make the most of the produce you have on hand—even if it's starting to wilt—try making a big batch of soup with your leftover vegetables at the end of each week. You can use nearly any combo of veggies and legumes with a low-salt, organic broth to create a delicious, healthy soup and give your sad-looking produce new life.

LENTIL-BROCCOLI RABE SOUP

PREP TIME: 10 MINUTES / TOTAL TIME: 40 MINUTES / **MAKES 6 SERVINGS**

2	teaspoons olive oil
2	carrots, chopped
2	cloves garlic, minced
I	yellow onion, chopped
4	cups low-sodium vegetable broth or water
I	cup dried red lentils
2	tablespoons no-salt-added tomato paste
I	tablespoon finely chopped fresh oregano or I teaspoon dried
I	teaspoon ground cumin
½	pound broccoli rabe, rinsed, trimmed, and chopped
2	tablespoons grated Parmesan cheese

1 In a large saucepan over medium heat, heat the oil. Cook the carrots, garlic, and onion until the vegetables start to soften, 5 minutes. Stir in the broth or water, lentils, tomato paste, oregano, and cumin. Cover and bring to a brisk simmer.

2 Reduce the heat to low and simmer, covered, for 20 minutes. Stir in the broccoli rabe. Cover and simmer until the lentils and broccoli rabe are tender, 5 minutes. Add more water, if necessary, to thin the soup to the desired consistency. Serve garnished with the cheese.

NUTRITION (PER SERVING): 182 calories, 11 g protein, 27 g carbohydrates, 6 g fiber, 4 g sugars, 3 g fat, 1 g saturated fat, 151 mg sodium

CURRIED BUTTERNUT SQUASH–LENTIL SOUP

PREP TIME: 15 MINUTES / TOTAL TIME: 1 HOUR / **MAKES 4 SERVINGS**

1	tablespoon olive oil
1	onion, chopped
2	teaspoons curry powder
½	teaspoon turmeric
⅛	teaspoon ground red pepper
6	cups water
1¼	cups dried red lentils (8 ounces), picked over
1	pound butternut squash, cut into ½" pieces
½	teaspoon salt
2	tablespoons fresh lime juice
¼	cup chopped cilantro

1 In a large saucepan over medium heat, heat the oil. Cook the onion, stirring, until softened, 4 minutes. Stir in the curry powder, turmeric, and ground red pepper and cook, stirring, for 1 minute. Add the water and lentils. Bring to a boil. Skim the top of the water to remove foam. Reduce the heat to low and simmer, partially covered, for 15 minutes. Add the squash and salt and simmer, partially covered, until the squash is tender, about 20 minutes.

2 In a blender or food processor, working in batches, puree the soup until smooth. Return the soup to the saucepan. Warm over medium heat, stirring, until heated through. Stir in the lime juice and cilantro. Add more water, if necessary, to thin the soup to the desired consistency.

NUTRITION (PER SERVING): 300 calories, 17 g protein, 51 g carbohydrates, 6 g fiber, 7 g sugars, 4 g fat, 1 g saturated fat, 218 mg sodium

CREAMY CAULIFLOWER AND PARMESAN SOUP

PREP TIME: 5 MINUTES / TOTAL TIME: 55 MINUTES / MAKES 2 SERVINGS

2   tablespoons grapeseed oil
2   cups chopped cauliflower
1   carrot, chopped
1   small onion, chopped
1   clove garlic, minced
1   cup water
1   cup 2% milk
¼   cup + 2 tablespoons grated Parmesan
1   tablespoon finely chopped fresh dill or 1 teaspoon dried

1 In a medium saucepan over medium-high heat, heat the oil. Cook the cauliflower, carrot, and onion, stirring frequently, until lightly browned, about 5 minutes. Stir in the garlic and cook until the garlic becomes fragrant, 1 minute. Add the water and bring to a boil. Reduce the heat, cover, and simmer until the vegetables are very tender, 20 minutes.

2 Use an immersion blender to puree the soup, adding the milk gradually to the pot (or transfer to a blender and puree). Stir in the cheese and dill.

NUTRITION (PER SERVING): 232 calories, 8 g protein, 11 g carbohydrates, 3 g fiber, 4 g sugars, 18 g fat, 4 g saturated fat, 351 mg sodium

HEALTHY HINT

Go ahead, give goat milk a whirl. It doesn't have a huge presence in the United States, but it does worldwide—and can hold its own against cow milk. With less lactose and a chemical structure similar to that of breast milk, it's often easier for sensitive stomachs to digest. Plus, it has more calcium, potassium, and vitamin A. Cow's milk, on the other hand, delivers more B vitamins and selenium with less fat and fewer calories.

CREAMY SPINACH AND MUSHROOM SOUP

PREP TIME: 15 MINUTES / TOTAL TIME: 1 HOUR 10 MINUTES / **MAKES 6 SERVINGS**

1	teaspoon olive oil
3	slices bacon
8	ounces mushrooms, trimmed and sliced
1	onion, chopped
½	cup dry white wine or vegetable broth
1	russet (baking) potato, peeled and cubed
5	cups water
2	cups frozen edamame, thawed
8	ounces baby spinach
2	tablespoons fresh lemon juice
¼	cup 2% plain Greek yogurt

1 In a large saucepot over medium heat, heat the oil. Cook the bacon until crisp, 6 minutes. Drain on paper towels. Crumble and set aside.

2 Remove all but 1 tablespoon of the bacon fat. Return the pot to medium heat and cook the mushrooms, stirring occasionally, until golden, 5 minutes. Add the onion and cook, stirring, until tender, about 4 minutes. Stir in the wine or broth and simmer until reduced by half, 4 minutes.

3 Stir in the potato and water. Bring to a boil, reduce the heat to low, and simmer until the potato is very tender, 15 minutes. Add the edamame and spinach and simmer, stirring occasionally, until the edamame is tender, 5 minutes.

4 In a blender or food processor, working in batches, puree the soup until smooth. Return the soup to the pot and bring to a simmer. Add more water, if necessary, to thin the soup to the desired consistency. Remove from the heat and stir in the lemon juice. Ladle into bowls, dollop with the yogurt, and sprinkle with the bacon.

HEALTHY HINT

Fight the flu naturally with this hearty soup. Give your infection-fighting white blood cells a boost with selenium from mushrooms and vitamin A from spinach. And as a bonus benefit, potatoes pack blood-pressure-lowering potassium and B vitamins that help support a healthy heart and brain.

NUTRITION (PER SERVING): 178 calories, 11 g protein, 18 g carbohydrates, 6 g fiber, 3 g sugars, 7 g fat, 2 g saturated fat, 359 mg sodium

ROASTED TOMATO AND GARLIC SOUP WITH MOZZARELLA TOASTS

PREP TIME: 20 MINUTES / TOTAL TIME: 1 HOUR 25 MINUTES / **MAKES 4 SERVINGS**

2   pounds small tomatoes (such as Campari) or plum tomatoes, halved

1   onion, cut into eighths

¼   teaspoon salt

¼   teaspoon black pepper

1   head garlic (unpeeled), separated

1   tablespoon tomato paste

2   cups low-sodium vegetable broth, divided

¼   cup chopped fresh basil + leaves for garnish

4   thin slices baguette, toasted

2   bocconcini (small balls of fresh mozzarella), sliced

1 Position a rack in the upper third of the oven, and preheat the oven to 375°F. On a large, shallow baking pan coated with cooking spray, arrange the tomatoes and onion, cut sides up. Coat the vegetables with cooking spray and sprinkle with the salt and pepper. Wrap the garlic in a small piece of foil and place in a corner of the pan.

2 Roast until the tomatoes and onion are wilted and golden brown and the garlic is very soft, 55 minutes. Keep the oven on.

3 Squeeze the garlic pulp out of the skin. In a food processor, combine the garlic, tomatoes, onion, and tomato paste. Pulse until almost smooth.

4 Transfer to a large saucepan and stir in 1½ cups of the broth. Over medium heat, bring to a simmer, adding some of the remaining ½ cup of broth, if necessary, to thin the soup to the desired consistency. Stir in the chopped basil. Remove from the heat and cover to keep warm.

5 Place the bread slices on a baking sheet. Top with the cheese. Bake until the cheese begins to melt, 4 minutes. Ladle the soup into bowls, top each with a cheese toast, and garnish with the basil leaves.

NUTRITION (PER SERVING): 170 calories, 8 g protein, 28 g carbohydrates, 5 g fiber, 9 g sugars, 4 g fat, 2 g saturated fat, 353 mg sodium

SWEET POTATO–BLACK BEAN SOUP

PREP TIME: 20 MINUTES / TOTAL TIME: 30 MINUTES / **MAKES 4 SERVINGS**

2 tablespoons extra-virgin olive oil

2 onions, chopped

2 red bell peppers, chopped

2 cloves garlic, minced

2½ cups water

2 cans (15 ounces each) low- or no-sodium black beans, rinsed and drained

1 medium sweet potato, peeled and cut into ½" cubes

1 cup tomato puree

1 teaspoon ground cumin

½ teaspoon salt

¼ teaspoon black pepper

¼ cup chopped cilantro

   Lime wedges, for serving (optional)

1 In a medium saucepan over medium heat, heat the oil. Cook the onions, bell peppers, and garlic, stirring, until tender, 10 minutes. Stir in the water, beans, sweet potato, tomato puree, cumin, salt, and black pepper. Bring to a boil over medium-high heat. Reduce the heat to low, cover, and simmer until the sweet potatoes are tender, 15 minutes.

2 Using a potato masher, lightly mash some of the beans and vegetables until the soup is thick and chunky. Stir in the cilantro and serve with the lime wedges, if using.

NUTRITION (PER SERVING): 280 calories, 10 g protein, 43 g carbohydrates, 11 g fiber, 11 g sugars, 7 g fat, 1 g saturated fat, 413 mg sodium

CREATE-YOUR-OWN
NO-CREAM SOUPS

What's the key to making a clean cream soup? Sweet, tender vegetables! Pureeing them with your favorite flavorful broth and a little bit of clean oil or butter yields a rich, velvety soup that rivals anything you'd find at a restaurant or deli. Best of all, the combinations are nearly endless. Follow this simple formula and get creative with your favorite flavors, or use one of our tried-and-true combos. Each recipe will take about 20 minutes of prep time, be ready in 1 hour, and make 6 servings.

- 1 tablespoon (total) clean fat (choose up to two): Unsalted butter, extra-virgin olive oil, avocado oil, grapeseed oil, canola oil, or coconut oil
- 1½ cups (total) aromatics, chopped (choose two to four): Onion, leek, shallot, carrot, celery (up to ¼ cup), grated ginger, or minced garlic (up to 1 tablespoon)
  Pinch of salt
- 1 to 2 teaspoons ground spice (choose one): Curry powder, ground cumin, smoked paprika, mustard seeds, ground fennel seeds, garam masala, ground cinnamon, or up to ¼ teaspoon of ground red pepper or chili powder
- 2 pounds vegetables, chopped (choose one): Broccoli, cauliflower, carrots, butternut squash, mushrooms, asparagus, peas, or tomatoes (if using canned, use whole tomatoes in juice)
- ¼ cup deglazing liquid (optional, choose one): Dry white wine, red wine, beer, dry vermouth, cooking sherry, apple cider, or fresh orange juice
- 2½ cups broth (choose one): Low-sodium vegetable broth, chicken broth, beef broth, or mushroom broth
- 2½ cups water
- 1 teaspoon acid (choose one): Fresh lemon or lime juice, red or white wine vinegar, sherry vinegar, balsamic vinegar, or rice wine vinegar
  Finishing touches (optional; choose one): Toasted sesame or extra-virgin olive oil (½ teaspoon), chopped toasted nuts or seeds (1 teaspoon), or chopped fresh herbs (1 to 2 tablespoons)

1 In a medium saucepan over medium-low heat, heat the fat until warm or melted. Add the aromatics and salt and cook, stirring, until softened, 8 minutes. Add the spice and cook for 1 minute.

2 Add the vegetables and cook, stirring, until lightly browned, 5 minutes. (For mushrooms, cook until golden, about 10 minutes.)

3 Add the deglazing liquid (if using) and scrape the bottom of the pan. Cook until the liquid has almost evaporated, about 3 minutes. Add the broth and water, and bring the soup to a boil over medium-high heat. Reduce the heat to low, cover, and simmer until the vegetables are very tender and the soup has developed a deep flavor, 10 to 25 minutes. (Harder vegetables, such as broccoli and butternut squash, will take longer to get tender than softer vegetables, such as tomatoes and mushrooms.)

4 Using an immersion blender, puree the soup until silky smooth. (If you're using a blender, work in batches to puree the soup. Return the soup to the pan as you complete each batch.) Continue cooking until the soup reaches the consistency of heavy cream.

5 Stir in the acid and season to taste with salt and pepper. Top with a finishing touch of your choice, if desired.

Favorite Flavor Combos

Broccoli Leek: Butter, leek + garlic, pinch of ground red pepper, broccoli, dry white wine, chicken broth, lemon juice, extra-virgin olive oil garnish

Curry Butternut Squash: Coconut oil, onion + carrot + celery + ginger, curry powder, butternut squash, orange juice, vegetable broth, lime juice, toasted sunflower seed garnish

Sherry Mushroom: Grapeseed oil, shallot + garlic, cumin, mushrooms, sherry, mushroom broth, sherry vinegar, rosemary and thyme garnish

Smoked Paprika Cauliflower: Avocado oil, onion + garlic, smoked paprika, cauliflower, chicken broth, white wine vinegar, toasted chopped pecan garnish

Tomato Basil: Extra-virgin olive oil, onion + carrot + garlic, fennel seed, tomatoes, red wine, water, balsamic vinegar, basil garnish

MAKE IT AHEAD! This soup will keep for up to 5 days in the refrigerator or 1 month in the freezer.

NOTE: In a rush? Opt for frozen, chopped vegetables. Use them straight out of the freezer, increasing the cooking time by a few minutes.

PROTEIN-PACKED CARROT-GINGER SOUP

PREP TIME: 20 MINUTES / TOTAL TIME: 55 MINUTES / **MAKES 4 SERVINGS**

Shown in photo insert pages.

I   tablespoon olive oil

I   large onion, chopped

I   rib celery, chopped

1½ tablespoons minced fresh ginger

2   cloves garlic, minced

4   cups low-sodium vegetable broth

4   cups chopped carrots (about 1½ pounds)

I   can (15 ounces) white beans, rinsed and drained

2   ounces (about ¼ cup) unflavored whey protein powder

½   teaspoon salt

½   teaspoon black pepper

2   tablespoons 0% plain Greek yogurt

2   tablespoons chopped fresh chives

1 In a Dutch oven or large saucepan over medium heat, heat the oil. Cook the onion and celery until soft, 10 minutes.

2 Add the ginger and garlic and cook until fragrant, 2 minutes. Add the broth, carrots, and beans and bring to a simmer. Cook until the carrots are soft, 25 minutes. Remove from the heat.

3 Stir the protein powder into the soup, 2 tablespoons at a time, until incorporated. Add the salt and pepper. With an immersion blender, blend the soup in the pot until smooth, or puree in a blender or food processor, working in batches.

4 Top each serving with the yogurt and chives.

NUTRITION (PER SERVING): 279 calories, 19 g protein, 39 g carbohydrates, 9 g fiber, 11 g sugars, 5 g fat, 1 g saturated fat, 517 mg sodium

CREAMY CHICKEN, GREEN GRAPE, AND FARRO SALAD

¾ cup farro, rinsed and drained

1 boneless, skinless chicken breast (6 ounces), butterflied

¼ teaspoon salt

⅛ teaspoon black pepper

¼ cup plain Greek yogurt

2 tablespoons red wine vinegar

1 tablespoon extra-virgin olive oil

1 small clove garlic, mashed into a paste

¼ teaspoon ground cumin

1 cup arugula

¾ cup green grapes, halved

½ cucumber, seeded and chopped

1 tablespoon chopped fresh dill

1 Prepare the farro according to package directions. Let cool slightly.

2 Meanwhile, season the chicken with the salt and pepper. Heat a cast-iron grill pan or skillet coated with cooking spray over medium-high heat. Cook the chicken, turning once, until no longer pink, about 8 minutes. Chop into bite-size pieces.

3 In a large bowl, whisk together the yogurt, vinegar, oil, garlic, and cumin. Add the farro, chicken, arugula, grapes, cucumber, and dill, and toss to coat.

NUTRITION (PER SERVING): 471 calories, 32 g protein, 63 g carbohydrates, 6 g fiber, 11 g sugars, 10 g fat, 2 g saturated fat, 639 mg sodium

CHANGE IT UP! To make this dish vegetarian, swap 1 cup of cooked chickpeas for the chicken. Want to experiment with another flavor profile? Substitute dried oregano for the ground cumin.

CHICKEN, QUINOA, AND PEACH SALAD

PREP TIME: 15 MINUTES / TOTAL TIME: 15 MINUTES / MAKES 4 SERVINGS

1 cup water

½ cup quinoa, rinsed and drained

2 tablespoons extra-virgin olive oil

2 tablespoons fresh lemon juice

2 teaspoons chopped fresh thyme

1 clove garlic, minced

1 teaspoon Dijon mustard

½ teaspoon grated lemon zest

¼ teaspoon salt

¼ teaspoon black pepper

2 cups chopped or shredded cooked chicken breasts

2 cups fresh or frozen and thawed sliced peaches, cut into ½" pieces

⅓ cup finely chopped unsalted dry-roasted almonds

1 In a small saucepan over high heat, bring the water and quinoa to a boil. Reduce the heat to low, cover, and simmer until tender, 15 minutes.

2 Meanwhile, in a large bowl, whisk together the oil, lemon juice, thyme, garlic, mustard, lemon zest, salt, and pepper.

3 Add the chicken, peaches, almonds, and quinoa to the bowl. Toss to coat well. Serve warm or chill to serve cold later.

NUTRITION (PER SERVING): 387 calories, 29 g protein, 30 g carbohydrates, 5 g fiber, 7 g sugars, 17 g fat, 2 g saturated fat, 186 mg sodium

CHANGE IT UP! Make this tasty salad with any leftover meat or fish. Vary the flavors more by using apples, grapes, plums, or apricots in place of the peaches.

TUNA AND CANNELLINI SALAD

PREP TIME: 15 MINUTES / TOTAL TIME: 20 MINUTES / **MAKES 2 SERVINGS**

2   tablespoons minced shallot

2   tablespoons fresh lemon juice

1   teaspoon Dijon mustard

⅛   teaspoon black pepper

1   whole wheat pita, split open and cut into 6 wedges

2   teaspoons extra-virgin olive oil

1   can or jar (5 ounces) clean tuna, drained and flaked

1   can (15 ounces) low- or no-sodium cannellini beans, rinsed and drained

½   cup peeled and chopped roasted red peppers*

1   carrot, chopped

¼   cup coarsely chopped fresh flat-leaf parsley

1 Preheat the oven to 400°F.

2 In a medium bowl, combine the shallot, lemon juice, mustard, and black pepper. Let stand to soften and mellow the shallot, 10 minutes.

3 Meanwhile, place the pita wedges on a baking sheet and bake until toasted and crisp, about 5 minutes.

4 When the shallot has mellowed, whisk in the oil until blended. Add the tuna, beans, roasted red peppers, carrot, and parsley. Toss to coat well.

5 Divide the tuna salad between 2 plates and serve with the pita wedges.

NUTRITION (PER SERVING): 382 calories, 26 g protein, 45 g carbohydrates, 10 g fiber, 6 g sugars, 11 g fat, 2 g saturated fat, 492 mg sodium

*TO MAKE HOMEMADE ROASTED RED PEPPERS: Place whole fresh red peppers over an open flame on the stove top or on a baking sheet under the broiler. Cook for 3 to 5 minutes per side, or until they're charred all over. Transfer the peppers to a bowl and cover with plastic wrap or an inverted plate until the peppers are cool enough to handle, about 10 minutes. (This steams the peppers, making it easier to remove the skins.) Use your fingers to carefully peel off the charred pepper skins and remove the stems and seeds. Stored in an airtight container, roasted red peppers will keep for up to 1 week in the refrigerator or up to 1 month in the freezer.

MAKE IT AHEAD! This recipe can easily be doubled or tripled to feed a larger group. Or prepare several servings for lunch later in the week. Store the pita wedges in a resealable plastic bag and refrigerate the tuna in a sealed container for up to 1 week.

CHANGE IT UP! Swap out the tuna for clean canned salmon or chicken. Or make a vegetarian version by subbing 2 chopped hard-cooked eggs.

TUNA AND TOMATO PASTA SALAD

PREP TIME: 10 MINUTES / TOTAL TIME: 20 MINUTES / **MAKES 4 SERVINGS**

Shown in photo insert pages.

3   cups whole grain rotini pasta

2   tablespoons fresh lime juice

1½ tablespoons olive oil

½   teaspoon honey

⅛   teaspoon red-pepper flakes
    Pinch of salt

2   cans (5 ounces each) low-sodium water-packed light tuna, drained and flaked

1   cup cherry tomatoes, halved

1   cup frozen green peas, thawed

2   tablespoons roughly chopped fresh cilantro (optional)

1 Prepare the pasta according to package directions.

2 Meanwhile, in a large bowl, whisk together the lime juice, oil, honey, red-pepper flakes, and salt.

3 Add the tuna, tomatoes, peas, cilantro (if desired), and pasta, and toss to coat well. Serve warm or chill to serve cold later.

NUTRITION (PER SERVING): 425 calories, 28 g protein, 58 g carbohydrates, 10 g fiber, 10 g sugars, 10 g fat, 1 g saturated fat, 258 mg sodium

HEALTHY HINT

It's time to ditch your fat-free dressing: Recent research shows that a little fat can go a long way toward helping you absorb more nutrients from your greens and other veggies, specifically boosting your absorption of carotenoids—antioxidants that have been linked to a reduced risk of cancer, heart disease, and macular degeneration. To get the most out of your next salad, dress your greens in olive oil and lemon juice or vinegar.

GREEK SALAD WITH SALMON

PREP TIME: 25 MINUTES / TOTAL TIME: 1 HOUR / **MAKES 4 SERVINGS**

1   cup short-grain brown rice

    Juice of 1 lemon

2   tablespoons olive oil

1   teaspoon dried oregano

¼   teaspoon salt

2   cans (6 ounces each) salmon, drained and flaked

1   cup grape tomatoes, halved

1   cucumber, peeled, seeded, and chopped

½   cup feta cheese, crumbled

10   pitted kalamata olives, quartered

1 Prepare the rice according to package directions.

2 Meanwhile, in a large bowl, whisk together the lemon juice, olive oil, oregano, and salt. Add the rice, salmon, tomatoes, cucumber, cheese, and olives. Toss to coat well. Serve warm or chill to serve cold later.

NUTRITION (PER SERVING): 390 calories, 20 g protein, 45 g carbohydrates, 4 g fiber, 3 g sugars, 16 g fat, 4 g saturated fat, 514 mg sodium

NOTE: To make this dish at the last minute, use 3 cups cooked organic brown rice. Look for cooked organic rice in the frozen foods section or on supermarket shelves.

FIESTA QUINOA WITH SHRIMP

PREP TIME: 15 MINUTES / TOTAL TIME: 30 MINUTES / **MAKES 4 SERVINGS**

⅓   cup white quinoa, rinsed and drained

1   lime

1   clove garlic, mashed into a paste

¼   teaspoon dried oregano

¼   teaspoon ground cumin

   Pinch of salt

   Pinch of black pepper

1½ tablespoons olive oil, divided

1   cup canned low- or no-sodium black beans, rinsed and drained

½   cup thawed frozen corn kernels

½   red bell pepper, minced

2   scallions, thinly sliced

½   pound jumbo shrimp, peeled and deveined

1   tablespoon chopped cilantro

1 Prepare the quinoa according to package directions.

2 Meanwhile, zest the lime, reserving ½ teaspoon of zest. Juice the lime, reserving 2 tablespoons of juice.

3 In a large bowl, whisk together the lime juice, garlic, cumin, oregano, salt, black pepper, and 1 tablespoon of the oil. Add the cooked quinoa, beans, corn, bell pepper, scallions, and toss to coat well.

4 In a medium nonstick skillet over medium heat, heat the remaining ½ tablespoon oil. Add the shrimp and cook, tossing occasionally, 4 minutes. Toss in the lime zest and cilantro. Stir into the quinoa mixture.

NUTRITION (PER SERVING): 421 calories, 26 g protein, 49 g carbohydrates, 10 g fiber, 4 g sugars, 14 g fat, 2 g saturated fat, 644 mg sodium

WARM RED POTATO SALAD

PREP TIME: 10 MINUTES / TOTAL TIME: 35 MINUTES / **MAKES 6 SERVINGS**

2   pounds red potatoes, cut into large chunks

3   strips organic uncured bacon, chopped

6   scallions, thinly sliced

5   ribs celery, sliced

3   tablespoons ground flaxseeds

3   tablespoons apple cider vinegar

3   tablespoons apple juice

1   tablespoon stone-ground mustard

3   sprigs parsley, finely chopped

½   teaspoon salt

1 Place a steamer basket in a large pot with 3" water. Place the potatoes in the steamer. Cover and bring to a boil over high heat. Reduce the heat to medium. Steam until tender, 15 minutes. Transfer to a large bowl and cool for 10 minutes.

2 In a medium skillet over medium heat, cook the bacon for 3 minutes. Add the scallions and celery. Cook, stirring, until the scallions are soft and the bacon is browned, 3 minutes. Reduce the heat to low. Add the flaxseeds and toss to coat. Add the vinegar, apple juice, mustard, parsley, and salt. Cook until heated through, 2 minutes. Pour over the potatoes and toss to evenly coat.

NUTRITION (PER SERVING): 178 calories, 5 g protein, 28 g carbohydrates, 5 g fiber, 4 g sugars, 6 g fat, 1 g saturated fat, 288 mg sodium

CHILLED CILANTRO–SOBA NOODLE SALAD

PREP TIME: 15 MINUTES / TOTAL TIME: 15 MINUTES + CHILLING TIME / **MAKES 6 SERVINGS**

8   ounces soba noodles

2   cups frozen shelled edamame

3   tablespoons sesame oil

2   tablespoons low-sodium soy sauce

2   tablespoons orange juice

1   teaspoon orange zest

½   teaspoon crushed red-pepper flakes

1   red bell pepper, thinly sliced

1   green bell pepper, thinly sliced

3   scallions, thinly sliced

¼   cup thinly sliced fresh cilantro

1 Prepare the soba noodles according to package directions, adding the edamame with the noodles. Drain and rinse under cold water. Drain well.

2 Meanwhile, in a large bowl, whisk together the oil, soy sauce, orange juice, orange zest, and red-pepper flakes. Add the noodles and edamame, bell peppers, scallions, and cilantro. Toss gently to coat.

3 Chill for 30 minutes to allow the flavors to blend. Serve cold or at room temperature.

NUTRITION (PER SERVING): 273 calories, 13 g protein, 37 g carbohydrates, 4 g fiber, 5 g sugars, 10 g fat, 1 g saturated fat, 436 mg sodium

HEALTHY HINT

Serve this with grilled or roasted shrimp, salmon, chicken, or turkey for a hearty meal in no time.

ARUGULA SALAD WITH ZUCCHINI RIBBONS

PREP TIME: 15 MINUTES / TOTAL TIME: 15 MINUTES / **MAKES 4 SERVINGS**

4   cups arugula

l   medium zucchini

¼   cup salted, roasted sunflower seeds

⅔   cup (2 ounces) pecan halves (optional: toasted)

l   ounce Parmesan cheese, shaved

l   lemon, halved

    Grated zest of l small orange

¼   cup extra-virgin olive oil

1 In a large bowl, place the arugula. Over the bowl, using a vegetable peeler, shave the zucchini on one side over and over to make ribbons, turning every few strokes to evenly distribute peel. Stop when you reach the seedy core and no more ribbons can be sliced.

2 Sprinkle with the sunflower seeds, pecans, and cheese. Squeeze the lemon juice over the salad. Sprinkle with the orange zest and drizzle with the oil. Toss to coat well.

NUTRITION (PER SERVING): 329 calories, 7 g protein, 7 g carbohydrates, 3 g fiber, 2 g sugars, 32 g fat, 5 g saturated fat, 155 mg sodium

NOTE: This salad makes the perfect accompaniment to roasted or grilled meat or fish.

HEALTHY HINT

Cutting out grains? That doesn't mean you have to ditch pasta altogether. Get a spiralizer and turn your veggies—zucchini, carrots, sweet potatoes, etc.—into low-carb, nutrient-dense noodles. Bonus: These "noodles" will be naturally low in calories, so you can get away with going for seconds.

SPINACH SALAD WITH LEMON-SHALLOT VINAIGRETTE

PREP TIME: 15 MINUTES / TOTAL TIME: 15 MINUTES / **MAKES 2 SERVINGS**

2   tablespoons extra-virgin olive oil

1½   tablespoons fresh lemon juice

1   teaspoon honey

2   teaspoons finely minced shallots

3   cups baby spinach

¾   cup chopped red grapes

½   cup chopped strawberries

½   cup blueberries

¼   cup chopped walnuts

1 In a large bowl, whisk together the oil, lemon juice, honey, and shallots.

2 Add the spinach, grapes, strawberries, blueberries, and walnuts. Toss to coat well.

NUTRITION (PER SERVING): 376 calories, 7 g protein, 29 g carbohydrates, 6 g fiber, 18 g sugars, 28 g fat, 6 g saturated fat, 331 mg sodium

HEALTHY HINT

Popeye was right: Spinach really can make you strong. The naturally occurring nitrates in spinach can actually elevate levels of specific proteins in your body that aid in muscle contraction, and researchers think that could help people with muscle weakness remain active. The best part is, you only need about a cup of raw spinach per day to get the boost.

SHAVED SALAD

PREP TIME: 15 MINUTES / TOTAL TIME: 15 MINUTES / **MAKES 2 SERVINGS**

Shown in photo insert pages.

2   teaspoons olive oil

1   teaspoon white wine vinegar

2   tablespoons fresh dill, chopped

1   teaspoon lemon zest

½   teaspoon salt

¼   teaspoon black pepper

2   medium carrots, peeled

1   broccoli stalk (no florets)

6   to 8 asparagus spears

1   medium zucchini

1 In a large bowl, whisk together the oil, vinegar, dill, lemon zest, salt, and pepper.

2 Over the bowl, using a vegetable peeler, shave the carrots, broccoli, asparagus, and zucchini lengthwise into long ribbons. Toss to coat well.

NUTRITION (PER SERVING): 105 calories, 4 g protein, 13 g carbohydrates, 5 g fiber, 6 g sugars, 5 g fat, 1 g saturated fat, 458 mg sodium

NOTE: This salad makes the perfect accompaniment to roasted or grilled meat or fish.

PANZANELLA

PREP TIME: 15 MINUTES / TOTAL TIME: 30 MINUTES / **MAKES 2 SERVINGS (ABOUT 2 CUPS EACH)**

Shown in photo insert pages.

I	tablespoon avocado oil
I	tablespoon red wine vinegar
I	tablespoon capers, drained and chopped
½	teaspoon Dijon mustard
¼	teaspoon black pepper
	Pinch of salt
2	slices multigrain or whole wheat bread
I	clove garlic, halved
I	cup cherry tomatoes, halved
I	small cucumber, peeled, seeded, and chopped
½	small red onion, halved and thinly sliced
I	yellow bell pepper, chopped
¼	cup fresh basil, chopped
8	ounces boneless, skinless chicken breast

1 In a large bowl, whisk together the oil, vinegar, capers, mustard, black pepper, and salt. Set aside.

2 Lightly coat a grill rack with oil. Preheat the grill to medium-high. Grill the bread until toasted and grill marks form, 1 to 2 minutes. Remove the bread from the grill and rub each slice thoroughly with the garlic. Cut the bread into cubes. Add the bread, tomatoes, cucumber, onion, bell pepper, and basil to the bowl with the vinaigrette. Toss to coat well. Set aside to let the flavors meld.

3 Grill the chicken, turning once, until browned and an instant-read thermometer inserted in the thickest part of the chicken registers 165°F, about 15 minutes. Let stand for 5 minutes, then cut into cubes. Toss with the salad.

NUTRITION (PER SERVING): 362 calories, 29 g protein, 33 g carbohydrates, 4 g fiber, 10 g sugars, 12 g fat, 3 g saturated fat, 558 mg sodium

CHANGE IT UP! Short on time? Use the breast from an organic rotisserie chicken. Or, to make a vegetarian version, swap out the chicken for one 15-ounce can of low-sodium white beans, rinsed and drained.

CLEAN COLESLAW

PREP TIME: 10 MINUTES / TOTAL TIME: 30 MINUTES / **MAKES 4 SERVINGS**

½   cup extra-virgin olive oil

⅓   cup white vinegar

2   teaspoons honey

1   teaspoon celery seed

1   teaspoon salt

1   teaspoon black pepper

1   head napa cabbage, finely shredded

2   medium carrots, shredded

1   small red onion, shredded or cut into very fine strips

1 In a large bowl, whisk together the oil, vinegar, honey, celery seed, salt, and pepper.

2 Add the cabbage, carrots, and onion to the bowl, and toss to coat. Chill for at least 30 minutes before serving.

NUTRITION (PER SERVING): 117 calories, 2 g protein, 11 g carbohydrates, 3 g fiber, 7 g sugars, 7 g fat, 1 g saturated fat, 428 mg sodium

MAIN DISHES

TRADITIONAL SLOW-COOKER POT ROAST

PREP TIME: 15 MINUTES / TOTAL TIME: 8 HOURS 15 MINUTES / **MAKES 4 SERVINGS**

6   carrots, cut into I" pieces

3   ribs celery, coarsely chopped

I   onion, sliced

I   potato, cut into I" pieces

I   cup low-sodium beef broth

½   cup no-salt-added tomato puree or sauce

2   teaspoons chopped fresh thyme or
     I teaspoon dried

I   pound boneless beef chuck roast, trimmed of
     all visible fat

½   teaspoon salt

I   teaspoon paprika

I   tablespoon olive oil

1 In a 4- to 6-quart slow cooker, combine the carrots, celery, onion, potato, broth, tomato puree or sauce, and thyme. Season the beef with the salt and paprika.

2 In a large skillet over medium-high heat, heat the oil. Cook the beef, turning once, until browned on all sides, 4 minutes. Place on the vegetables. Cover and cook on low until the beef is fork-tender, 8 hours.

3 Remove the beef to a cutting board. Let stand for 10 minutes before slicing. Serve with the vegetables.

NUTRITION (PER SERVING): 268 calories, 26 g protein, 22 g carbohydrates, 5 g fiber, 8 g sugars, 8 g fat, 2 g saturated fat, 446 mg sodium

HEALTHY HINT

If "grass-fed" is the gold standard, then "grass-fed, grain-finished" sure sounds like a close second. But nutritionally, it's nothing more than a trick of words. Basically, anything you buy that's not 100% grass-fed is grass-fed, grain-finished. Most calves actually start out on pasture but then get shipped to feedlots to fatten up on grain, and within weeks, the nutritional perks of grass feeding are lost.

SIZZLIN' BEEF FAJITAS

PREP TIME: 10 MINUTES / TOTAL TIME: 30 MINUTES + MARINATING TIME / **MAKES 4 SERVINGS**

1   tablespoon olive oil

4   cloves garlic, minced

2   tablespoons fresh lime juice

1   teaspoon ground cumin

¾   pound lean flank steak, trimmed of all visible fat

1   green bell pepper, cut into ¼" strips

1   red bell pepper, cut into ¼" strips

1   small onion, cut into ¼" slices

4   whole wheat tortillas (6" diameter)

¼   cup salsa

1   In a resealable plastic bag, combine the oil, garlic, lime juice, and cumin. Add the steak and toss to coat well. Refrigerate for 4 hours or overnight.

2   Coat a grill rack or broiler pan rack with cooking spray. Preheat the grill or broiler to medium-high. Remove the steak from the marinade. Grill or broil 4" from the heat, turning once, until a thermometer inserted in the center registers 145°F for medium-rare, 10 minutes. Transfer to a cutting board and cover loosely with foil.

3   Meanwhile, heat a skillet coated with cooking spray over medium-high heat. Cook the green and red bell peppers and onion, stirring, until the vegetables are softened, 10 minutes. Warm the tortillas according to the package directions. Thinly slice the steak across the grain on a slight angle.

4   Place 1 tortilla on 4 plates and top each with one-quarter of the steak, one-quarter of the vegetable mixture, and 1 tablespoon of the salsa.

NUTRITION (PER SERVING): 239 calories, 22 g protein, 26 g carbohydrates, 3 g fiber, 3 g sugars, 7 g fat, 3 g saturated fat, 288 mg sodium

BEEF STROGANOFF

PREP TIME: 10 MINUTES / TOTAL TIME: 40 MINUTES / **MAKES 4 SERVINGS**

4   ounces whole wheat egg noodles

I   tablespoon olive oil

5   ounces white or cremini mushrooms, stems removed, halved

8   ounces asparagus, trimmed and cut into I" pieces

I   pound lean sirloin steak, trimmed of visible fat, cut into thin strips

I   teaspoon salt

I   yellow onion, finely chopped

2   cloves garlic, minced

½   cup low-sodium beef broth

2   teaspoons cornstarch

I   tablespoon tomato paste

⅓   cup reduced-fat sour cream

2   sprigs fresh parsley, chopped

1 Prepare the noodles according to package directions.

2 Meanwhile, in a large skillet over medium heat, heat the oil. Cook the mushrooms and asparagus until the asparagus is lightly golden and the mushrooms are caramelized, 5 minutes. Remove to a large bowl and set aside.

3 Season the steak with the salt. Add more oil to the skillet if necessary, and cook the steak, turning once, until browned, 5 minutes. Remove and set aside.

4 In the same skillet, cook the onion and garlic until softened, 5 minutes. Stir in the broth, scraping the pan to release any browned bits. Transfer ¼ cup of the broth into a small glass measuring cup and stir in the cornstarch until smooth. Add the tomato paste and broth mixture to the skillet and stir until combined. Reduce the heat to low and simmer until the liquid thickens and reduces by half, 10 minutes.

5 Return the asparagus, mushrooms, and steak to the skillet and cook until heated through, 2 minutes. After the liquid cools just slightly, stir in the sour cream. Serve over the noodles and sprinkle with the parsley.

NUTRITION (PER SERVING): 372 calories, 33 g protein, 30 g carbohydrates, 2 g fiber, 5 g sugars, 13 g fat, 4 g saturated fat, 241 mg sodium

STEAK BURRITO BOWL

PREP TIME: 10 MINUTES / TOTAL TIME: 30 MINUTES / **MAKES 6 SERVINGS**

Shown in photo insert pages.

1¼ cups instant brown rice

¾ pound sirloin steak, trimmed

1 teaspoon chipotle seasoning

½ teaspoon black pepper

1 teaspoon olive oil

1 can (15 ounces) black beans, rinsed and drained

3 hearts romaine lettuce, shredded

¼ cup salsa

¼ cup guacamole

¼ cup reduced-fat shredded Cheddar cheese

1 Prepare the rice according to package directions. Set aside.

2 On a plate, rub the steak with the chipotle seasoning and pepper. Rub the oil onto the steak.

3 Coat a grill rack with cooking spray, and preheat the grill over medium-high heat. Grill the steak, turning once, until a thermometer inserted in the center registers 145°F for medium-rare, 10 minutes.

4 Transfer the steak to a cutting board and let stand for 5 minutes. Slice into thin strips. Evenly divide the rice, steak, beans, lettuce, salsa, guacamole, and cheese among 6 bowls.

NUTRITION (PER SERVING): 247 calories, 19 g protein, 26 g carbohydrates, 5 g fiber, 3 g sugars, 7 g fat, 2 g saturated fat, 305 mg sodium

BEEF AND SWEET POTATO STEW

PREP TIME: 15 MINUTES / TOTAL TIME: 1 HOUR 35 MINUTES / **MAKES 2 SERVINGS**

1   tablespoon olive oil

1   rib celery, chopped

1   carrot, chopped

¼   yellow onion, chopped

½   large sweet potato, chopped

½   pound lean beef stew meat

½   cup chopped cremini mushrooms

2   cloves garlic, minced

1¼   cups beef broth

1   cup water

2   teaspoons tomato paste

1   bay leaf

1 In a medium saucepan over medium-high heat, heat the oil. Cook the celery, carrot, onion, and sweet potato until the onion becomes translucent, 10 minutes.

2 Add the beef and mushrooms and cook, stirring frequently, until the beef is browned and the mushrooms are softened, 10 minutes. Add the garlic and cook for 1 minute.

3 Add the broth, water, tomato paste, and bay leaf. Bring the mixture to a boil. Reduce the heat to low, cover, and simmer for 1 hour. Remove and discard the bay leaf before serving.

NUTRITION (PER SERVING): 358 calories, 31 g protein, 29 g carbohydrates, 5 g fiber, 11 g sugars, 12 g fat, 3 g saturated fat, 720 mg sodium

MOM'S MEAT LOAF

PREP TIME: 15 MINUTES / TOTAL TIME: 1 HOUR 25 MINUTES / **MAKES 8 SERVINGS**

GLAZE

¼   **cup organic ketchup**

2   **cloves garlic**

1   **teaspoon mustard powder**

1   **tablespoon Worcestershire sauce**

MEATLOAF

1½   **pounds 95% lean ground beef**

½   **cup ground flaxseeds**

1   **teaspoon dried oregano**

2   **tablespoons Worcestershire sauce**

1   **small onion, finely chopped**

1   **egg**

1 Preheat the oven to 350°F. Coat a 9" x 5" loaf pan with cooking spray.

2 *To make the glaze:* In a small bowl, stir together the ketchup, garlic, mustard, and Worcestershire sauce. Set aside.

3 *To make the meat loaf:* In a large bowl, mix together the beef, flaxseeds, oregano, Worcestershire sauce, onion, egg, and 2 tablespoons of the reserved glaze. Press the mixture into the prepared loaf pan. Bake until a thermometer inserted in the center registers 160°F and the meat is no longer pink, 1 hour.

4 Spread the top of the meat loaf with the remaining glaze and bake for 10 minutes.

NUTRITION (PER SERVING): 147 calories, 20 g protein, 4 g carbohydrates, 0 g fiber, 3 g sugars, 5 g fat, 2 g saturated fat, 236 mg sodium

SALISBURY STEAK

PREP TIME: 10 MINUTES / TOTAL TIME: 35 MINUTES / **MAKES 4 SERVINGS**

1   pound 95% lean ground beef

¼   cup ground flaxseeds

1   clove garlic, minced

½   teaspoon onion powder

3   tablespoons Worcestershire sauce, divided

1   tablespoon tomato paste

2   egg whites

½   onion, halved and thinly sliced

4   ounces cremini mushrooms, sliced

1½   cups low-sodium beef broth, divided

1½   tablespoons cornstarch

1   In a large bowl, combine the beef, flaxseeds, garlic, onion powder, 2 tablespoons of the Worcestershire sauce, tomato paste, and egg whites. Mix well. Form into 4 patties.

2   Heat a large nonstick skillet coated with cooking spray over medium-high heat. Cook the patties, turning once, until browned, 8 minutes. Transfer to a plate.

3   In the same skillet over medium-high heat, cook the onion and mushrooms until tender and golden brown, 5 minutes. Stir in 1¼ cups of the broth.

4   In a small bowl, whisk together the remaining ¼ cup broth and the cornstarch until the cornstarch has dissolved. Add to the skillet and bring to a boil, whisking continuously. Reduce the heat to low and simmer, whisking often, until thickened, 5 minutes. Stir in the remaining 1 tablespoon Worcestershire sauce.

5   Return the patties to the skillet and cook until a thermometer inserted in the center registers 160°F and the meat is no longer pink, 5 minutes.

NUTRITION (PER SERVING): 318 calories, 30 g protein, 27 g carbohydrates, 5 g fiber, 3 g sugars, 9 g fat, 3 g saturated fat, 290 mg sodium

ZESTY ITALIAN CHEESEBURGERS

PREP TIME: 11 MINUTES / TOTAL TIME: 22 MINUTES / **MAKES 4 SERVINGS**

Shown in photo insert pages.

1	egg
1	pound ground beef
2	cloves garlic, minced
¼	cup no-salt-added tomato sauce
1	teaspoon dried basil
⅛	teaspoon salt
4	whole wheat hamburger buns
4	slices part-skim mozzarella cheese
2	cups fresh spinach
1	plum tomato, sliced
2	tablespoons pesto

1 In a large bowl, beat the egg. Add the beef, garlic, tomato sauce, basil, and salt, mixing with your hands until all ingredients are combined. Form into 4 burgers.

2 Heat a grill pan or large skillet coated with cooking spray over medium-high heat. Cook the burgers, turning once, until a thermometer inserted in the center registers 145°F for medium-rare, 10 minutes.

3 Place each burger on a bun and top each with 1 slice of cheese, ½ cup of spinach, tomato slices, and ½ tablespoon of pesto.

NUTRITION (PER SERVING): 389 calories, 36 g protein, 27 g carbohydrates, 4 g fiber, 6 g sugars, 16 g fat, 6 g saturated fat, 643 mg sodium

BEEF GOULASH

PREP TIME: 15 MINUTES / TOTAL TIME: 55 MINUTES / MAKES 4 SERVINGS

l   **package (8 ounces) shirataki noodles**

¼   **cup plain 0% Greek yogurt**

1½   **tablespoons all-purpose flour**

l   **tablespoon canola oil**

l   **onion, chopped**

l   **red bell pepper, chopped**

l   **green bell pepper, chopped**

1¼   **teaspoons paprika**

¾   **pound 95% lean ground beef**

l   **can (14.5 ounces) no-salt-added petite-diced tomatoes**

½   **cup fat-free reduced-sodium beef broth**

¼   **teaspoon salt**

1 Preheat the oven to 350°F. Prepare the noodles according to package directions. In a small bowl, whisk together the yogurt and flour. Set aside.

2 Meanwhile, in an ovenproof Dutch oven over medium-high heat, heat the oil. Cook the onion, red and green peppers, and paprika, stirring, for 3 minutes. Crumble the beef into the pan. Cook, stirring, until the beef is no longer pink, 4 minutes. Stir in the tomatoes (with juice), noodles, broth, and salt. Bring to a simmer. Reduce the heat to low. Stir in the yogurt mixture and cook until thickened, 2 minutes.

3 Cover and bake for 15 minutes. Carefully remove the cover and stir. Bake, uncovered, for 10 minutes.

NUTRITION (PER SERVING): 224 calories, 22 g protein, 15 g carbohydrates, 3 g fiber, 8 g sugars, 8 g fat, 2 g saturated fat, 294 mg sodium

GROUND BEEF RAGU OVER BARLEY

PREP TIME: 15 MINUTES / TOTAL TIME: 1 HOUR 15 MINUTES / MAKES 4 SERVINGS

1	cup barley
3	cups water
2	tablespoons olive oil
½	small onion, finely chopped
1	red bell pepper, chopped
1	yellow bell pepper, chopped
4	ounces cremini mushrooms, chopped
1	clove garlic, minced
1	pound lean ground beef
1	teaspoon Italian seasoning
¼	teaspoon salt
2	cups canned crushed tomatoes
2	tablespoons tomato paste

1 In a medium saucepan, combine the barley and water. Bring to a boil, reduce to a low simmer, cover, and cook until the barley is tender, about 35 minutes. Drain any excess water from the barley.

2 Meanwhile, in a large saucepan over medium heat, heat the oil. Cook the onion, red and yellow peppers, and mushrooms until soft, 10 minutes. Add the garlic and cook, stirring constantly, for 1 minute.

3 Push the veggies to the edges of the pan and place the beef in the center. Break the beef apart and cook until browned, about 5 minutes.

4 Add the Italian seasoning and salt. Stir the veggies and seasonings into the beef and cook for 1 minute. Add the tomatoes and tomato paste. Cover and simmer until the mixture thickens, 10 minutes.

5 Serve the ragu over the barley.

NUTRITION (PER SERVING): 312 calories, 23 g protein, 36 g carbohydrates, 8 g fiber, 7 g sugars, 9 g fat, 3 g saturated fat, 250 mg sodium

LAMB BURGERS WITH LEMON-YOGURT SAUCE

PREP TIME: 10 MINUTES / TOTAL TIME: 20 MINUTES / MAKES 4 SERVINGS

¼ cup plain 0% Greek yogurt

2 tablespoons fresh lemon juice

5 mint leaves, finely chopped

½ teaspoon honey

3 cups fresh spinach leaves, divided

1 pound lean ground lamb

1 small red onion, finely chopped

¼ cup crumbled feta cheese

¼ teaspoon ground cumin

1 egg white

2 whole wheat pitas, halved

1 plum tomato, thinly sliced

1 In a small bowl, whisk together the yogurt, lemon juice, mint, and honey. Set aside.

2 Chop 1 cup of the spinach. In a large bowl, mix together the chopped spinach, lamb, onion, cheese, cumin, and egg white. Form into 4 burgers.

3 In a large nonstick skillet over medium-high heat, cook the burgers, turning once, until a thermometer inserted in the center registers 160°F and the meat is no longer pink, 10 minutes.

4 Open half of a pita pocket and spread a spoonful of the yogurt sauce inside. Cut a burger in half and place 2 halves into each pita pocket half. Fill each with ½ cup of the remaining spinach leaves and a few tomato slices.

NUTRITION (PER SERVING): 283 calories, 32 g protein, 23 g carbohydrates, 3 g fiber, 3 g sugars, 8 g fat, 3 g saturated fat, 401 mg sodium

SLOW-COOKER PULLED PORK SANDWICH

PREP TIME: 15 MINUTES / TOTAL TIME: 15 MINUTES + 6 TO 8 HOURS IN A SLOW COOKER / MAKES 4 SERVINGS

1 teaspoon light brown sugar

1 teaspoon chili powder

½ teaspoon ground cumin

¼ teaspoon ground cinnamon

1 pound pork tenderloin

½ small onion, finely chopped

¼ cup low-sodium vegetable broth

Double batch of Citrus Garlic Aioli (page 273)

8 slices whole wheat bread (optional: toasted)

1 In a small bowl, combine the sugar, chili powder, cumin, and cinnamon.

2 Rub the pork with the seasoning mix and place in a slow cooker. Sprinkle the onion over the pork. Pour in the vegetable broth. Cover and cook on low until very tender, 6 to 8 hours. Use a fork to pull apart and shred the pork.

3 Place 1 slice of bread on 4 plates. Divide the pork on the slices. Top each with ¼ of the Citrus Garlic Aioli and 1 slice of bread.

NUTRITION (PER SERVING): 362 calories, 34 g protein, 33 g carbohydrates, 5 g fiber, 7 g sugars, 10 g fat, 3 g saturated fat, 371 mg sodium

HEALTHY HINT

Walk through any natural food store and you'll see that sprouted-grain breads are super popular—and super pricey, too. They're made by soaking and sprouting grains and then grinding them into a flour that can be used for baking. This purportedly makes breads easier to digest and the grains' nutrients easier to absorb. And while many experts agree that this is true to an extent, their advantages over unsprouted whole grain breads are nominal.

PORK TENDERLOIN WITH ROASTED VEGETABLES AND APPLES

PREP TIME: 15 MINUTES / TOTAL TIME: 1 HOUR / MAKES 2 SERVINGS

Shown in photo insert pages.

½ pound baby Yukon Gold potatoes, halved

½ pound carrots, peeled and cut into I" chunks

2 leeks, trimmed, halved lengthwise, and cut into I" chunks

I teaspoon chopped fresh rosemary or ½ teaspoon dried

2 teaspoons olive oil, divided

¼ teaspoon salt, divided

½ teaspoon black pepper, divided

I½ teaspoons Dijon mustard

I teaspoon pure maple syrup

½ teaspoon chopped fresh sage or ¼ teaspoon dried

½ teaspoon chopped fresh thyme or ¼ teaspoon dried

I small clove garlic, mashed into a paste

8 ounces pork tenderloin, trimmed of all visible fat

I sweet, tart apple, such as Honeycrisp or Jonagold, cored and cut into ¾" wedges

1 Position a rack in the upper third of the oven, and preheat the oven to 425°F. In a 13" x 9" baking dish, toss the potatoes, carrots, leeks, rosemary, 1 teaspoon of the oil, ⅛ teaspoon of the salt, and ¼ teaspoon of the pepper. Roast until the vegetables begin to soften, about 12 minutes.

2 In a small bowl, combine the mustard, maple syrup, sage, thyme, garlic, and the remaining 1 teaspoon oil, ⅛ teaspoon salt, and ¼ teaspoon pepper. Rub the pork with the mustard mixture.

3 Add the apple wedges to the baking dish, stir to combine, and top with the pork. Roast, turning the tenderloin once, until a thermometer registers 145°F for rare when inserted into the thickest part of the tenderloin, 18 minutes.

4 Transfer the pork to a cutting board and let stand 5 minutes. Serve with the vegetables.

NUTRITION (PER SERVING): 407 calories, 27 g protein, 58 g carbohydrates, 9 g fiber, 22 g sugars, 8 g fat, 2 g saturated fat, 508 mg sodium

EVOLUTION OF THE DINNER PLATE

Fun fact: In the 1960s, the diameter of the average American dinner plate was 9 inches. In the 1980s, 10 inches. And today, 12 whopping inches. So is it a coincidence that the average American today is 24 pounds heavier than in 1960 or that obesity rates have more than doubled in the past 35 years? Well, we're not saying plate size is everything, but it's certainly something to think about.

PORK CHOPS WITH APPLE SALAD

PREP TIME: 15 MINUTES / TOTAL TIME: 25 MINUTES / **MAKES 4 SERVINGS**

2 tablespoons balsamic vinegar

1 tablespoon Dijon mustard

2 apples, cored and thinly sliced lengthwise

1 head Bibb lettuce, chopped

2 cups fresh spinach

1 rib celery, sliced

½ small onion, sliced

¼ cup reduced-fat blue cheese crumbles

4 pork chops (6 ounces each)

⅛ teaspoon salt

1 tablespoon chopped fresh thyme or 1 teaspoon dried

1 clove garlic, minced

1 In a large bowl, whisk together the vinegar and mustard. Add the apples, lettuce, spinach, celery, and onion. Toss to coat. Sprinkle with the blue cheese and set aside.

2 Combine the salt, thyme, and garlic then season each pork chop.

3 Heat a large nonstick skillet coated with cooking spray over medium heat. Cook the pork chops, turning once, until lightly browned, a thermometer inserted in the center of a chop registers 145°F for rare, and the juices run clear, 8 minutes. Serve with the apple salad.

NUTRITION (PER SERVING): 328 calories, 42 g protein, 18 g carbohydrates, 3 g fiber, 12 g sugars, 9 g fat, 4 g saturated fat, 404 mg sodium

GRILLED PORK TACOS WITH MANGO SALSA

PREP TIME: 10 MINUTES / TOTAL TIME: 55 MINUTES / **MAKES 4 SERVINGS**

Shown in photo insert pages.

1   mango, peeled, pitted, and diced

2   plum tomatoes, diced

¼   cup diced fresh cilantro

1   jalapeño chile pepper, seeded and finely chopped (wear plastic gloves when handling)

2   cloves garlic, minced

1½   teaspoons chipotle seasoning

¼   teaspoon salt

1¼   pounds trimmed pork tenderloin

1   tablespoon olive oil

8   soft corn tortillas (6" diameter)

1   cup shredded lettuce

1 In a medium bowl, stir together the mango, tomatoes, cilantro, and pepper. Set aside.

2 Coat a grill rack with cooking spray. Preheat the grill to medium.

3 In a small bowl, combine the garlic, chipotle seasoning, and salt. Rub the pork with the garlic mixture. Rub the oil into the pork.

4 Grill the pork, turning occasionally, until a thermometer inserted in the center reaches 145°F for rare and the juices run clear, 25 minutes. Let stand for 10 minutes.

5 Meanwhile, stack the tortillas and wrap in foil. Place on a cool corner of the grill to warm for 10 minutes.

6 Slice the pork. Place 1 tortilla on 4 plates. Evenly divide the pork, lettuce, and salsa among the tortillas.

NUTRITION (PER SERVING): 350 calories, 34 g protein, 36 g carbohydrates, 5 g fiber, 13 g sugars, 8 g fat, 2 g saturated fat, 223 mg sodium

PORK AND BROCCOLI STIR-FRY

PREP TIME: 10 MINUTES / TOTAL TIME: 20 MINUTES / **MAKES 4 SERVINGS**

3 tablespoons low-sodium soy sauce

2 tablespoons fresh lime juice

1 tablespoon Asian chili paste

1 teaspoon honey

1 tablespoon sesame oil, divided

1 pound pork tenderloin, cut into ¼" strips

1 tablespoon grated fresh ginger or 1 teaspoon dried

1 clove garlic, minced

3 cups broccoli florets

2 carrots, sliced

1 red bell pepper, thinly sliced

3 tablespoons water

½ cup (1 ounce) snap peas

2 cups cooked brown rice

1 In a small bowl, combine the soy sauce, lime juice, chili paste, and honey. Set aside.

2 In a large nonstick skillet over medium-high heat, heat 1 teaspoon of the oil. Working in batches if necessary, cook the pork, stirring often, until lightly browned, 3 minutes. Transfer to a plate and set aside.

3 Add the remaining 2 teaspoons oil to the skillet. Cook the ginger and garlic until fragrant, 30 seconds. Stir in the broccoli and cook for 1 minute.

4 Add the carrots, pepper, and water. Cover and simmer until tender-crisp, 3 minutes. Uncover and stir in the peas, reserved soy sauce mixture, and pork. Cook, stirring, until thickened, 2 minutes. Serve over the rice.

NUTRITION (PER SERVING): 322 calories, 29 g protein, 34 g carbohydrates, 5 g fiber, 5 g sugars, 7 g fat, 2 g saturated fat, 713 mg sodium

SALAMI AND HAM FLATBREAD

PREP TIME: 15 MINUTES / TOTAL TIME: 35 MINUTES / **MAKES 6 SERVINGS**

1   envelope (2¼ teaspoons) rapid rise yeast

1½ cups whole wheat flour, divided

1   teaspoon dried oregano

1   tablespoon sugar

⅛   teaspoon salt

½   cup warm (not hot) water

2   tablespoons extra-virgin olive oil

2   ounces uncured salami, sliced

2   ounces uncured sliced ham, rolled into straws

¼   cup kalamata olives

1   large roasted red pepper, thinly sliced

¾   cup water-packed canned artichoke hearts, drained

2   ounces sliced mozzarella cheese

1   cup chopped romaine lettuce

3   tablespoons fresh basil leaves, roughly chopped

1 Preheat the oven to 425°F.

2 In a large bowl, combine the yeast, 1 cup of the flour, the oregano, sugar, and salt. Stir in the water until well blended. (The dough will be wet.) Lightly flour a work surface with the remaining ½ cup flour and transfer the dough to the surface. Knead in enough additional flour so the dough is no longer sticky. Continue to knead to develop gluten, 4 minutes. Place in a warm place for 5 minutes.

3 On a baking sheet, stretch the dough into a rough 14" square. Brush or drizzle with the oil and bake for 10 minutes. Reduce the oven temperature to 375°F. Remove from the oven and top with the salami, ham, olives, roasted pepper, artichokes, and cheese. Bake until heated through, 10 minutes.

4 Garnish with the lettuce and basil.

NUTRITION (PER SERVING): 291 calories, 12 g protein, 30 g carbohydrates, 5 g fiber, 3 g sugars, 15 g fat, 4 g saturated fat, 668 mg sodium

MEDITERRANEAN CHICKEN WRAPS

PREP TIME: 5 MINUTES / TOTAL TIME: 5 MINUTES / MAKES 2 SERVINGS

½   small cucumber

4   tablespoons roasted garlic hummus

2   whole wheat tortillas (8" diameter)

¼   cup (I ounce) crumbled feta cheese

4   ounces roasted chicken breast

I   small tomato, sliced

I   cup fresh spinach

2   sprigs fresh dill

1 With a vegetable peeler, shave ribbons the length of the cucumber, turning to shave ribbons from all sides.

2 Spread 2 tablespoons of hummus over each tortilla. Sprinkle each with half of the cheese. Divide the cucumber, chicken, tomato, spinach, and dill between the two. Fold the side over to wrap.

NUTRITION (PER SERVING): 269 calories, 24 g protein, 30 g carbohydrates, 4 g fiber, 4 g sugars, 9 g fat, 3 g saturated fat, 542 mg sodium

SLOW-COOKER BBQ PULLED CHICKEN FLATBREADS

PREP TIME: 15 MINUTES / TOTAL TIME: 3 HOURS 45 MINUTES / MAKES 4 SERVINGS

Shown in photo insert pages.

1½ cups crushed tomatoes or tomato puree

¼ cup apple cider vinegar

2 tablespoons molasses

2 teaspoons smoked or sweet paprika

½ teaspoon salt

½ teaspoon black pepper, divided

2 teaspoons Dijon mustard, divided

1 red onion, thinly sliced, divided

1 pound boneless, skinless chicken breasts

3 cups shredded green cabbage (about ½ head)

2 large carrots, grated

2 tablespoons dill pickle juice

2 tablespoons mayonnaise

4 corn tortillas, whole wheat flatbreads, or pitas (6" diameter; use corn tortillas for gluten-free)

1 In a slow cooker, whisk together the tomatoes or puree, vinegar, molasses, paprika, salt, ⅛ teaspoon of the pepper, and 1 teaspoon of the mustard. Add half of the onion. Add the chicken, spooning some of the tomato mixture over the top. Cover and cook on low until the chicken is very tender and reaches an internal temperature of 165°F, 3½ hours.

2 Meanwhile, in a large bowl, combine the cabbage, carrots, pickle juice, mayonnaise, the remaining ⅛ teaspoon pepper, the remaining 1 teaspoon mustard, and the remaining red onion. Cover and refrigerate the coleslaw until ready to serve.

3 Remove the chicken from the sauce and place on a cutting board. Shred with two forks and stir into the sauce in the slow cooker. Place 1 tortilla, flatbread, or pita on 4 plates. Evenly divide the chicken and slaw over each.

NUTRITION (PER SERVING): 420 calories, 30 g protein, 53 g carbohydrates, 7 g fiber, 18 g sugars, 11 g fat, 2 g saturated fat, 581 mg sodium

TIP: If you don't like the taste of raw onion in salads like this slaw, soak the onion slices in cold water for 10 minutes and drain well before adding to the salad.

MAKE IT AHEAD! Pulled chicken freezes well, and this recipe doubles easily. Make a big batch and freeze half for a fast weeknight dinner.

CHICKEN CACCIATORE

PREP TIME: 10 MINUTES / TOTAL TIME: 50 MINUTES / **MAKES 4 SERVINGS**

4   ounces whole wheat egg noodles

2   teaspoons olive oil

1   pound boneless, skinless chicken breasts

1   package (8 ounces) cremini mushrooms, sliced

1   green bell pepper, sliced

1   red bell pepper, sliced

2   carrots, sliced

1   small onion, sliced

2   cloves garlic, minced

1   can (8 ounces) diced tomatoes

1   teaspoon dried oregano

¾   cup dry white wine

1 Prepare the noodles according to package directions.

2 Meanwhile, in a large nonstick skillet over medium-high heat, heat the oil. Cook the chicken, turning occasionally, until browned on all sides, 6 minutes. Transfer to a plate.

3 Stir the mushrooms, green and red peppers, carrots, onion, and garlic into the skillet. Reduce the heat to medium, cover, and cook, stirring occasionally, until the mushrooms begin to release liquid, 7 minutes. Uncover and cook until the liquid evaporates.

4 Add the tomatoes (with juice), oregano, wine, and the reserved chicken. Reduce the heat to low and simmer until a thermometer inserted in the thickest portion of the chicken registers 165°F and the juices run clear, 30 minutes. Serve the chicken over the noodles.

NUTRITION (PER SERVING): 367 calories, 31 g protein, 37 g carbohydrates, 5 g fiber, 9 g sugars, 7 g fat, 1 g saturated fat, 180 mg sodium

QUICK, CREAMY CHICKEN LASAGNA

PREP TIME: 15 MINUTES / TOTAL TIME: 1 HOUR 25 MINUTES / **MAKES 12 SERVINGS**

15 **oven-ready, rippled-style lasagna noodles**

4 **cups shredded cooked chicken**

1½ **teaspoons dried basil**

12 **ounces cream cheese, softened, divided**

½ **cup chicken or vegetable broth, divided**

3 **cups marinara sauce (no-sugar-added or low-sugar), divided**

4 **cups shredded mozzarella cheese**

¾ **cup grated Parmesan cheese**

1 Preheat the oven to 400°F. Coat a 13" x 9" baking dish with cooking spray. Place the noodles in a large shallow bowl. Cover with very hot tap water and soak for 10 minutes. Drain.

2 In a large bowl, combine the chicken, basil, 8 ounces of the cream cheese, and ¼ cup of the broth.

3 Meanwhile, in a medium bowl, stir together the remaining 4 ounces cream cheese and ¼ cup broth. Spread ⅓ cup of the marinara on the bottom of the prepared baking dish. Layer 3 of the noodles, ⅔ cup of the sauce, 1 cup of the chicken mixture, ¾ cup of the mozzarella, and 2 tablespoons of the Parmesan in the dish. Repeat these layers 3 more times. Top with the remaining noodles, the cream cheese mixture, and the remaining cheese.

4 Cover with foil and bake for 35 minutes. Remove the foil and bake until golden brown and heated through, 15 minutes. Let stand 10 minutes.

NUTRITION (PER SERVING): 418 calories, 33 g protein, 27 g carbohydrates, 2 g fiber, 4 g sugars, 20 g fat, 13 g saturated fat, 626 mg sodium

CHICKEN POT PIE

PREP TIME: 10 MINUTES / TOTAL TIME: 45 MINUTES / MAKES 6 SERVINGS

Shown in photo insert pages.

2   tablespoons olive oil, divided

1¼ pounds boneless, skinless chicken breasts, cut into ½" cubes

2   carrots, thinly sliced

2   ribs celery, thinly sliced

1   teaspoon dried rosemary, crushed

2   cups frozen corn, bean, and pea mix, thawed

2   cups low-sodium chicken broth, divided

1   tablespoon cornstarch

8   sheets whole wheat phyllo dough

1 Preheat the oven to 350°F. Coat a 9" x 9" baking dish with cooking spray.

2 In a large skillet over medium-high heat, heat 1 tablespoon of the oil. Cook the chicken, stirring, until no longer pink, 8 minutes. Transfer to a bowl and set aside.

3 In the same skillet, heat the remaining 1 tablespoon oil. Cook the carrots, celery, and rosemary, stirring, until tender, 5 minutes. Stir in the chicken and the corn mix. Transfer to the prepared baking dish.

4 Add 1½ cups of the broth to the skillet, reduce the heat to medium-low, and bring to a boil. Reduce the heat to low.

5 In a small bowl, whisk together the cornstarch and the remaining ½ cup broth until smooth. Add to the skillet and whisk until thickened, 3 minutes. Pour over the chicken and vegetable mixture in the baking dish.

6 Lay 2 sheets of phyllo dough across the top of the dish, tucking the edges into the pan. Lightly coat the sheets with cooking spray. Repeat to make 3 more layers. Bake until golden and bubbling, 20 minutes.

NUTRITION (PER SERVING): 248 calories, 24 g protein, 20 g carbohydrates, 3 g fiber, 1 g sugars, 8 g fat, 1 g saturated fat, 256 mg sodium

BAKED CHICKEN WITH MUSTARD SAUCE

PREP TIME: 10 MINUTES / TOTAL TIME: 35 MINUTES / **MAKES 4 SERVINGS**

2 tablespoons olive oil, divided

I large egg

¼ cup + 3 tablespoons honey mustard

½ teaspoon black pepper

¼ teaspoon paprika

4 boneless, skinless chicken breasts

¾ cup whole wheat panko bread crumbs

3 tablespoons plain 0% Greek yogurt

2 tablespoons orange juice

1 Preheat the oven to 375°F. Coat a rimmed baking sheet with 1 tablespoon of the oil.

2 In a large bowl, whisk the egg until foamy. Whisk in ¼ cup mustard, the pepper, and paprika. Add the chicken and turn to coat.

3 Place the bread crumbs in a shallow dish or pie plate. Place the chicken in the bread crumbs, turning and pressing to adhere. Place on the prepared baking sheet. Drizzle the chicken with the remaining 1 tablespoon oil. Bake, turning once, until crispy and browned, a thermometer inserted in the thickest portion registers 165°F, and the juices run clear, 25 minutes.

4 Meanwhile, in a small bowl, whisk together the 3 tablespoons of the mustard, the yogurt, and the orange juice. Serve with the chicken.

NUTRITION (PER SERVING): 347 calories, 40 g protein, 17 g carbohydrates, 2 g fiber, 2 g sugars, 12 g fat, 2 g saturated fat, 503 mg sodium

PARMESAN CHICKEN FINGERS

PREP TIME: 10 MINUTES / TOTAL TIME: 25 MINUTES / **MAKES 4 SERVINGS**

1 pound boneless, skinless chicken breast tenderloins

¼ teaspoon black pepper

2 eggs

¾ cup bran flakes cereal, finely crushed

¼ cup grated Parmesan cheese

2½ tablespoons ground flaxseeds

1 teaspoon dried basil

½ teaspoon garlic powder

1 Preheat the oven to 450°F. Lightly coat a baking sheet with cooking spray.

2 Season the chicken with the pepper.

3 In a shallow bowl, whisk the eggs. In a shallow dish or pie plate, combine the bran flakes, cheese, flaxseeds, basil, and garlic powder.

4 Dip the chicken in the egg, shaking off any excess, and toss in the bran flake mixture. Place on the prepared baking sheet. Bake until no longer pink and the juices run clear, 12 minutes.

NUTRITION (PER SERVING): 200 calories, 33 g protein, 8 g carbohydrates, 3 g fiber, 2 g sugars, 5 g fat, 1 g saturated fat, 238 mg sodium

CHICKEN PAD THAI

Shown in photo insert pages.

4   ounces flat brown rice noodles

2   tablespoons low-sodium soy sauce

2   tablespoons peanut butter

1   tablespoon Sriracha sauce

1   teaspoon low-sodium fish sauce

1   tablespoon peanut oil

¾   pound boneless, skinless chicken breast, cut into 1½" strips

2   cloves garlic, minced

3   scallions, sliced

1   cup bean sprouts, for garnish

¼   cup peanuts, chopped, for garnish

1   lime, quartered, for garnish (optional)

1 Prepare the noodles according to package directions. Reserve 2 tablespoons of the cooking water.

2 In a small bowl, whisk together the soy sauce, peanut butter, Sriracha sauce, fish sauce, and the reserved noodle water.

3 In a large nonstick skillet over medium-high heat, heat the oil. Cook the chicken, stirring often, until no longer pink and the juices run clear, 5 minutes. Add the garlic and cook for 30 seconds. Stir in the noodles and cook until hot, 1 minute.

4 Add the soy sauce mixture and cook, tossing, for 1 minute. Stir in the scallions and remove from the heat.

5 Divide among 4 plates, garnishing each with ¼ cup of the bean sprouts and sprinkling with the peanuts, if using. Serve with the lime wedges, if using.

NUTRITION (PER SERVING): 504 calories, 30 g protein, 55 g carbohydrates, 7 g fiber, 4 g sugars, 20 g fat, 4 g saturated fat, 628 mg sodium

BROCCOLI-CHICKEN CASSEROLE

PREP TIME: 10 MINUTES / TOTAL TIME: 1 HOUR / **MAKES 6 SERVINGS**

1½ **cups wild rice**

1 **tablespoon canola oil**

¾ **pound boneless, skinless chicken breasts**

1 **package (10 ounces) frozen chopped broccoli, thawed**

1 **small onion, chopped**

2 **cloves garlic, minced**

1¼ **cups 1% milk, divided**

¾ **cup light sour cream**

¾ **cup reduced-fat shredded Cheddar cheese**

2 **tablespoons whole wheat panko bread crumbs**

2 **tablespoons ground flaxseeds**

1 Preheat the oven to 350°F. Lightly coat an 8" x 8" baking dish with cooking spray.

2 In a saucepan, prepare the rice according to package directions. Place in the prepared dish.

3 Meanwhile, in a large nonstick skillet over medium-high heat, heat the oil. Cook the chicken, turning once, until browned, a thermometer inserted in the thickest portion registers 165°F, and the juices run clear, 10 minutes. Transfer to a clean cutting board and let stand 5 minutes. Using a fork, shred the chicken into small pieces. Add to the rice in the baking dish.

4 In the same skillet, cook the broccoli, onion, and garlic until the onion softens, 5 minutes. Add to the rice and chicken mixture.

5 In the same skillet over medium-low heat, bring ¾ cup of the milk to a simmer. Whisk the sour cream, cheese, and the remaining ½ cup milk into the skillet and cook, stirring constantly, until thickened, 5 minutes. Stir into the chicken mixture until well blended.

6 In a small bowl, combine the bread crumbs and flaxseeds. Sprinkle over the chicken mixture. Bake until heated through, 20 minutes.

NUTRITION (PER SERVING): 267 calories, 24 g protein, 19 g carbohydrates, 3 g fiber, 6 g sugars, 11 g fat, 4 g saturated fat, 229 mg sodium

ORANGE-SAGE BRAISED CHICKEN THIGHS

PREP TIME: 10 MINUTES / TOTAL TIME: 55 MINUTES / **MAKES 4 SERVINGS**

2 tablespoons sunflower oil

4 bone-in, skinless chicken thighs

4 teaspoons grated orange zest

1 cup orange juice

2 tablespoons balsamic vinegar

1 medium onion, sliced

1 teaspoon ground dried sage

1 teaspoon salt

1 Preheat the oven to 375°F.

2 In a small Dutch oven or ovenproof lidded saucepan over medium-high heat, heat the oil. Cook the chicken, turning until browned, 8 minutes.

3 In the Dutch oven, stir in the orange zest, orange juice, vinegar, onion, sage, and salt. Bring to a simmer. Cover and transfer to the oven. Roast for 40 minutes, removing the cover halfway through the cooking time.

NUTRITION (PER SERVING): 314 calories, 29 g protein, 11 g carbohydrates, 1 g fiber, 8 g sugars, 17 g fat, 3 g saturated fat, 104 mg sodium

TURKEY CUBAN WRAP WITH BLACK BEAN SALAD

PREP TIME: 25 MINUTES / TOTAL TIME: 25 MINUTES / **MAKES 2 SERVINGS**

SALAD

- 2 **tablespoons fresh lime juice**
- 1 **teaspoon extra-virgin olive oil**
- 2 **tablespoons diced red onion**
- ½ **teaspoon ground cumin**
- 1 **can (15 ounces) black beans, rinsed and drained**
- 1 **cup cherry or grape tomatoes, halved**
- 1 **head butter lettuce, torn into bite-size pieces**
  Pinch of salt
  Pinch of black pepper

WRAPS

- 2 **teaspoons coarse grain Dijon mustard**
- 2 **whole wheat tortillas (8" diameter)**
- 1½ **ounces thinly sliced Swiss cheese (about 2 slices), halved**
- 5 **ounces roast turkey breast, thinly sliced (about 6 slices)**
- 8 **dill pickle slices**

1 *To make the salad:* In a medium bowl, whisk together the lime juice, oil, onion, and cumin. Add the beans and tomatoes and let stand for 10 minutes. Toss in the lettuce and season with the salt and pepper.

2 *To make the wraps:* Spread the mustard over the tortillas. Lay 1 half slice of the cheese in the center of each tortilla. Top each with 3 slices of turkey breast and 4 dill pickle slices. Top with the remaining cheese. Fold the sides of the tortillas in toward the center and roll up from the bottom.

3 Heat a griddle or skillet over medium heat and cook the wraps with their seam sides down. Press down with another pot or skillet to gently flatten the wraps. Cook, turning once, until crisp and golden, 5 minutes.

4 Serve with the black bean salad.

NUTRITION (PER SERVING): 404 calories, 36 g protein, 42 g carbohydrates, 11 g fiber, 5 g sugars, 10 g fat, 4 g saturated fat, 651 mg sodium

SWEET POTATO AND TURKEY SHEPHERD'S PIE

PREP TIME: 10 MINUTES / TOTAL TIME: 50 MINUTES / **MAKES 6 SERVINGS**

2 sweet potatoes (8 ounces), peeled and cut into ½" pieces

l tablespoon olive oil

l cup low-sodium chicken broth

3 tablespoons whole wheat flour

l onion, chopped

2 teaspoons dried thyme

l2 ounces 99% fat-free, lean ground turkey

3 carrots, chopped

l cup frozen peas, thawed

l cup frozen corn, thawed

l cup frozen cut green beans, thawed

¼ cup dried cranberries

1 Fill a large saucepan halfway with water and bring to a boil over high heat. Cook the sweet potatoes until tender, 15 minutes. Remove from the heat. Drain. Place the potatoes back in the saucepan and drizzle with the oil. Using a potato masher, mash the potatoes until smooth. Set aside.

2 Preheat the oven to 350°F. Coat an 8" x 8" baking dish with cooking spray. In a measuring cup, whisk together the broth and flour.

3 Heat a nonstick skillet coated with cooking spray over medium-high heat. Cook the onion and thyme, stirring, until starting to soften, 4 minutes. Add the turkey and cook until no longer pink, 5 minutes. Add the broth mixture and cook, stirring constantly, until thickened, 5 minutes. Stir in the carrots, peas, corn, beans, and cranberries. Pour into the baking dish. Spread the mashed sweet potatoes over the top of the mixture. Bake until the top is browned and the filling is hot and bubbly, 20 minutes.

NUTRITION (PER SERVING): 228 calories, 15 g protein, 29 g carbohydrates, 5 g fiber, 9 g sugars, 7 g fat, 1 g saturated fat, 118 mg sodium

TURKEY MEAT LOAF WITH CRANBERRY CHUTNEY

PREP TIME: 10 MINUTES / TOTAL TIME: 1 HOUR 45 MINUTES / MAKES 8 SERVINGS

½ cup quinoa, rinsed and drained

1½ tablespoons olive oil, divided

1 shallot, finely chopped

2 cups cranberries

1 cup water

1 onion, chopped

2 cloves garlic, minced

3 pounds 99% fat-free, lean ground turkey

¼ cup organic ketchup

2 egg whites, lightly beaten

2 tablespoons ground flaxseeds

1 Preheat the oven to 350°F. Lightly coat a 13" x 9" baking dish with cooking spray. Prepare the quinoa according to package directions.

2 In a small saucepan over medium-high heat, heat ½ tablespoon of the oil. Cook the shallot for 5 minutes. Add the cranberries and cook for 10 minutes. Set aside.

3 In a skillet over medium heat, heat the remaining 1 tablespoon oil. Cook the onion and garlic until lightly browned, 5 minutes. Transfer to a large bowl.

4 Add the turkey, prepared quinoa, ketchup, egg whites, and flaxseeds to the bowl. Stir until well blended. Transfer the meat loaf to the baking dish and loosely form into a rectangular log. Cover with half of the cranberry mixture. Bake the meat loaf until a thermometer inserted in the center registers 165°F and the meat is no longer pink, 60 minutes. Serve the meat loaf with the remaining cranberry mixture.

NUTRITION (PER SERVING): 291 calories, 46 g protein, 16 g carbohydrates, 3 g fiber, 4 g sugars, 7 g fat, 1 g saturated fat, 192 mg sodium

BAKED ZITI WITH TURKEY

PREP TIME: 10 MINUTES / TOTAL TIME: 55 MINUTES / **MAKES 4 SERVINGS**

Shown in photo insert pages.

1½ cups (5 ounces) whole wheat penne pasta

6 ounces lean Italian-style turkey sausage (sweet or mild), cut into I`` slices

8 ounces 99% fat-free, lean ground turkey

I large green bell pepper, chopped

I small onion, chopped

4 ounces button mushrooms, chopped

3 cloves garlic, minced

I teaspoon Italian seasoning

2 cups low-sodium pasta sauce

½ pound baby kale

¾ cup shredded part-skim mozzarella cheese (3 ounces)

1. Preheat the oven to 375°F. Coat a shallow 3-quart baking dish with cooking spray.

2. Prepare the pasta according to package directions. Drain.

3. Heat a large nonstick skillet over medium heat. Cook the sausage and ground turkey until browned and no longer pink, 10 minutes. Transfer the meat to a clean plate and set aside.

4. In the same skillet, cook the pepper, onion, mushrooms, garlic, and Italian seasoning, stirring occasionally, until the onion is soft, 5 minutes. Stir in the pasta sauce and kale. Return the meat to the skillet and cook until heated through, 5 minutes.

5. Stir in the pasta. Place in the prepared baking dish. Sprinkle with the cheese. Bake until heated through and the cheese is melted, 20 minutes.

NUTRITION (PER SERVING): 418 calories, 36 g protein, 45 g carbohydrates, 7 g fiber, 9 g sugars, 12 g fat, 2 g saturated fat, 575 mg sodium

SALMON SALAD LETTUCE WRAPS

PREP TIME: 15 MINUTES / TOTAL TIME: 15 MINUTES / MAKES 2 SERVINGS

3   tablespoons plain 2% Greek yogurt

½   tablespoon low-sodium soy sauce

I   tablespoon rice vinegar

¼   teaspoon ground ginger

2   cans (5 ounces each) wild salmon, drained

3   tablespoons finely chopped celery

2   tablespoons shredded carrot

2   tablespoons chopped cashews

I   tablespoon chopped scallion

½   medium cucumber, thinly sliced into coins

6   large Bibb or butterhead lettuce leaves

1 In a large bowl, whisk together the yogurt, soy sauce, vinegar, and ginger. Add the salmon, celery, carrot, cashews, and scallion, tossing to coat well.

2 Evenly divide the salmon mixture and cucumber among the lettuce leaves.

NUTRITION (PER SERVING): 249 calories, 28 g protein, 8 g carbohydrates, 2 g fiber, 3 g sugars, 12 g fat, 2 g saturated fat, 563 mg sodium

HEALTHY HINT

The easiest way to figure out which seafood is safest (and which to avoid) is to download the Monterey Bay Aquarium Seafood Watch guide from seafoodwatch.org. The easy-to-read chart provides convenient color-coded info on best choices, good alternatives, and fish to avoid, based on the region of the country that you live in. Print it out and tuck it in a reusable shopping bag or your purse so you always have it at the store. You can also download an app for your phone from the same site.

SALMON CROQUETTES

PREP TIME: 15 MINUTES / TOTAL TIME: 45 MINUTES / **MAKES 2 SERVINGS**

1   can (14 ounces) wild salmon, drained

1   large egg

½   cup frozen spinach, thawed, drained of
    excess water, and chopped

2   tablespoons chopped garlic or 1 teaspoon
    garlic powder

1   teaspoon onion powder

¾   cup whole wheat bread crumbs, divided

1 Preheat the oven to 350°F. Line a baking sheet with parchment paper.

2 In a large bowl, combine the salmon, egg, spinach, garlic, onion powder, and ½ cup of the bread crumbs. Stir until well blended.

3 Place the remaining ¼ cup bread crumbs on a shallow plate. Shape the salmon mixture into 4 balls, then roll in the bread crumbs. Place on the prepared baking sheet and bake until lightly browned, about 30 minutes.

NUTRITION (PER SERVING): 445 calories, 49 g protein, 27 g carbohydrates, 5 g fiber, 1 g sugars, 15 g fat, 4 g saturated fat, 250 mg sodium

SALMON PASTA CASSEROLE

PREP TIME: 10 MINUTES / TOTAL TIME: 50 MINUTES / **MAKES 4 SERVINGS**

6   ounces whole grain farfalle pasta (bow ties)

2   pouches (5 ounces each) wild pink salmon, drained

1   package (10 ounces) frozen artichoke hearts, thawed and chopped

1   package (10 ounces) frozen chopped spinach, thawed and drained

¼   cup mayonnaise

¼   cup grated Parmesan cheese, divided

1   tablespoon fresh lemon juice

¼   cup ground golden flaxseeds

1 Preheat the oven to 350°F. Coat an 8" x 8" baking dish with cooking spray.

2 Prepare the pasta according to package directions.

3 Meanwhile, in a large bowl, combine the salmon, artichoke hearts, spinach, mayonnaise, 2 tablespoons of the cheese, and the lemon juice. Toss gently until well blended. Stir in the pasta, and place in the prepared baking dish. Top with the flaxseeds and the remaining 2 tablespoons cheese. Bake until heated through, 30 minutes.

NUTRITION (PER SERVING): 414 calories, 25 g protein, 41 g carbohydrates, 11 g fiber, 2 g sugars, 19 g fat, 2 g saturated fat, 458 mg sodium

ASIAN FISH PACKETS

PREP TIME: 15 MINUTES / TOTAL TIME: 25 MINUTES / **MAKES 4 SERVINGS**

4   **baby bok choy**

2   **carrots, cut into matchsticks**

1   **onion, cut into thin wedges**

2   **teaspoons low-sodium soy sauce, divided**

1   **teaspoon rice wine vinegar, divided**

2   **teaspoons freshly grated ginger, divided**

4   **wild cod fillets (6 ounces each)**

1 Preheat the oven to 450°F. Cut 4 sheets of parchment, each 20" x 12". Coat 1 side of each with cooking spray.

2 Divide the bok choy, carrots, and onion among 1 side of each the sheets of parchment. Drizzle each with ½ teaspoon soy sauce, ¼ teaspoon vinegar, and ½ teaspoon ginger. Add 1 fillet to each.

3 Fold the other half of each sheet over the filling and fold the edges all the way around to make a tight seal. Place the packets on a large baking sheet. Bake until the packets are puffed, 10 minutes.

4 Transfer each packet to a serving plate. Carefully slit the top of each to allow the steam to escape. After 1 minute, peel back the paper.

NUTRITION (PER SERVING): 205 calories, 34 g protein, 11 g carbohydrates, 4 g fiber, 5 g sugars, 2 g fat, 1 g saturated fat, 297 mg sodium

TUNA TETRAZZINI

PREP TIME: 15 MINUTES / TOTAL TIME: 1 HOUR / MAKES 4 SERVINGS

Shown in photo insert pages.

8   ounces multigrain spaghetti

4   cups broccoli florets

¼   pound mushrooms, sliced

I   onion, chopped

¼   cup water

I   jar (2 ounces) diced pimientos, drained

1½   teaspoons Italian seasoning

¼   cup whole grain pastry flour

2½   cups I% milk

¼   cup grated Parmesan cheese

2   cans (5 ounces each) light tuna packed in water, drained

1 Preheat the oven to 350°F. Coat an 8" x 8" baking dish with cooking spray.

2 Prepare the pasta according to package directions.

3 Meanwhile, in a large saucepan coated with cooking spray over medium-high heat, cook the broccoli, mushrooms, onion, and water, stirring occasionally, until the broccoli is tender-crisp, 5 minutes. Stir in the pimientos and Italian seasoning. Place in a large bowl.

4 In the same saucepan, add the flour. Gradually add the milk, whisking constantly, until smooth. Cook over medium heat, whisking constantly, until slightly thickened and bubbling, 6 minutes. Remove from the heat. Stir in the cheese, tuna, the reserved broccoli mixture, and the spaghetti. Toss to mix. Place in the prepared baking dish.

5 Cover with foil and bake for 30 minutes, removing the foil during the last 10 minutes of baking. Let stand for 5 minutes before serving.

HEALTHY HINT

A couple of smaller brands, such as Wild Planet and Safe Catch, are leading the charge in canning low-mercury, high-omega-3 products. Wild Planet purposefully selects smaller, younger tuna that have had less time to accumulate mercury, while Safe Catch actually tests each and every fish to make sure its mercury levels are safe. Bonus: Both brands use a "once-cooked" method that preserves the maximum amount of omega-3s, fatty acids that may actually help counteract mercury's damaging effects.

NUTRITION (PER SERVING): 276 calories, 22 g protein, 41 g carbohydrates, 6 g fiber, 9 g sugars, 5 g fat, 2 g saturated fat, 260 mg sodium

SWEET AND SOUR SHRIMP

PREP TIME: 5 MINUTES / TOTAL TIME: 10 MINUTES / MAKES 2 SERVINGS

2   teaspoons canola oil

2   cups (half of a 16-ounce package) frozen bell
    pepper strips

¼   cup apricot all-fruit jam

2   teaspoons red wine vinegar

6   ounces cooked, peeled, and deveined shrimp

4   cups steamed broccoli

1 In a large nonstick skillet over medium-high heat, heat the oil. Cook the peppers, stirring, until lightly browned, 3 minutes.

2 Stir in the jam, vinegar, and shrimp. Cook until bubbly, 2 minutes. Serve with the broccoli.

NUTRITION (PER SERVING): 272 calories, 24 g protein, 30 g carbohydrates, 3 g fiber, 16 g sugars, 6 g fat, 0 g saturated fat, 272 mg sodium

SHRIMP SCAMPI FETTUCCINE

PREP TIME: 10 MINUTES / TOTAL TIME: 20 MINUTES / MAKES 4 SERVINGS

Shown in photo insert pages.

I   package (8 ounces) shirataki fettuccine

2   tablespoons canola oil

I   pound medium shrimp, peeled and deveined

4   cloves garlic, minced

½   teaspoon red-pepper flakes

I   pint cherry tomatoes, halved

½   cup dry white wine

2   tablespoons fresh lemon juice

4   cups baby spinach

I   can (15 ounces) lentils, rinsed and drained

1 Prepare the fettuccine according to package directions.

2 Meanwhile, in a large skillet over medium heat, heat the oil. Cook the shrimp, garlic, and red-pepper flakes, stirring, until the shrimp start to turn pink, 2 minutes.

3 Add the tomatoes, wine, and lemon juice. Cook until the tomatoes start to soften, 2 minutes. Add the spinach and lentils and cook, stirring, until the spinach wilts, 1 minute. Stir in the fettuccine and toss to coat well. Divide among 4 plates.

NUTRITION (PER SERVING): 232 calories, 17 g protein, 18 g carbohydrates, 7 g fiber, 4 g sugars, 8 g fat, 1 g saturated fat, 607 mg sodium

BLACK BEAN AND MUSHROOM BURGERS

PREP TIME: 10 MINUTES / TOTAL TIME: 25 MINUTES / **MAKES 2 SERVINGS**

8   ounces mushrooms, minced

2   scallions, minced

½   cup cilantro leaves, minced

1   can (15 ounces) black beans, rinsed and drained

½   cup dry bread crumbs

     Pinch of salt

1 Position a rack 6" from the heating element, and preheat the broiler. Line a baking sheet with parchment paper.

2 In a medium bowl, combine the mushrooms, scallions, cilantro, and half of the black beans, mashing to combine. Add the bread crumbs, salt, and the remaining beans. Shape into 4 burgers.

3 Arrange the burgers a few inches apart on the prepared baking sheet. Broil, turning once, until browned and crisp, 15 minutes.

NUTRITION (PER SERVING): 274 calories, 17 g protein, 52 g carbohydrates, 12 g fiber, 6 g sugars, 3 g fat, 0 g saturated fat, 391 mg sodium

HEALTHY HINT

Instantly boost the nutrition and flavor profile of your best veggie burger by topping it with slices of avocado or a dollop of guacamole. Not only does avocado in all its forms add a delicious richness, but the healthy monounsaturated fats in this fruit (yep, it's technically a large berry) actually help you absorb more nutrients from your vegetables.

SWEET POTATO LENTIL BURGERS

PREP TIME: 10 MINUTES / TOTAL TIME: 50 MINUTES / MAKES 2 SERVINGS

½   cup red lentils

1   cup low-sodium vegetable broth

1   medium sweet potato, skin on, diced

1   tablespoon smoked paprika

1   teaspoon ground cumin

2   tablespoons minced onion

⅓   cup whole wheat panko bread crumbs

2   roasted red peppers, diced

    Pinch of salt

1   tablespoon extra-virgin olive oil

1 In a small saucepan over medium heat, cook the lentils and broth, covered, until softened but still firm, 10 minutes.

2 In a covered microwaveable bowl, microwave the sweet potato on high until soft enough to mash easily, 6 to 7 minutes.

3 Position a rack in the top third of the oven and preheat the broiler. Line a baking sheet with parchment or foil.

4 In a medium bowl, combine the lentils, sweet potato, paprika, cumin, and onion. Mash with a potato masher or fork until the mixture becomes sticky. Fold in the bread crumbs and roasted peppers. Form into 4 burgers.

5 Arrange the burgers on the prepared baking sheet and sprinkle with the salt and oil. Broil, turning once, until golden brown and crisp, 10 minutes.

NUTRITION (PER SERVING): 373 calories, 17 g protein, 57 g carbohydrates, 12 g fiber, 6 g sugars, 9 g fat, 1 g saturated fat, 463 mg sodium

STUFFED PORTOBELLO MUSHROOMS

PREP TIME: 20 MINUTES / TOTAL TIME: 2 HOURS 15 MINUTES / **MAKES 2 SERVINGS**

I   tablespoon grapeseed oil or unsalted butter

I   large onion, chopped

½   teaspoon balsamic vinegar

1¼   cups vegetable broth

½   cup semi-pearled farro

I   egg, lightly beaten

3   tablespoons low-fat plain yogurt

   Pinch of salt

   Pinch of black pepper

2   portobello mushroom caps, stemmed

½   cup crumbled feta cheese (2 ounces)

1   In a cast-iron skillet over low heat, heat the oil or butter. Cook the onion, stirring occasionally, until caramelized, about 45 minutes. Stir in the vinegar.

2   Meanwhile, in a medium saucepan, bring the broth and farro to a boil. Reduce the heat to medium-low, cover, and simmer until the farro is tender, about 30 minutes. Transfer to a medium bowl and set aside.

3   Preheat the oven to 350°F. Line a baking sheet with foil and lightly oil.

4   Stir the egg, yogurt, salt, pepper, and onions into the bowl of farro.

5   Set the mushroom caps on the prepared baking sheet and scoop the farro stuffing into each of the mushroom caps. Bake until the stuffing is set, 35 minutes.

6   Sprinkle with the cheese before serving.

NUTRITION (PER SERVING): 400 calories, 20 g protein, 52 g carbohydrates, 7 g fiber, 10 g sugars, 13 g fat, 7 g saturated fat, 694 mg sodium

HEALTHY HINT

Whole-milk yogurt may be healthier for you than fat-free and low-fat varieties. A recent study links the consumption of full-fat yogurt (but not low-fat) to a reduced risk of diabetes, while another study finds that low-fat dairy wasn't any better at helping people lose weight than whole-fat dairy is. In fact, people eating the low-fat stuff were more likely to eat more carbs to make up for the difference in calories.

VEGETARIAN CHILI

PREP TIME: 30 MINUTES / TOTAL TIME: 2 HOURS 40 MINUTES / **MAKES 4 SERVINGS**

Shown in photo insert pages.

I   cup dried beans (a mixture of black, kidney, white, and pinto)

I   tablespoon olive oil

½   medium yellow onion, chopped

I   large bell pepper, chopped

I   clove garlic, minced

½   cup dark beer or vegetable broth

I   cup canned fire-roasted diced tomatoes

½   teaspoon ground cumin

½   teaspoon salt

2½   cups vegetable broth

½   cup quinoa, rinsed and drained

I   cup water

     Chopped cilantro (optional)

1 In a medium saucepan, combine the beans with enough water to cover by 1" or 2". Bring to a boil, and boil for 10 minutes. Turn off the heat, cover, and let soak for 1 hour. Drain.

2 In a large saucepan over medium heat, warm the oil. Cook the onion, bell pepper, and garlic until browned, 5 minutes. Stir in the beer or broth and simmer until the liquid is evaporated.

3 Stir in the tomatoes, cumin, salt, broth, and soaked beans. Bring to a boil. Reduce to a simmer, cover, and cook until the beans are tender, about 1 hour. Add more water if the mixture looks dry.

4 Add the quinoa and water and cook until heated through, 15 minutes. Serve garnished with the cilantro, if using.

NUTRITION (PER SERVING): 320 calories, 14 g protein, 51 g carbohydrates, 14 g fiber, 6 g sugars, 5 g fat, 1 g saturated fat, 481 mg sodium

WHAT IS MINDFUL EATING?

There's been a lot of buzz about mindful eating—that whole, "it's not all about what you eat, but how you eat it" mentality that emphasizes slowing down and enjoying your meal. The perks: It may actually help you eat less and achieve your optimal weight. But what exactly does it consist of? There are many helpful tips from the brightness of the lights and using a specific plate color, but essentially, it's all about slowing down to smell the pasta sauce. Head back to page 56 for more practical steps to being mindful at mealtime.

PASTA WITH SUMMER VEGETABLES

PREP TIME: 15 MINUTES / TOTAL TIME: 35 MINUTES / **MAKES 4 SERVINGS**

8   ounces whole grain shell pasta

I   tablespoon olive oil

I   small red onion, thinly sliced

2   cloves garlic, sliced

I   medium zucchini, cut into I" chunks

I   yellow squash, cut into I" chunks

I   cup cherry tomatoes, halved

I   cup small fresh mozzarella balls (ciliegini), halved

¼   cup chopped fresh basil or 8 teaspoons dried

1   Prepare the pasta according to package directions.

2   Meanwhile, in a large nonstick skillet over medium-high heat, heat the oil. Cook the onion and garlic, stirring, until softened, 2 minutes. Stir in the zucchini and squash. Cook, stirring, until the vegetables are tender-crisp, 8 minutes. Stir in the tomatoes and cook just until the tomatoes begin to burst, 3 minutes.

3   Stir in the pasta and mozzarella. Cook, stirring, until the pasta is hot and the mozzarella just begins to melt, 2 minutes. Remove the skillet from the heat and stir in the basil.

NUTRITION (PER SERVING): 351 calories, 31 g protein, 50 g carbohydrates, 8 g fiber, 6 g sugars, 5 g fat, 1 g saturated fat, 425 mg sodium

ROASTED VEGETABLE MAC AND CHEESE

PREP TIME: 20 MINUTES / TOTAL TIME: 1 HOUR 15 MINUTES / **MAKES 6 SERVINGS**

Shown in photo insert pages.

I   head cauliflower, cut into large florets

I   large onion, cut into wedges

I   yellow or red bell pepper, cut into eighths

2   teaspoons canola oil

8   ounces whole grain elbow pasta

2   cups 1% milk

2   tablespoons whole wheat flour

½   teaspoon dried mustard

¼   teaspoon salt

1½   cups shredded reduced-fat sharp Cheddar cheese

2   tablespoons grated Romano cheese

1   Preheat the oven to 350°F. Coat an 11" x 7" baking dish with cooking spray.

2   On a rimmed baking sheet, toss the cauliflower, onion, and bell pepper with the oil. Roast, stirring once, until the cauliflower is golden brown, 30 minutes. Remove from the oven to a cutting board, and chop the roasted vegetables coarsely. Place in the prepared baking dish.

3   Meanwhile, prepare the pasta according to package directions. Place in the dish with the roasted vegetables.

4   In a medium saucepan, whisk together the milk, flour, mustard, and salt. Cook, whisking constantly, until the mixture begins to thicken, 4 minutes. Stir in the cheeses and cook until melted, 2 minutes. Pour over the pasta and vegetables, tossing to coat. Bake until bubbling, 20 minutes.

NUTRITION (PER SERVING): 311 calories, 19 g protein, 42 g carbohydrates, 6 g fiber, 10 g sugars, 10 g fat, 5 g saturated fat, 372 mg sodium

VEGETABLE LO MEIN

PREP TIME: 15 MINUTES / TOTAL TIME: 20 MINUTES / **MAKES 4 SERVINGS**

8   ounces whole wheat spaghetti

½   cup low-sodium vegetable broth

2   cloves garlic, minced

3   tablespoons low-sodium soy sauce

2   tablespoons rice wine vinegar

2   teaspoons cornstarch

1   teaspoon toasted sesame oil

1   tablespoon canola oil

1   red onion, thinly sliced

3   baby bok choy, thinly sliced

2   carrots, thinly sliced

4   ounces snow peas, sliced lengthwise

1 Prepare the pasta according to package directions. In a small bowl, whisk together the broth, garlic, soy sauce, vinegar, cornstarch, and sesame oil.

2 Meanwhile, in a large skillet over medium-high heat, heat the canola oil. Cook the onion, bok choy, and carrots until tender-crisp, 3 minutes. Add the broth mixture and peas. Cook, stirring constantly, until the sauce is thickened, 3 minutes. Add the pasta and toss to combine.

NUTRITION (PER SERVING): 293 calories, 11 g protein, 50 g carbohydrates, 11 g fiber, 5 g sugars, 6 g fat, 1 g saturated fat, 458 mg sodium

BEAN ENCHILADAS

PREP TIME: 15 MINUTES / TOTAL TIME: 1 HOUR 5 MINUTES / **MAKES 4 SERVINGS**

2   teaspoons canola oil

1   onion, chopped

2   cloves garlic, minced

½   teaspoon ground cumin

3   cups chopped fresh kale

1   can (15 ounces) black beans, rinsed and drained

2   tablespoons ground flaxseeds

1   can (15 ounces) diced tomatoes, drained

½   cup loosely packed chopped cilantro

8   corn tortillas (6" diameter)

4   slices reduced-sodium pepper Jack cheese, halved

½   avocado, thinly sliced into 8 pieces

1 Preheat the oven to 350°F. Coat a 13" x 9" baking dish with cooking spray.

2 In a large nonstick skillet over medium heat, heat the oil. Cook the onion, garlic, and cumin, stirring occasionally, until the onion has softened, 3 minutes. Add the kale and cook, stirring, until wilted, 5 minutes. Stir in the beans and flaxseeds. Cook until heated through, 5 minutes. Mash some of the beans with the back of a spoon to thicken the mixture.

3 In a medium bowl, combine the tomatoes and cilantro. Set aside.

4 Wrap the tortillas in paper towels and microwave until softened, 1 minute. Remove to a work surface. Evenly divide the bean mixture down the center of each tortilla. Roll each into a tube. Place seam sides down in the prepared baking dish. Spoon the tomato mixture over the enchiladas. Cover tightly with foil.

5 Bake for 20 minutes. Carefully remove the foil and place 1 piece of the cheese on each enchilada. Bake until the cheese melts, 10 minutes. Let stand 5 minutes before serving with the avocado.

NUTRITION (PER SERVING): 419 calories, 17 g protein, 48 g carbohydrates, 10 g fiber, 5 g sugars, 19 g fat, 6 g saturated fat, 220 mg sodium

WHEAT-FREE PIZZA

PREP TIME: 20 MINUTES / TOTAL TIME: 45 MINUTES / **MAKES 2 SERVINGS**

Shown in photo insert pages.

3 teaspoons olive oil, divided

3 cups chopped cauliflower (1 medium to large head)

1 egg, beaten

½ cup grated Parmesan cheese

3 tablespoons soft goat cheese

½ teaspoon dried oregano

1 cup sliced cremini mushrooms

¼ cup low-sugar pizza sauce

½ cup fresh mozzarella cheese, cut into thin slices

¼ cup fresh basil leaves

1 Preheat the oven to 400°F and place a baking sheet in the oven to heat. Cut a piece of parchment paper to fit the baking sheet, and coat with 1 teaspoon of the oil. Set the parchment paper aside.

2 In a food processor or blender, pulse the cauliflower until the size of seeds.

3 In a loosely covered microwaveable dish, microwave the cauliflower until lightly steamed, about 4 minutes. Drain in a fine-mesh sieve. Press with the back of a wooden spoon to remove all excess moisture. Transfer to a large bowl and stir in the egg, Parmesan, goat cheese, and oregano.

4 Divide the mixture in half and form two compact balls. Place on the parchment paper and press into 2 circles, each 6" in diameter and ¼" thick. Move the parchment to the preheated baking sheet. Bake until the crusts begin to turn golden, 10 minutes, then flip and bake until lightly golden and firm, 7 minutes.

5 In a medium skillet over medium-high heat, heat the remaining 2 teaspoons oil. Cook the mushrooms until tender, about 5 minutes.

6 Evenly divide the tomato sauce, mozzarella, basil, and mushrooms over the crusts. Bake until the cheese melts, 5 to 10 minutes.

NUTRITION (PER SERVING): 357 calories, 22 g protein, 14 g carbohydrates, 5 g fiber, 6 g sugars, 25 g fat, 11 g saturated fat, 576 mg sodium

VEGETABLE PIZZA

PREP TIME: 20 MINUTES / TOTAL TIME: 1 HOUR 20 MINUTES / MAKES 8 SERVINGS

⅔ cup warm water (105°–115°F)

1 envelope (¼ ounce or 2¼ teaspoons) active dry yeast

2 teaspoons + 1 tablespoon olive oil, divided

2 cups whole wheat pastry or white whole wheat flour, divided

¼ teaspoon salt

1½ cups frozen mixed bell peppers, thawed

1 package (10 ounces) frozen chopped spinach, thawed and well drained

1 clove garlic, minced

1 can (14.5 ounces) diced tomatoes, well drained

4 ounces fresh mozzarella cheese, shredded

NUTRITION (PER SERVING): 196 calories, 8 g protein, 26 g carbohydrates, 5 g fiber, 2 g sugars, 7 g fat, 2 g saturated fat, 192 mg sodium

1 Coat a large bowl with cooking spray. Set aside.

2 In a glass measuring cup, stir together the water and yeast until the yeast dissolves. Stir in 2 teaspoons of the oil.

3 In a food processor, pulse 1¾ cups of the flour and the salt to combine. With the machine running, add the yeast mixture through the feed tube. Process until the mixture forms a moist ball, 2 minutes. Lightly flour a work surface with some of the remaining ¼ cup flour and transfer the dough to the surface. Knead until the dough is smooth, 1 minute. Place the dough in the prepared bowl. Coat lightly with cooking spray, and cover with plastic wrap. Place in a warm place to rise until doubled in size, about 30 minutes.

4 Coat a 14" round pizza pan with cooking spray. Punch down the dough. Lightly flour a work surface with some of the remaining flour and transfer the dough to the surface. Let stand for 5 minutes. With floured hands or a rolling pin, pat or roll into a 14" circle. Transfer to the prepared pan. Pinch the edges to make a border. Cover with plastic wrap and let stand for 15 minutes. Preheat the oven to 375°F.

5 In a large skillet over medium-high heat, warm the remaining 1 tablespoon oil. Cook the peppers until lightly browned, 3 minutes. Stir in the spinach and garlic and cook, stirring, for 3 minutes. Add the tomatoes and cook, stirring, until the liquid evaporates, 3 minutes.

6 Spread the tomato mixture over the crust. Sprinkle with the cheese. Bake until golden and bubbly, 15 minutes. Cut into 8 slices.

SIDE DISHES

ROASTED BROCCOLI WITH A KICK

PREP TIME: 10 MINUTES / TOTAL TIME: 30 MINUTES / MAKES 4 SERVINGS

I   head broccoli (12 ounces), chopped into bite-size florets and spears, stalks peeled

I   tablespoon olive oil

¼   teaspoon crushed red-pepper flakes

¼   teaspoon salt

I   teaspoon lemon zest

Lemon wedges, to serve (optional)

1   Preheat the oven to 425°F.

2   On a baking sheet with sides, toss the broccoli, oil, red-pepper flakes, and salt. Roast until browned, 20 minutes. Remove from the oven and toss with the lemon zest before serving with lemon wedges, if desired.

NUTRITION (PER SERVING): 59 calories, 2 g protein, 6 g carbohydrates, 2 g fiber, 1 g sugars, 4 g fat, 1 g saturated fat, 127 mg sodium

GREEN BEAN CASSEROLE

PREP TIME: 15 MINUTES / TOTAL TIME: 1 HOUR 5 MINUTES / **MAKES 8 SERVINGS**

½ cup buttermilk

½ cup whole wheat panko bread crumbs

I medium onion, cut crosswise into ¼"-thick slices and separated into rings

½ pound mushrooms, sliced

I small onion, chopped

½ teaspoon dried thyme

¼ teaspoon salt

¼ cup whole wheat pastry flour

3 cups I% milk

I bag (16 ounces) frozen French-cut green beans, thawed and drained

¼ cup slivered almonds

1 Preheat the oven to 500°F. Coat a baking sheet with cooking spray. Coat a medium baking dish with cooking spray.

2 In a shallow bowl, place the buttermilk. In a shallow dish or pie plate, place the bread crumbs. Dip the onion rings into the buttermilk, coat with the bread crumbs, and place on the prepared baking sheet. Coat lightly with cooking spray. Bake until tender and golden brown, 20 minutes.

3 Meanwhile, heat a large saucepan coated with cooking spray over medium heat. Add the mushrooms, chopped onion, thyme, and salt. Coat with cooking spray. Cook, stirring occasionally, until the mushrooms are browned and begin to release liquid, about 5 minutes. Sprinkle with the flour. Cook, stirring, for 1 minute. Add the milk. Cook, stirring constantly, until thickened, 4 minutes. Stir in the green beans and almonds.

4 Reduce the oven temperature to 400°F. Pour the bean mixture into the prepared baking dish. Scatter the onion rings over the top. Bake until hot and bubbly, 30 minutes.

NUTRITION (PER SERVING): 122 calories, 7 g protein, 19 g carbohydrates, 3 g fiber, 9 g sugars, 3 g fat, 1 g saturated fat, 139 mg sodium

CREAMED SPINACH AND ARTICHOKES

PREP TIME: 10 MINUTES / TOTAL TIME: 20 MINUTES / MAKES 4 SERVINGS

1 tablespoon olive oil

1 onion, chopped

1 clove garlic, minced

¼ cup vegetable broth

1 pound baby spinach

1 box (9 ounces) frozen artichokes, thawed and chopped

3 ounces reduced-fat cream cheese, cubed

⅛ teaspoon ground nutmeg

1 In a large nonstick skillet over medium-high heat, heat the oil. Cook the onion and garlic, stirring occasionally, until softened, 5 minutes. Add the broth and bring to a simmer. Add the spinach and cook, tossing frequently, just until wilted, 4 minutes.

2 Stir in the artichokes, cream cheese, and nutmeg. Cook, stirring, until the cream cheese melts and is hot, 1 minute.

NUTRITION (PER SERVING): 176 calories, 7 g protein, 21 g carbohydrates, 10 g fiber, 3 g sugars, 9 g fat, 3 g saturated fat, 323 mg sodium

HONEY-GLAZED RADISHES

PREP TIME: 10 MINUTES / TOTAL TIME: 30 MINUTES / **MAKES 2 SERVINGS**

¼ cup water

1 tablespoon honey

1 teaspoon grapeseed oil

1 bunch radishes (about ½ pound), quartered, with greens reserved

½ teaspoon caraway seeds

Pinch of salt

⅛ teaspoon black pepper

½ teaspoon champagne vinegar or white wine vinegar

1 In a medium skillet over low heat, heat the water, honey, and oil. When the honey has melted, add the radishes and stir to coat. Raise the heat to medium-low, cover, and cook, stirring often, until the radishes are tender-crisp, 20 minutes.

2 Stir in the reserved radish greens, caraway seeds, salt, and pepper. Cook, stirring constantly, until the greens have wilted, 3 minutes. Stir in the vinegar.

NUTRITION (PER SERVING): 78 calories, 2 g protein, 14 g carbohydrates, 3 g fiber, 11 g sugars, 3 g fat, 0 g saturated fat, 107 mg sodium

HEALTHY HINT

Dietary cholesterol found in butter, beef, and other animal-based foods isn't as bad for heart health as we have been told for decades. After reviewing piles of research, the group that advises the US government on dietary guidelines recently reported that it's "not a nutrient of concern for overconsumption," meaning that on its own the cholesterol you eat isn't likely to raise your heart disease risk. Excess sugars and trans fats seem to be bigger culprits in heart disease.

LOADED REFRIED BEANS

PREP TIME: 5 MINUTES / TOTAL TIME: 20 MINUTES / **MAKES 3 SERVINGS**

2 tablespoons olive oil

½ yellow onion, chopped

2 cloves garlic, minced

2 large tomatoes, chopped

3 cups cooked pinto beans

1 cup reduced-sodium vegetable broth, divided

1 In a medium skillet over medium heat, heat the oil. Cook the onion until soft, 5 minutes.

2 Add the garlic and tomatoes and cook until most of the water from the tomatoes evaporates, about 8 minutes.

3 Meanwhile, in a blender or food processor, combine the beans and ½ cup of the broth. Pulse until most of the beans are smooth, adding additional broth if needed to achieve the right consistency.

4 Stir the beans into the skillet with the tomatoes and cook, stirring, until thickened and heated through, 3 minutes.

NUTRITION (PER SERVING): 181 calories, 8 g protein, 26 g carbohydrates, 9 g fiber, 2 g sugars, 5 g fat, 1 g saturated fat, 27 mg sodium

HEALTHY HINT

Beans aren't just for savory meals. Instantly up the health cred of your favorite boxed brownie mix or homemade recipe by substituting pureed black beans for the oil and eggs. Use one 15-ounce can of undrained black beans, pureed, in place of 1 egg plus ⅓ to ½ cup oil. The result will be perfectly fudgy brownies (that don't taste like beans) with far fewer calories and lots of plant-based protein and fiber.

HERB ROASTED SWEET POTATOES

PREP TIME: 10 MINUTES / TOTAL TIME: 30 MINUTES / **MAKES 2 SERVINGS**

2   large sweet potatoes, peeled and cut into
     ¾" cubes

1   tablespoon coconut oil, melted

1   tablespoon chopped fresh rosemary, thyme,
     or sage

1   clove garlic, minced

¼   teaspoon salt

¼   teaspoon black pepper

1 Preheat the oven to 425°F. Coat a large rimmed baking sheet with cooking spray.

2 On the baking sheet, toss the sweet potatoes, oil, rosemary (thyme or sage), garlic, salt, and pepper. Roast, turning halfway through, until the sweet potatoes are browned and tender, about 20 minutes.

NUTRITION (PER SERVING): 112 calories, 2 g protein, 19 g carbohydrates, 3 g fiber, 6 g sugars, 3 g fat, 3 g saturated fat, 153 mg sodium

HEALTHY HINT

It may seem a bit counterintuitive, but a tiny pinch of salt can enhance the natural sweetness of many ingredients and dishes, allowing you to use less sweetener. The trick works especially well with fresh fruit, so before you add something to sweeten that smoothie, try a sprinkle of salt and taste it again. The natural sweetness will be more pronounced.

TWICE-BAKED SWEET POTATOES

PREP TIME: 15 MINUTES / TOTAL TIME: 55 MINUTES / MAKES 4 SERVINGS

Shown in photo insert pages.

4   medium sweet potatoes, pierced

2   tablespoons pure maple syrup

¼   cup unsweetened plain almond milk

1   teaspoon ground cinnamon

1   teaspoon ground ginger

½   teaspoon ground nutmeg

¼   teaspoon salt

¼   cup + 2 tablespoons chopped walnuts, divided

¼   cup + 2 tablespoons chopped pecans, divided

1 Preheat the oven to 400°F.

2 Microwave the sweet potatoes on high, turning once, until soft, about 6 minutes. Let cool.

3 Make a slice lengthwise across the top of each baked sweet potato. Carefully scoop out the flesh and add to a medium bowl. Place the shells on a baking sheet.

4 Add the maple syrup, milk, cinnamon, ginger, nutmeg, salt, ¼ cup of the walnuts, and ¼ cup of the pecans to the bowl. Using a potato masher, mash the ingredients until combined.

5 Evenly spoon the sweet potato mixture back into the empty sweet potato shells. Sprinkle with the remaining 2 tablespoons walnuts and 2 tablespoons pecans. Bake until heated through and flavors blend, 40 minutes.

NUTRITION (PER SERVING): 285 calories, 5 g protein, 36 g carbohydrates, 6 g fiber, 13 g sugars, 15 g fat, 1 g saturated fat, 182 mg sodium

GARLIC OVEN FRIES

PREP TIME: 10 MINUTES / TOTAL TIME: 40 MINUTES / **MAKES 4 SERVINGS**

1 pound russet (baking) potatoes, cut into 3½" x ½" sticks

3 carrots, quartered lengthwise and cut into sticks

2 tablespoons canola oil

¼ teaspoon garlic salt

¼ teaspoon black pepper

1 Preheat the oven to 450°F. Coat 2 large baking sheets with cooking spray.

2 In a large bowl, combine the potatoes, carrots, oil, garlic salt, and pepper, tossing to coat well. On the baking sheets, arrange the potatoes and carrots in a single layer. Bake, turning once, until golden and crisp, 30 minutes.

NUTRITION (PER SERVING): 221 calories, 4 g protein, 36 g carbohydrates, 5 g fiber, 6 g sugars, 7 g fat, 1 g saturated fat, 204 mg sodium

CREAMY MASHED POTATOES

PREP TIME: 10 MINUTES / TOTAL TIME: 30 MINUTES / **MAKES 6 SERVINGS**

1   pound russet (baking) potatoes, peeled and halved

1   small head cauliflower, cut into florets

¼   cup vegetable broth

2   tablespoons olive oil

½   cup plain 0% Greek yogurt

1 In a large saucepan over high heat, combine the potatoes and cauliflower and cover with water. Over high heat, bring to a boil. Reduce the heat to medium and simmer until the potatoes and cauliflower are tender, 20 minutes. Drain.

2 In a large bowl, combine the potatoes, cauliflower, broth, and oil. With an electric mixer on medium speed, beat until smooth and creamy. Add the yogurt and beat just until blended.

NUTRITION (PER SERVING): 198 calories, 8 g protein, 29 g carbohydrates, 5 g fiber, 5 g sugars, 7 g fat, 1 g saturated fat, 84 mg sodium

SCALLOPED RED POTATOES

PREP TIME: 20 MINUTES / TOTAL TIME: 1 HOUR 5 MINUTES / **MAKES 4 SERVINGS**

Shown in photo insert pages.

3 tablespoons whole wheat flour

2 tablespoons white chia seeds

¼ teaspoon ground nutmeg

6 medium red potatoes, scrubbed and cut into
   ½" slices, divided

6 scallions, chopped, divided

1 cup shredded 4-cheese Italian blend, divided

1 cup 1% milk

1 Preheat the oven to 400°F. Coat an 11" x 7" baking dish with cooking spray.

2 In a small bowl, stir together the flour, chia seeds, and nutmeg.

3 Arrange one-third of the potatoes in the prepared dish. Sprinkle with one-third of the flour mixture, one-third of the scallions, and one-third of the cheese. Repeat the layers two more times. Pour the milk over the top. Cover and bake for 25 minutes.

4 Uncover and bake until the potatoes are tender and browned, 20 minutes.

NUTRITION (PER SERVING): 255 calories, 12 g protein, 42 g carbohydrates, 6 g fiber, 5 g sugars, 5 g fat, 3 g saturated fat, 206 mg sodium

WHIPPED SWEET POTATO CASSEROLES

PREP TIME: 10 MINUTES / TOTAL TIME: 35 MINUTES / MAKES 6 SERVINGS

1½ pounds sweet potatoes, peeled and cut into ½" cubes

8 tablespoons walnuts, finely chopped, divided

2 tablespoons ground flaxseeds

2½ tablespoons canola oil, divided

¼ cup orange juice

2 tablespoons Greek yogurt

½ teaspoon pumpkin pie spice

⅛ teaspoon salt

1 Preheat the oven to 400°F. Coat six 4-ounce ramekins with cooking spray. Place on a baking sheet.

2 Place a steamer basket in a large pot with 2" of water. Bring to a boil over high heat. Add the sweet potatoes, cover, and reduce the heat to medium. Cook until very tender, 15 minutes.

3 Meanwhile, in a small bowl, combine 6 tablespoons of the walnuts, the flaxseeds, and 1½ tablespoons of the oil until blended. Divide the mixture among the ramekins and press with a fork to cover the bottoms of the ramekins.

4 In a medium bowl, combine the potatoes, orange juice, yogurt, pie spice, salt, and the remaining 1 tablespoon oil. With an electric mixer, beat the mixture until smooth. Divide among the ramekins. Sprinkle with the remaining 2 tablespoons walnuts.

5 Bake until golden brown, 10 minutes.

NUTRITION (PER SERVING): 222 calories, 4 g protein, 24 g carbohydrates, 5 g fiber, 8 g sugars, 13 g fat, 1 g saturated fat, 115 mg sodium

BUTTERNUT SQUASH WITH MILLET AND PISTACHIOS

PREP TIME: 20 MINUTES / TOTAL TIME: 1 HOUR 15 MINUTES / **MAKES 2 SERVINGS**

Shown in photo insert pages.

- 1 **pound butternut squash, peeled and cut into ½" cubes**
- 1 **red onion, cut into thin strips**
- 1 **tablespoon grapeseed oil**
- 1 **tablespoon finely chopped fresh rosemary**
- 1 **tablespoon finely chopped fresh sage**
- ¼ **teaspoon salt**
- ¼ **teaspoon black pepper**
- ½ **cup millet**
- 1¼ **cups low-sodium vegetable broth**
- ½ **cup finely chopped unsalted, dry-roasted pistachios**

1 Preheat the oven to 400°F.

2 On a large baking sheet with sides, combine the butternut squash and onion. Drizzle with the oil and sprinkle with the rosemary, sage, salt, and pepper. Toss to coat well. Arrange in a single layer. Roast until browned, turning once, for 45 minutes.

3 Meanwhile, in a medium saucepan over medium-low heat, cook the millet until golden brown and fragrant, 4 minutes. Carefully stir in the broth. Increase the heat to high, and bring to a boil. Reduce the heat to low, cover, and simmer until the broth is absorbed, 10 minutes. Remove from the heat and let stand for 10 minutes.

4 Place the millet in a large bowl and add the roasted squash mixture. Top with the pistachios.

NUTRITION (PER SERVING): 259 calories, 7 g protein, 34 g carbohydrates, 6 g fiber, 4 g sugars, 11 g fat, 1 g saturated fat, 234 mg sodium

BARLEY PILAF WITH ARTICHOKES AND KALE

PREP TIME: 15 MINUTES / TOTAL TIME: 1 HOUR 5 MINUTES / MAKES 6 SERVINGS

1	tablespoon olive oil
1	onion, chopped
1	carrot, chopped
1	rib celery, chopped
½	cup barley
1	clove garlic, minced
2½	cups reduced-sodium vegetable or chicken broth
½	cup water
¼	cup bulgur wheat
4	cups chopped kale
1	package (9 ounces) frozen artichoke hearts
½	teaspoon lemon zest

1 In a medium saucepan over medium-high heat, heat the oil. Cook the onion, carrot, and celery, stirring, until softened, 5 minutes. Add the barley and garlic and cook, stirring, until fragrant, 3 minutes.

2 Stir in the broth and water and bring to a boil over high heat. Reduce the heat to low, cover, and simmer for 25 minutes. Stir in the bulgur and kale and cook for 5 minutes. Stir in the artichokes and lemon zest and cook until the broth is absorbed and the barley is al dente, 10 minutes.

NUTRITION (PER SERVING): 162 calories, 6 g protein, 29 g carbohydrates, 8 g fiber, 3 g sugars, 4 g fat, 0 g saturated fat, 259 mg sodium

QUINOA PILAF

PREP TIME: 10 MINUTES / TOTAL TIME: 35 MINUTES / **MAKES 6 SERVINGS**

Shown in photo insert pages.

2   tablespoons olive oil

1   cup quinoa, rinsed and drained

4   scallions, chopped

1   clove garlic, minced

1½ cups water

1   cup vegetable broth

¼   teaspoon ground cardamom

½   cup pistachios, chopped

1 In a medium saucepan over medium-high heat, heat the oil. Cook the quinoa, scallions, and garlic, stirring, until the vegetables are softened, 3 minutes.

2 Add the water, broth, and cardamom, and bring to a boil. Reduce the heat to low, cover, and simmer until the quinoa is tender, 20 minutes. Remove from the heat and let stand, covered, 5 minutes. With a fork, fluff the quinoa. Stir in the pistachios.

NUTRITION (PER SERVING): 226 calories, 7 g protein, 24 g carbohydrates, 9 g fiber, 3 g sugars, 12 g fat, 1 g saturated fat, 88 mg sodium

SQUASH STUFFED WITH WILD RICE AND RAISINS

PREP TIME: 10 MINUTES / TOTAL TIME: 1 HOUR 10 MINUTES / **MAKES 4 SERVINGS**

1½ cups water

½ cup wild rice

¼ teaspoon salt

2 small dumpling or acorn squash

4 ounces mushrooms, finely diced

2 tablespoons golden raisins

½ cup shredded Gruyère cheese (2 ounces)

3 tablespoons roughly chopped walnuts

1 egg

1 In a small saucepan over high heat, combine the water, rice, and salt. Bring to a boil. Reduce the heat to low, cover, and simmer until the rice is tender, 45 to 50 minutes.

2 Preheat the oven to 350°F.

3 Cut each squash in half lengthwise, and scoop out the seeds with a spoon. Discard.

4 Place the squash halves on a baking sheet, cut sides up, and bake until just tender but still firm, about 30 minutes.

5 In a medium bowl, combine the warm rice, mushrooms, raisins, cheese, and walnuts. Stir in the egg to coat. Divide the stuffing among the squash halves.

6 Bake until the filling is heated through and the squash is fork-tender, 15 minutes.

NUTRITION (PER SERVING): 292 calories, 12 g protein, 43 g carbohydrates, 5 g fiber, 9 g sugars, 10 g fat, 4 g saturated fat, 174 mg sodium

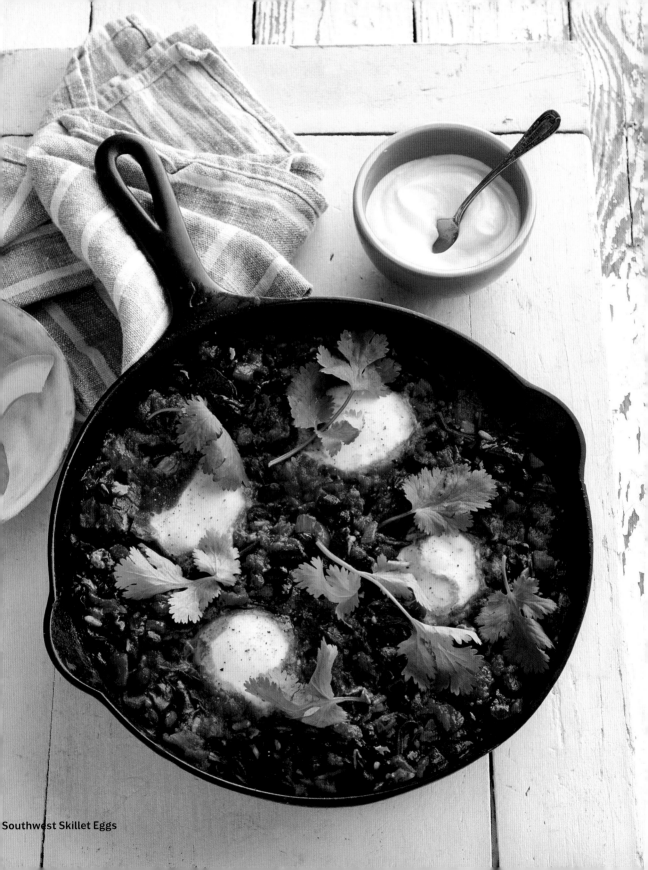

Southwest Skillet Eggs

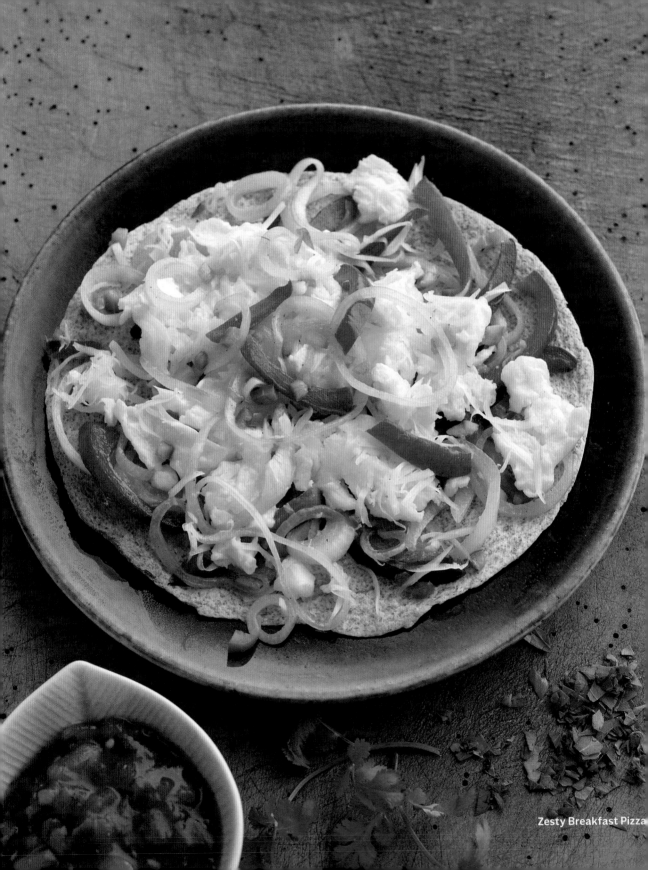

Zesty Breakfast Pizza

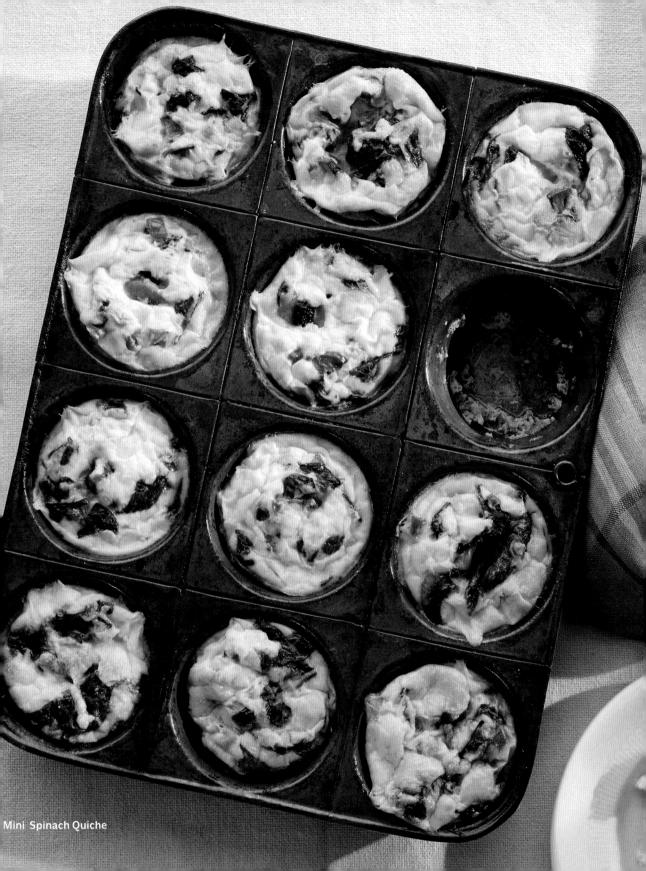
Mini Spinach Quiche

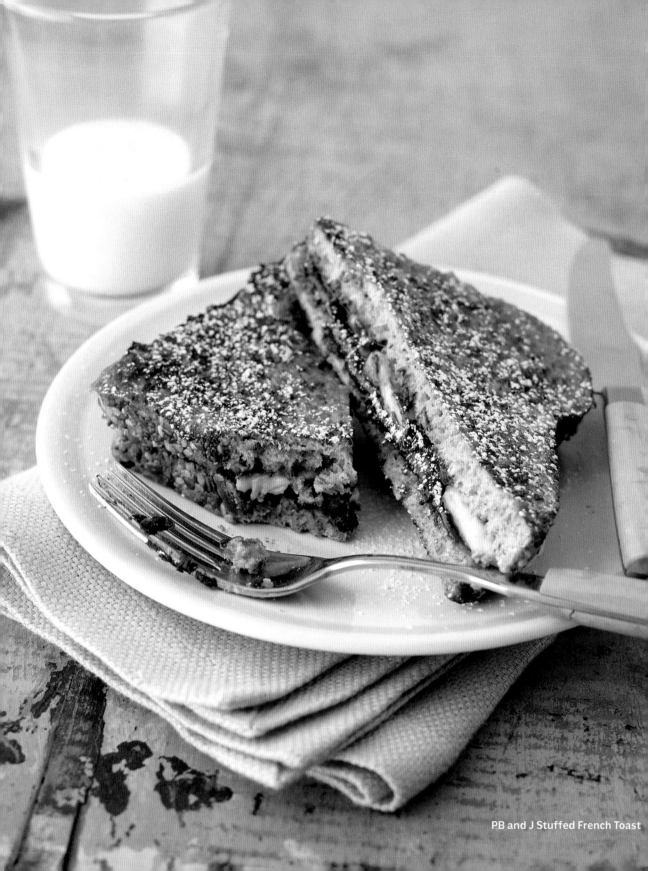

PB and J Stuffed French Toast

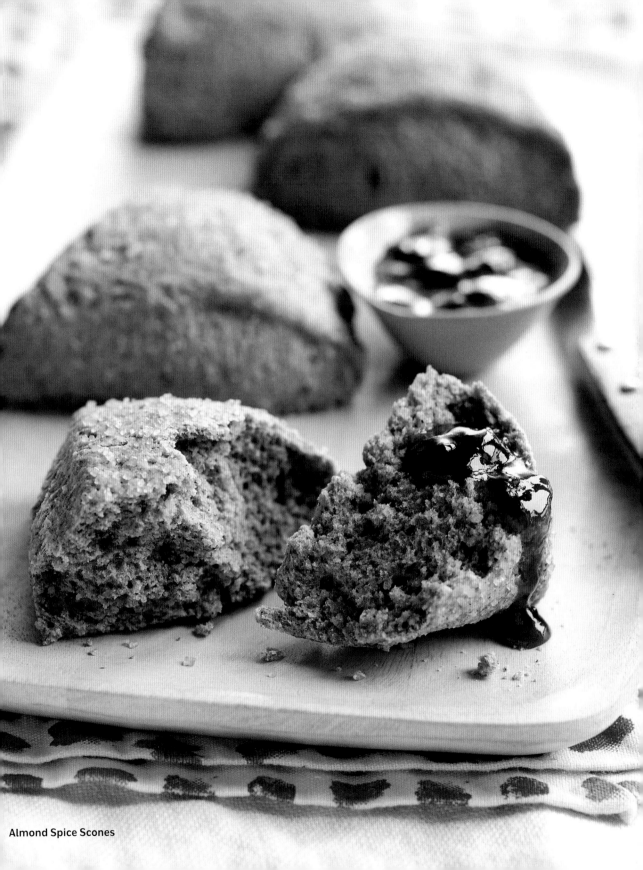

Almond Spice Scones

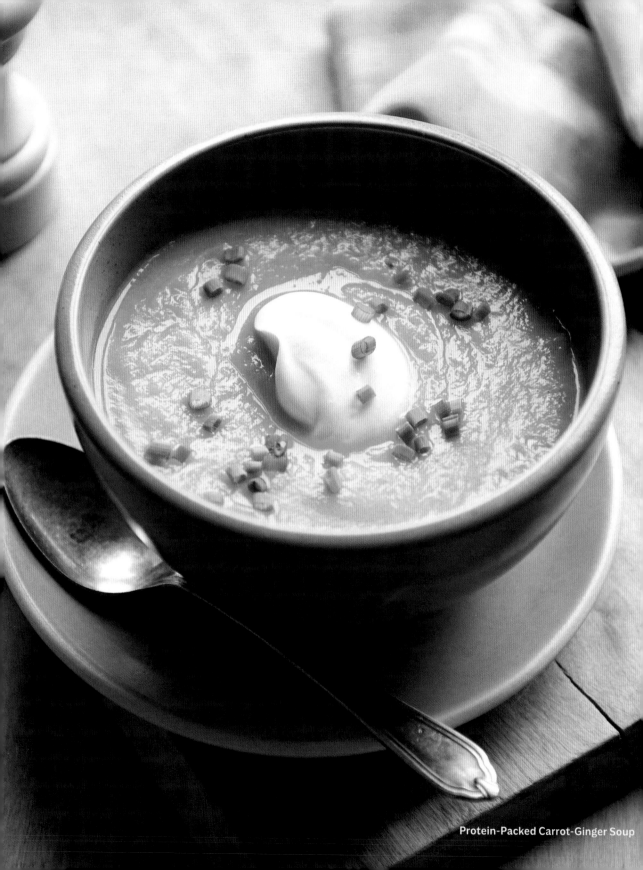

Protein-Packed Carrot-Ginger Soup

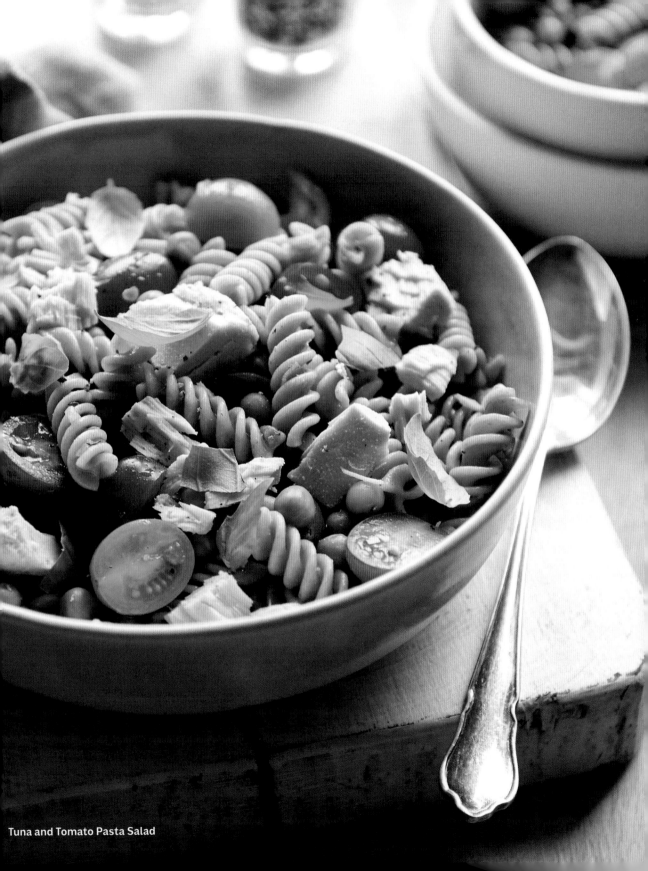

Tuna and Tomato Pasta Salad

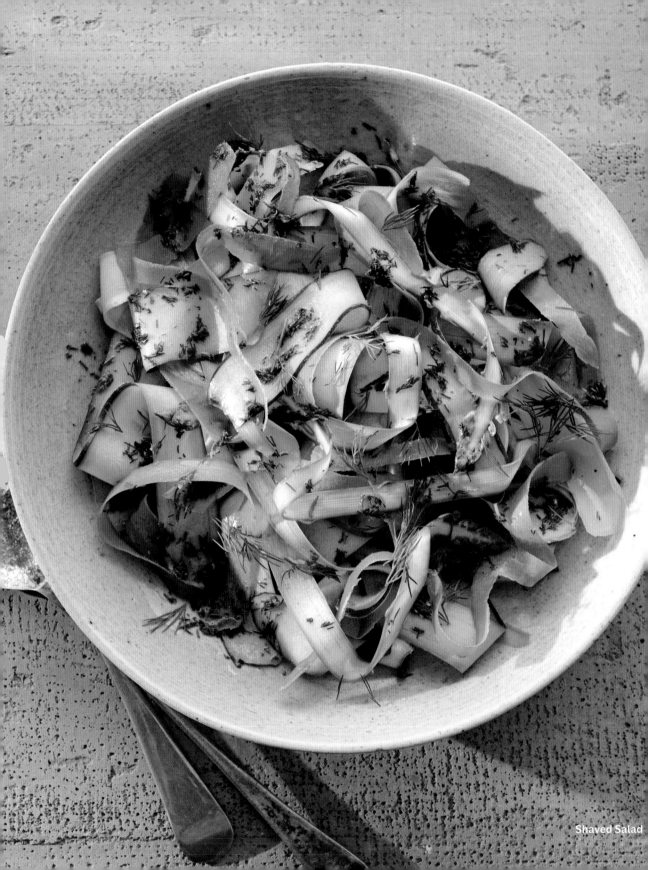

Shaved Salad

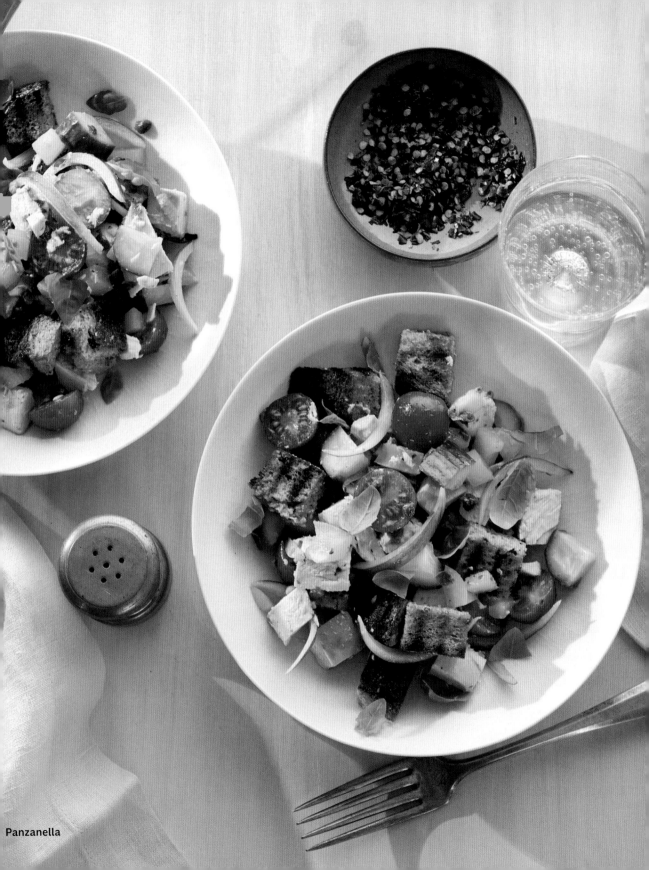

Panzanella

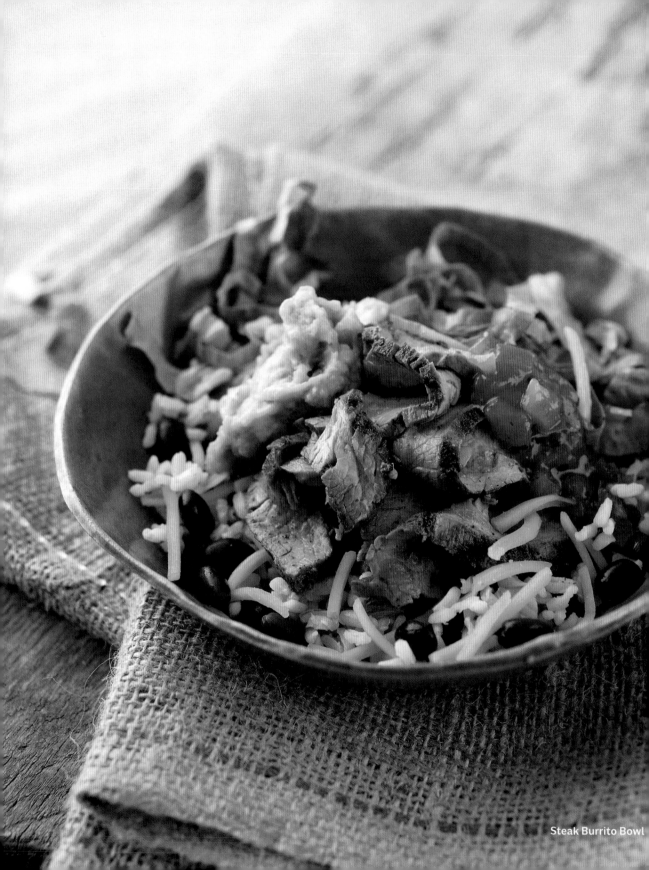

Steak Burrito Bowl

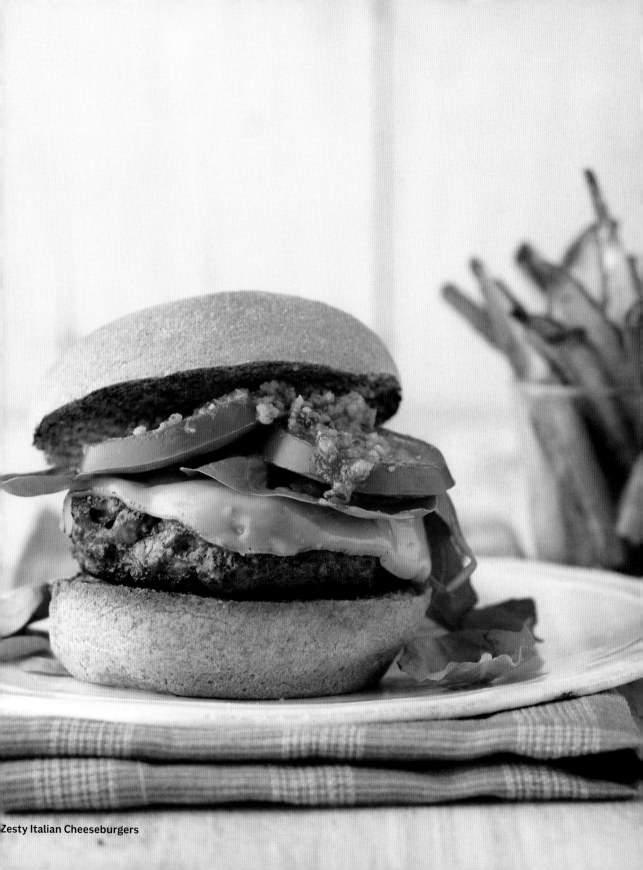

Zesty Italian Cheeseburgers

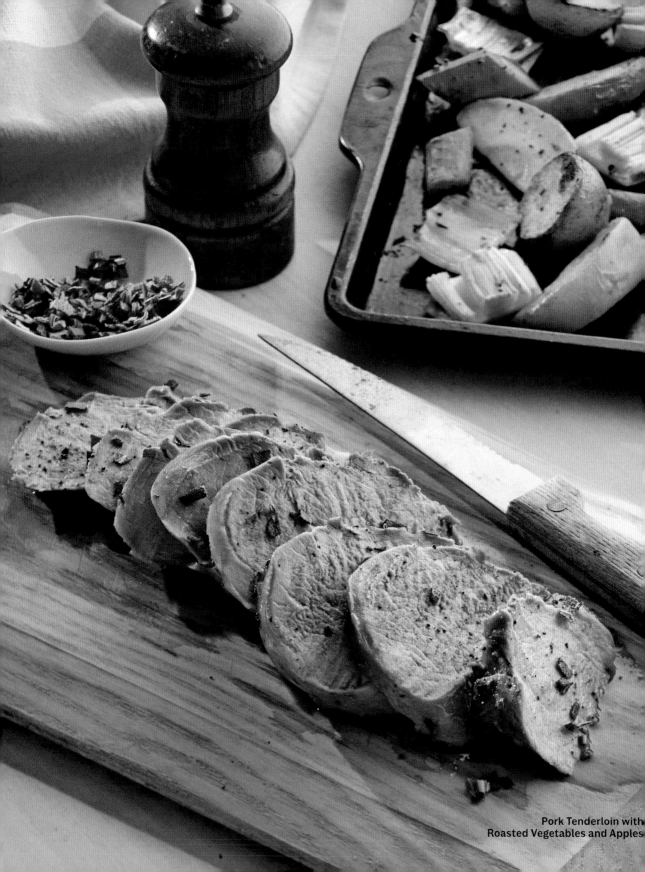

**Pork Tenderloin with
Roasted Vegetables and Apples**

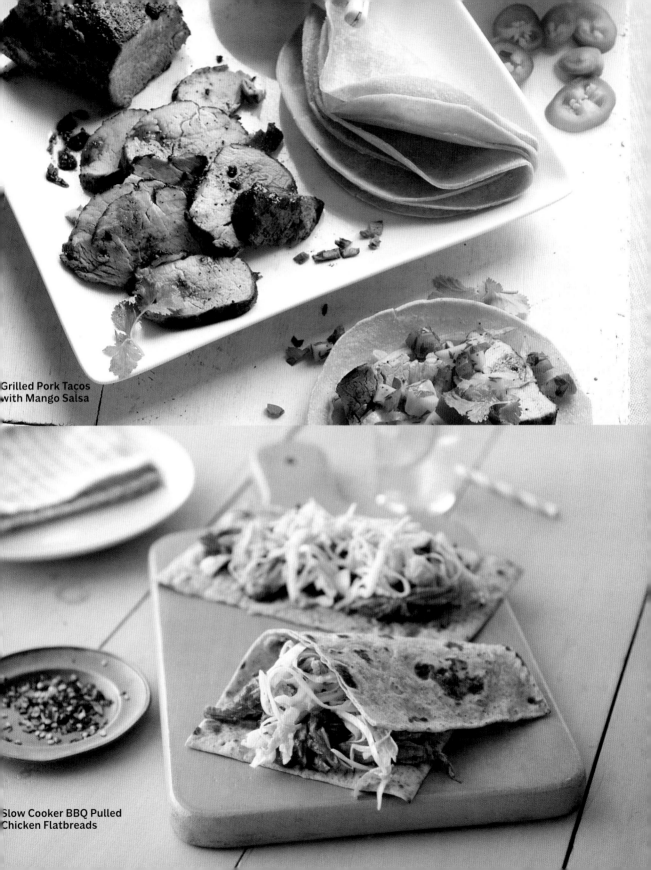

Grilled Pork Tacos
with Mango Salsa

Slow Cooker BBQ Pulled
Chicken Flatbreads

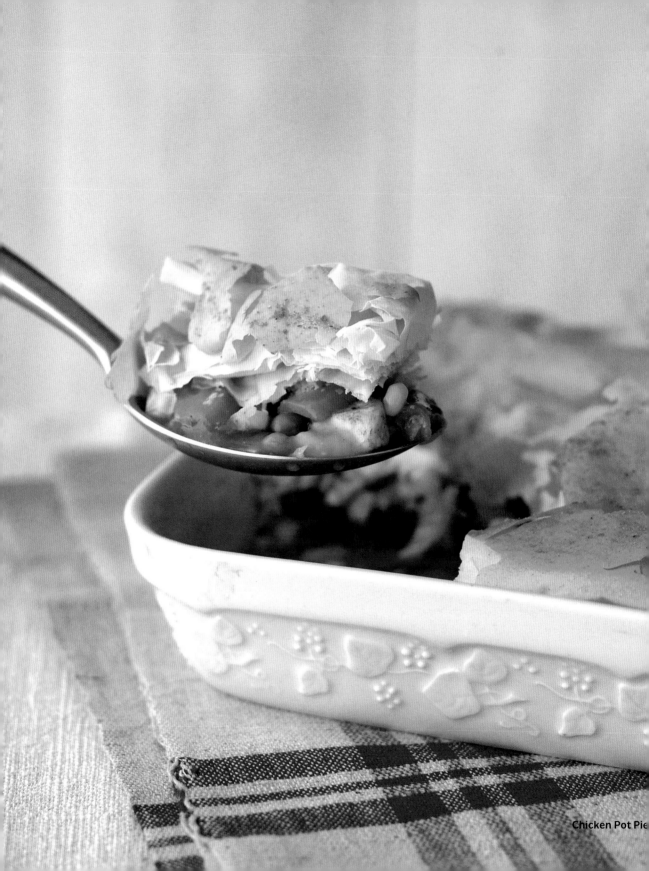

Chicken Pot Pie

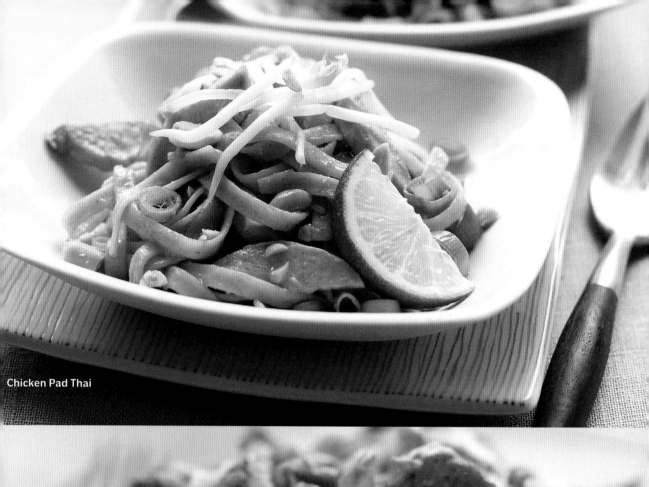

Chicken Pad Thai

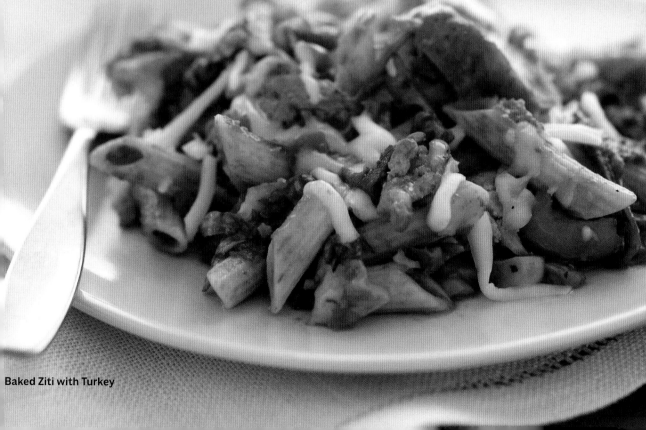

Baked Ziti with Turkey

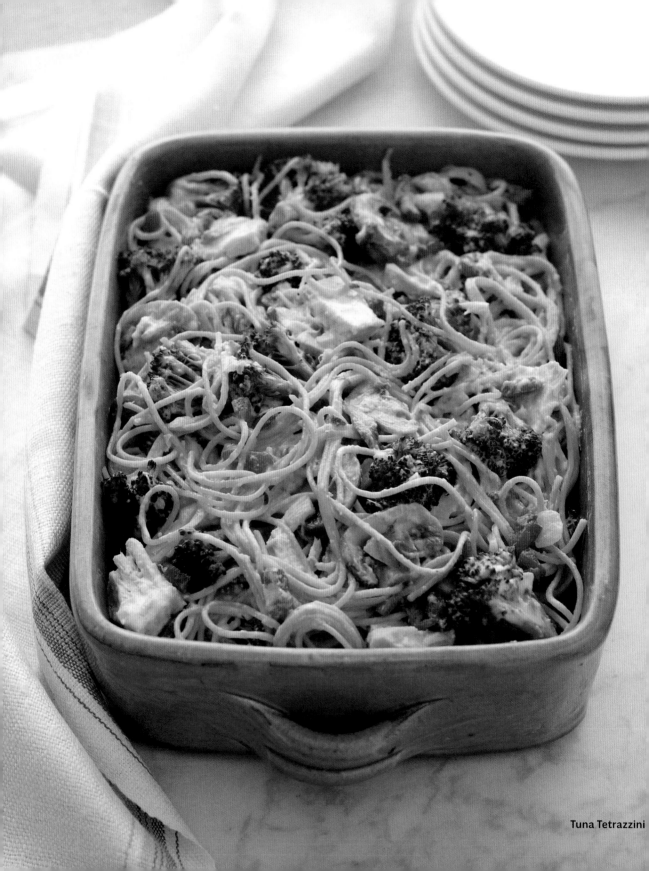

Tuna Tetrazzini

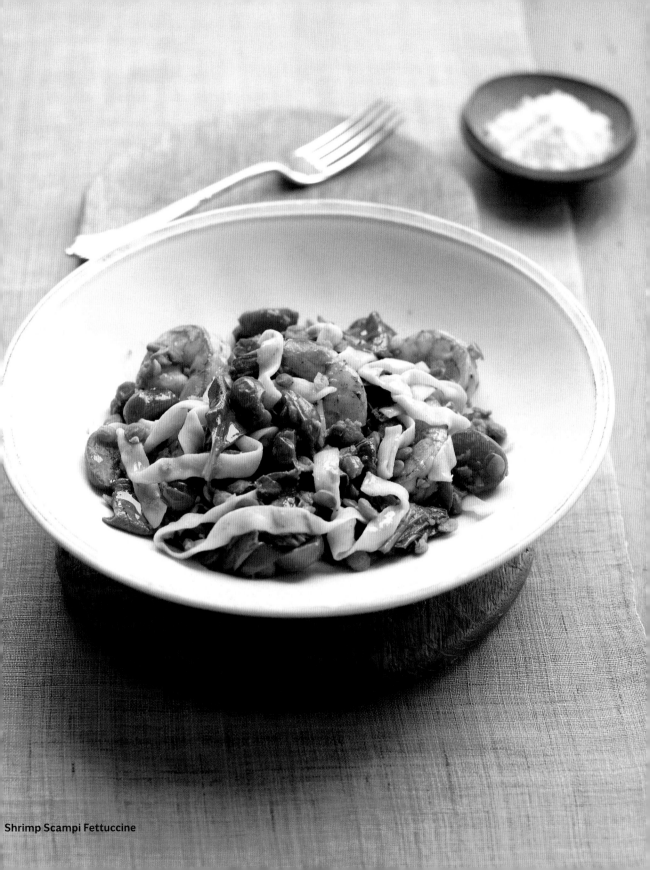

Shrimp Scampi Fettuccine

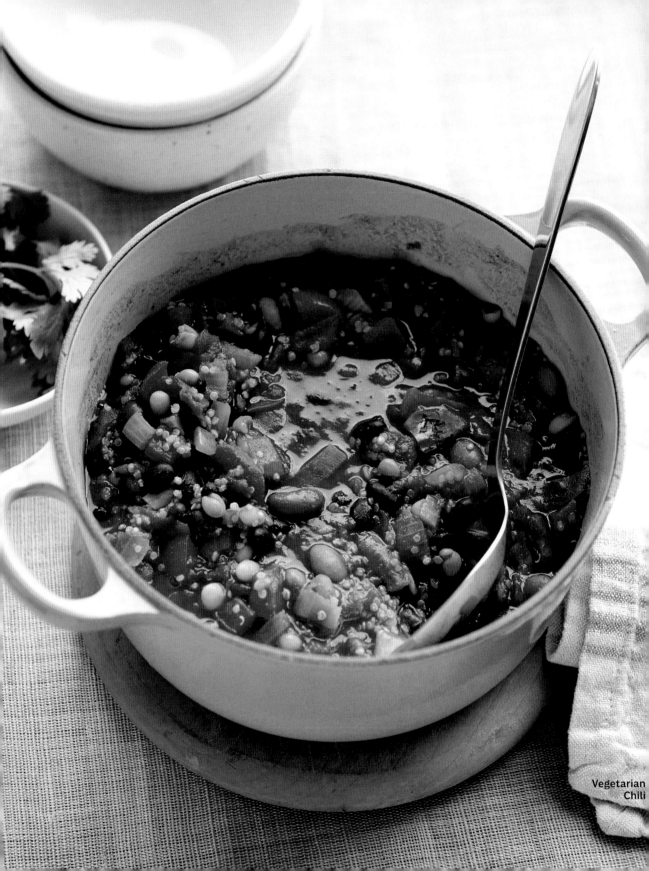

Vegetarian
Chili

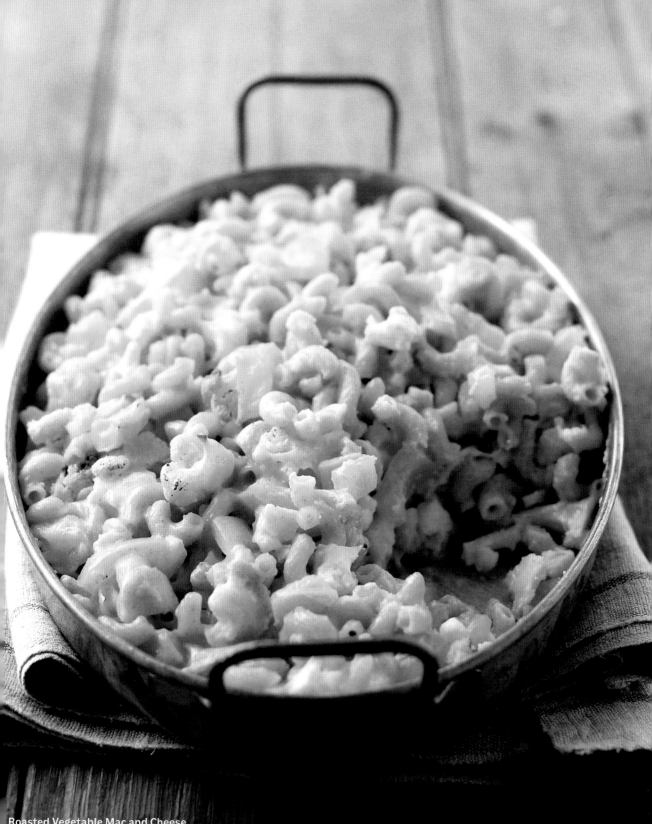

Roasted Vegetable Mac and Cheese

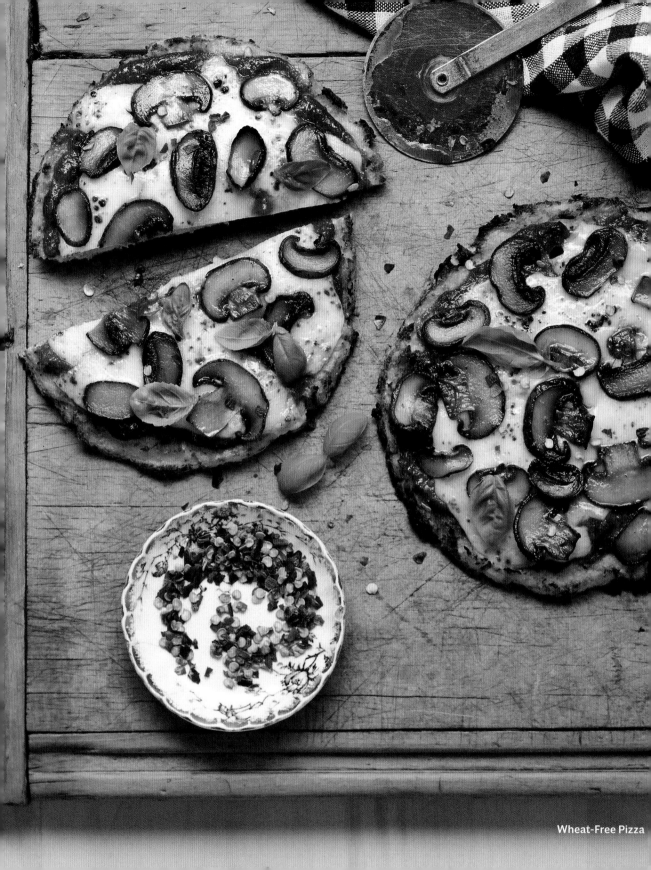

Wheat-Free Pizza

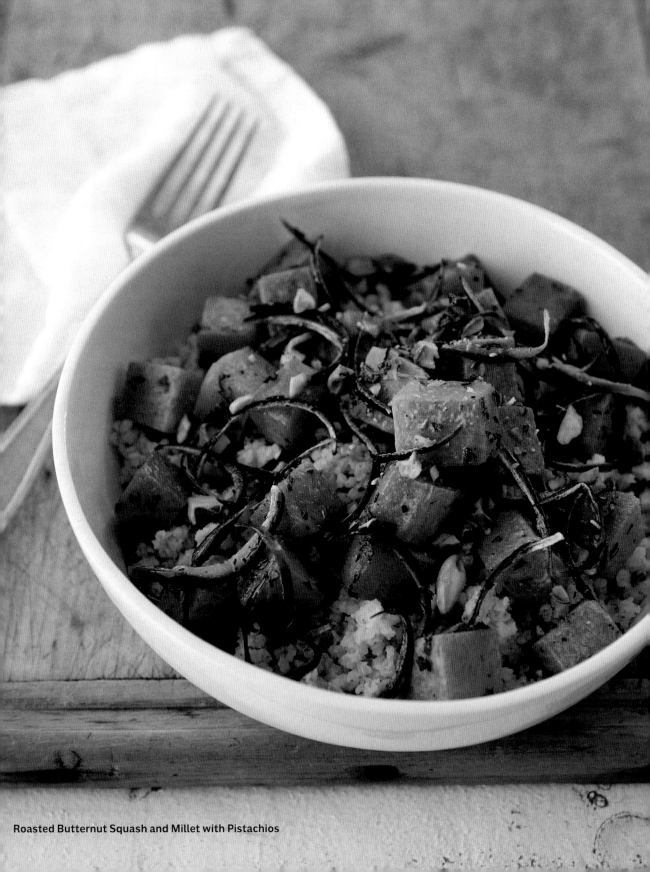

Roasted Butternut Squash and Millet with Pistachios

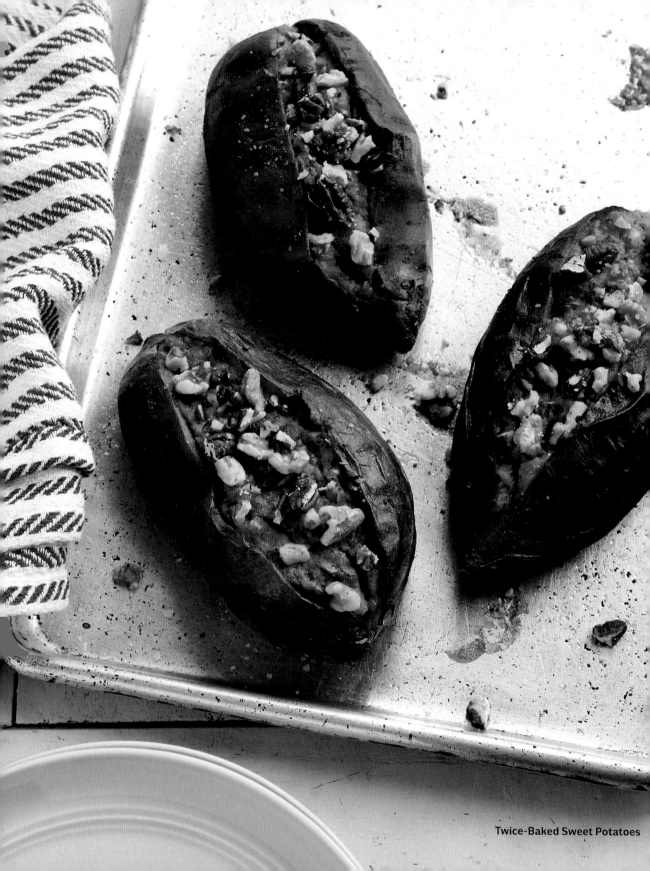

Twice-Baked Sweet Potatoes

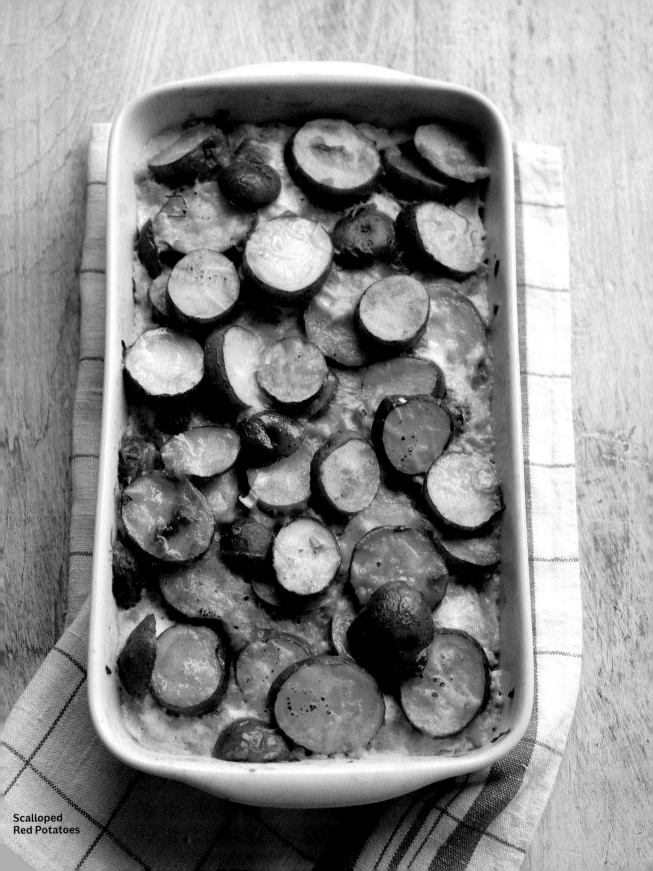

Scalloped
Red Potatoes

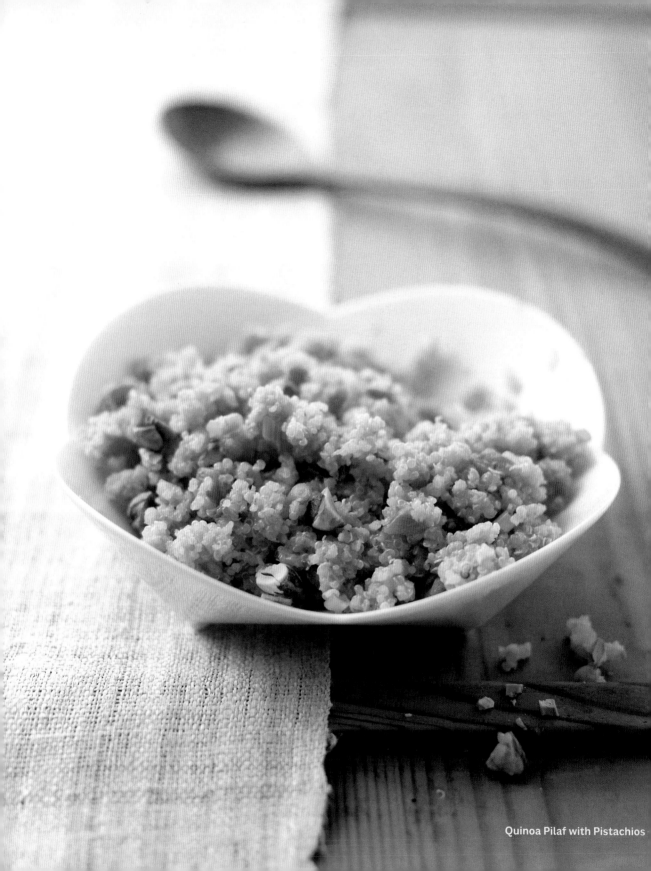

Quinoa Pilaf with Pistachios

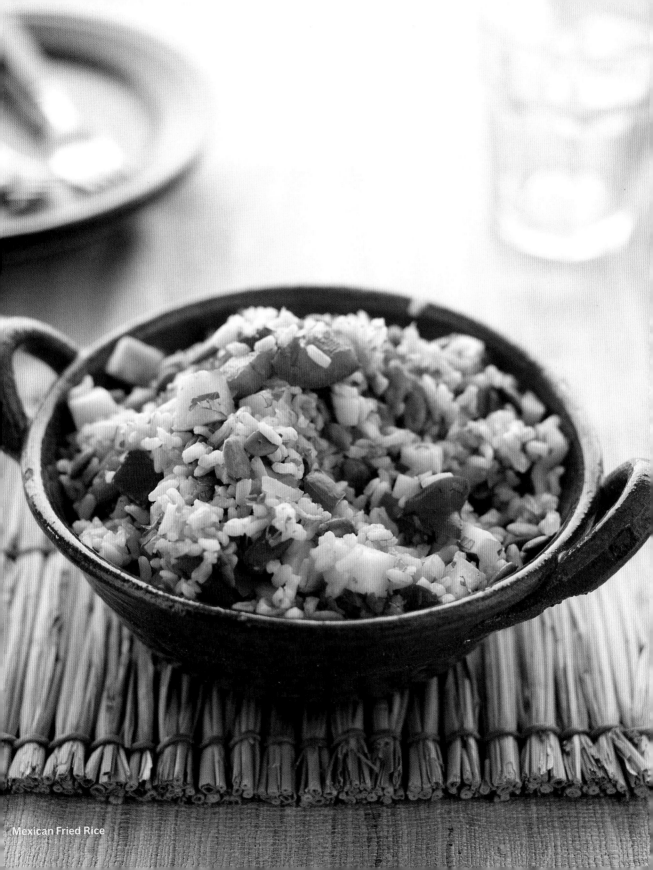

Mexican Fried Rice

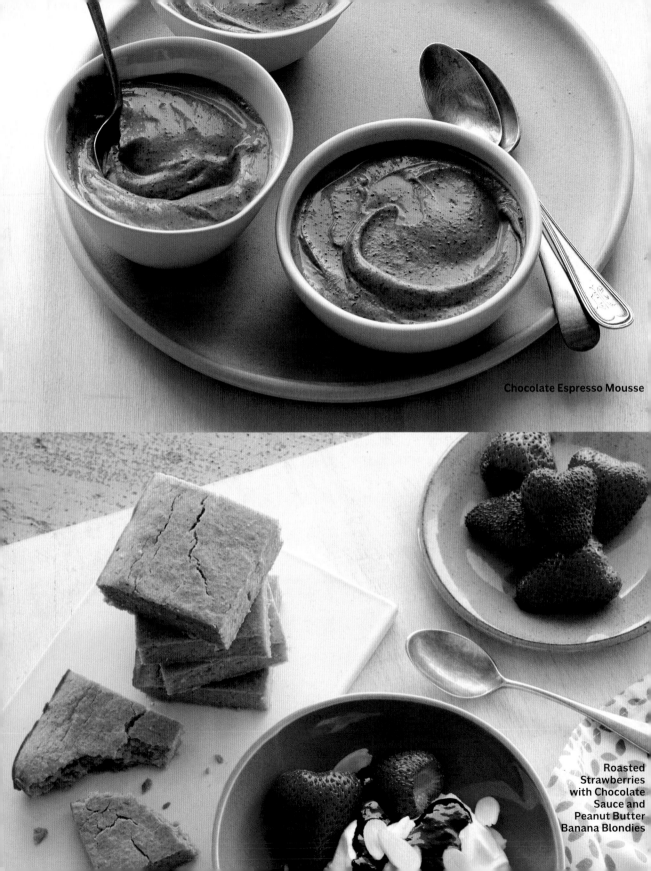

Chocolate Espresso Mousse

Roasted
Strawberries
with Chocolate
Sauce and
Peanut Butter
Banana Blondies

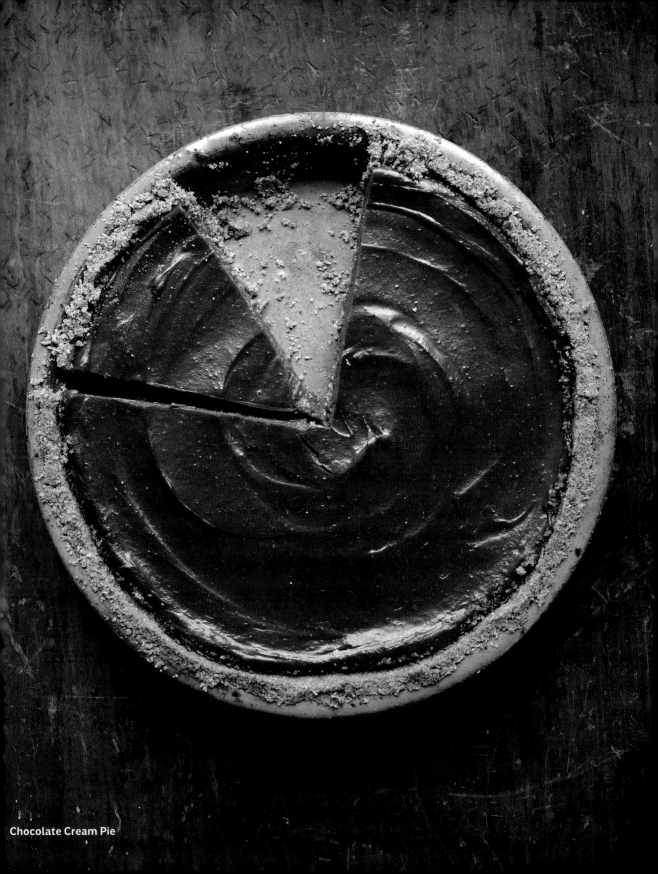

Chocolate Cream Pie

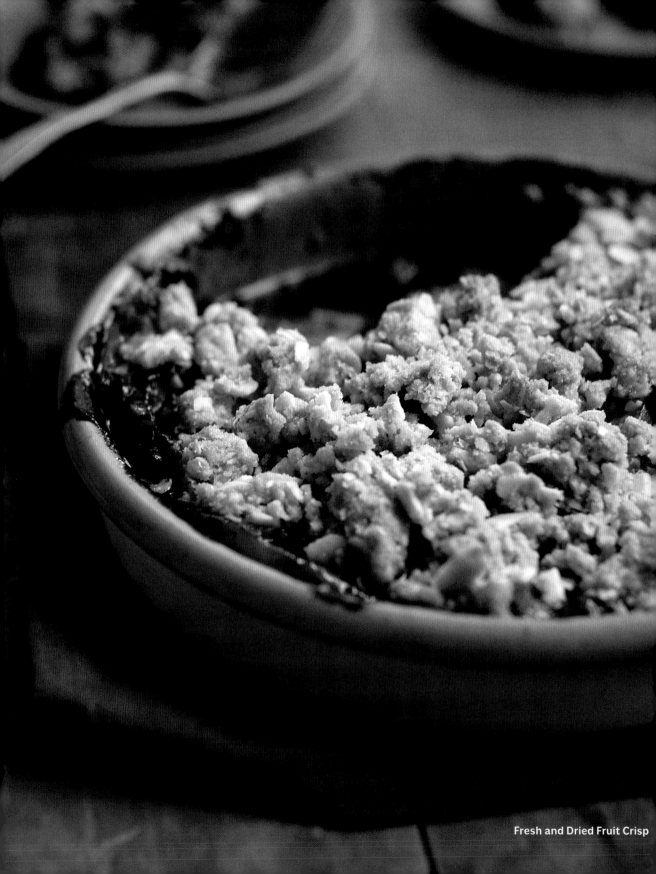

Fresh and Dried Fruit Crisp

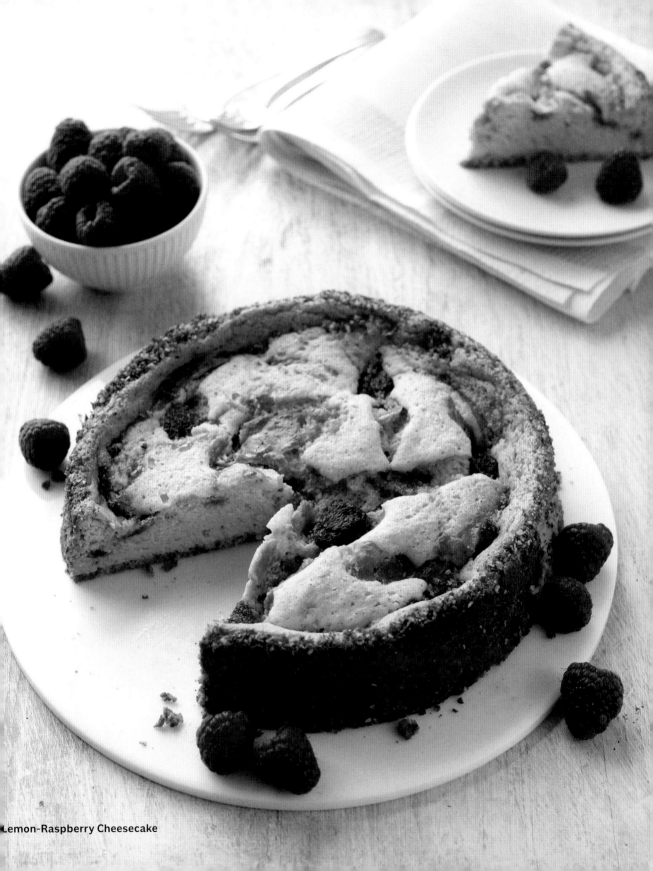

Lemon-Raspberry Cheesecake

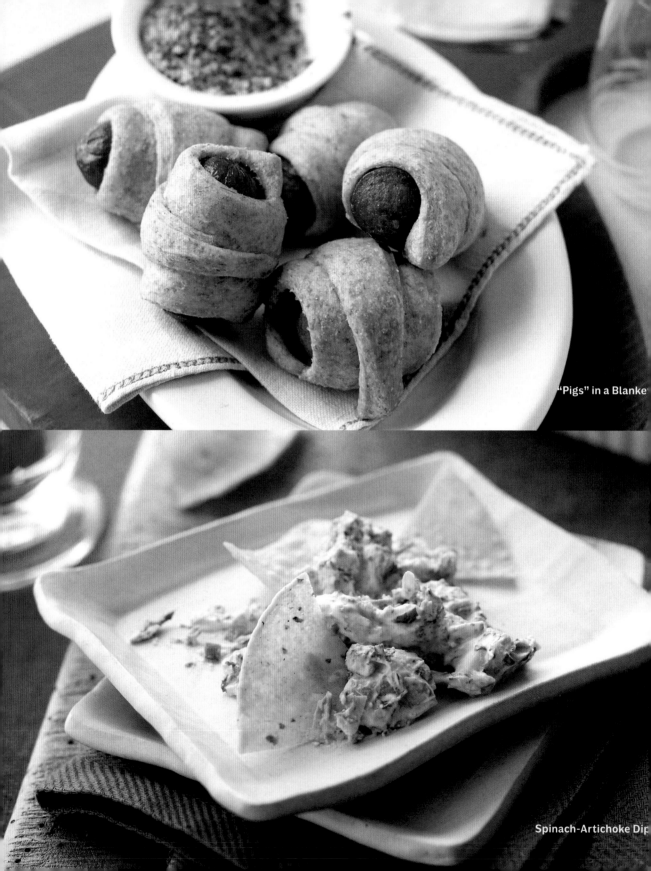

"Pigs" in a Blanket

Spinach-Artichoke Dip

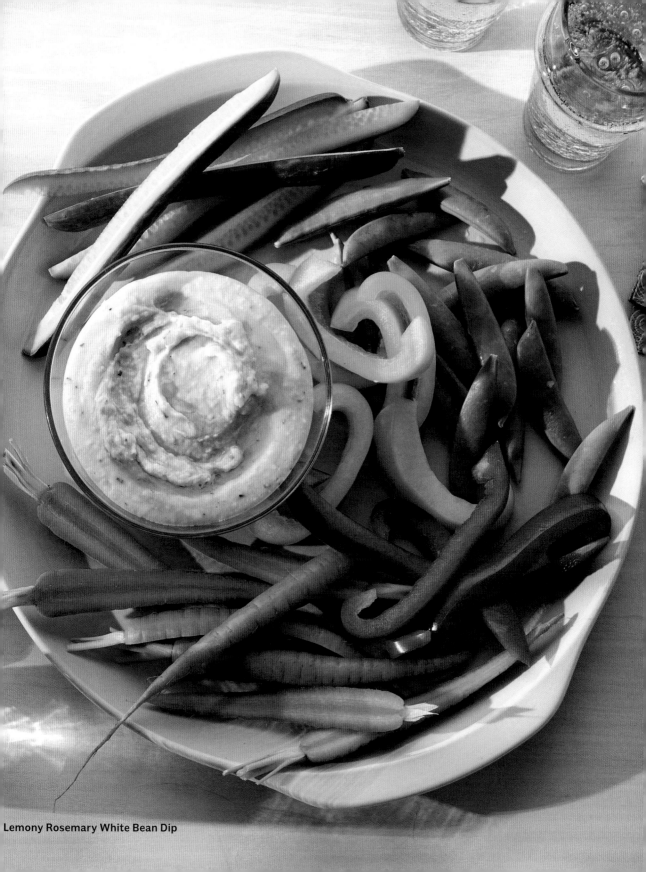

Lemony Rosemary White Bean Dip

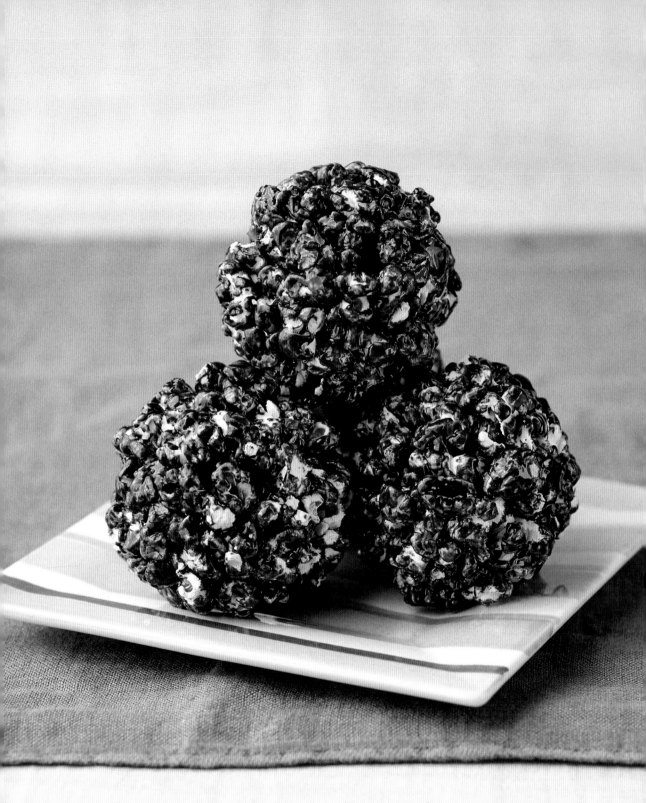

Mexican Chocolate Popcorn Balls

WILD RICE CASSEROLE

I   cup wild rice

I   cup brown rice

8   cups low-sodium vegetable or chicken broth, divided

I   large onion, chopped

2   cups baby spinach

I   cup shredded Cheddar cheese (4 ounces)

I   cup fresh whole wheat bread crumbs

2   large eggs, beaten

I   tablespoon olive oil

½   cup grated Parmesan cheese

1 In a large saucepan over high heat, combine the wild rice, brown rice, and 6 cups of the broth. Bring to a boil. Reduce the heat to low, cover, and simmer until the liquid is absorbed, about 45 minutes. Remove from the heat and let stand, uncovered, for 5 minutes.

2 Preheat the oven to 350°F. Grease a covered 3-quart baking dish.

3 Stir in the onion, spinach, Cheddar, bread crumbs, and eggs to the saucepan with the rice, tossing until well blended. Spread in the prepared baking dish. Sprinkle with the remaining 2 cups broth. Cover and bake for 20 minutes. Uncover and top with the Parmesan. Bake uncovered until the cheese is golden, 15 minutes. Let stand for 15 minutes before serving.

NUTRITION (PER SERVING): 291 calories, 13 g protein, 41 g carbohydrates, 4 g fiber, 2 g sugars, 8 g fat, 4 g saturated fat, 357 mg sodium

BAKED RISOTTO

2 tablespoons olive oil

l onion, chopped

l medium red bell pepper, chopped

½ cup brown rice, preferably short or medium grain

½ cup wild rice

l clove garlic, minced

3 cups vegetable broth

l cup frozen peas, thawed

¼ cup grated Romano cheese

1 Preheat the oven to 425°F.

2 In a large ovenproof saucepan or Dutch oven over medium-high heat, heat the oil. Cook the onion and pepper until softened, 3 minutes. Add the brown rice, wild rice, and garlic. Cook, stirring, until the rice is coated, 2 minutes.

3 Add the broth and bring to a boil. Cover and place in the oven. Bake until the broth is absorbed and the rice is just tender, 55 minutes. Remove from the oven and stir in the peas and cheese. Cover and let stand for 5 minutes.

NUTRITION (PER SERVING): 236 calories, 8 g protein, 32 g carbohydrates, 3 g fiber, 4 g sugars, 8 g fat, 2 g saturated fat, 383 mg sodium

MEXICAN FRIED RICE

PREP TIME: 15 MINUTES / TOTAL TIME: 25 MINUTES / **MAKES 8 SERVINGS**

Shown in photo insert pages.

1	tablespoon olive oil
1	onion, chopped
1	medium zucchini, chopped
1	chayote squash, peeled, seeded, and chopped
1	red bell pepper, chopped
1	teaspoon ground cumin
1½	cups cooked brown rice, chilled
1	cup pumpkin seeds, toasted
½	teaspoon salt
2	tablespoons chopped cilantro
1	teaspoon freshly grated lime zest

1 In a large nonstick skillet over medium-high heat, heat the oil. Cook the onion, zucchini, squash, pepper, and cumin, stirring, until tender-crisp, 5 minutes.

2 Add the rice and cook, stirring often, until lightly toasted, 2 minutes.

3 Stir in the pumpkin seeds and salt and cook for 1 minute. Remove from the heat and stir in the cilantro and lime zest.

NUTRITION (PER SERVING): 160 calories, 6 g protein, 15 g carbohydrates, 3 g fiber, 3 g sugars, 10 g fat, 2 g saturated fat, 154 mg sodium

BROCCOLI-WALNUT FARFALLE TOSS

PREP TIME: 10 MINUTES / TOTAL TIME: 25 MINUTES / **MAKES 4 SERVINGS**

4   ounces whole grain farfalle pasta (bow ties)
I   bunch broccoli, cut into florets
2   tablespoons olive oil
I   small red onion, thinly sliced
¼   teaspoon salt
⅛   teaspoon black pepper
1½ ounces crumbled goat cheese
¼   cup walnuts, toasted and coarsely chopped

1 Prepare the pasta according to package directions, adding the broccoli during the last 4 minutes of cooking time. Drain, reserving ¼ cup of the cooking water. Transfer the pasta and broccoli to a bowl.

2 In the same saucepan, over medium heat, heat the oil. Cook the onion, stirring occasionally, until softened, 5 minutes.

3 Stir in the pasta and broccoli, reserved pasta cooking water, salt, and pepper. Cook, stirring, until heated through, 1 minute. Remove from the heat and stir in the cheese. Sprinkle with the walnuts.

NUTRITION (PER SERVING): 296 calories, 12 g protein, 32 g carbohydrates, 7 g fiber, 4 g sugars, 16 g fat, 3 g saturated fat, 243 mg sodium

FETTUCCINE WITH BASIL-WALNUT SAUCE

PREP TIME: 10 MINUTES / TOTAL TIME: 20 MINUTES / MAKES 4 SERVINGS

1   package (8 ounces) shirataki fettuccine
½   cup walnuts, toasted and coarsely chopped
½   cup fresh basil
2   cloves garlic
2   tablespoons olive oil
3   cups baby spinach
½   cup plain 1% Greek yogurt
¼   cup grated Romano cheese

1 In a medium saucepan, prepare the fettuccine according to package directions. Drain and return to the saucepan.

2 Meanwhile, in a food processor or blender, combine the walnuts, basil, and garlic. Process until blended. Add the oil and pulse until well blended.

3 Add the walnut mixture and spinach to the pan with the fettuccine. Cook over low heat, stirring, until the spinach wilts, 3 minutes. Remove from the heat and stir in the yogurt and cheese.

NUTRITION (PER SERVING): 209 calories, 7 g protein, 6 g carbohydrates, 2 g fiber, 2 g sugars, 18 g fat, 3 g saturated fat, 154 mg sodium

NOTE: Shirataki noodles are a Japanese noodle made from a fiber-rich yam. This fiber slows digestion, keeping you satisfied longer. Available in the refrigerated section of your supermarket, these water-packed noodles are free of carbohydrates and are practically calorie-free, too. (Noodles made from tofu have a very small amount of carbs.) Use shirataki noodles as a substitute for pasta in simple sauce-tossed recipes.

TEX-MEX PASTA AND BEANS

PREP TIME: 10 MINUTES / TOTAL TIME: 25 MINUTES / MAKES 4 SERVINGS

I   cup whole wheat rotelle pasta

I   red onion, chopped

I   green bell pepper, chopped

½   teaspoon ground cumin

I   cup canned black beans, rinsed and drained

¾   cup salsa

2   tablespoons chopped cilantro

½   avocado, peeled, seeded, and chopped

1 Prepare the pasta according to package directions.

2 Meanwhile, heat a large nonstick skillet coated with cooking spray over medium-high heat. Cook the onion and pepper, stirring occasionally, until softened, 5 minutes. Add the cumin and cook, stirring, until fragrant, 1 minute.

3 Stir in the pasta, beans, salsa, and cilantro. Cook until hot, 1 minute. Top with the avocado.

NUTRITION (PER SERVING): 230 calories, 8 g protein, 42 g carbohydrates, 8 g fiber, 7 g sugars, 5 g fat, 1 g saturated fat, 274 mg sodium

DILL AND BASIL YOGURT BREAD

PREP TIME: 15 MINUTES / TOTAL TIME: 55 MINUTES + 1 HOUR RISE TIME / **MAKES 12 SERVINGS**

1½ cups spelt flour

1½ cups whole wheat flour

1½ teaspoons minced onion (optional)

2 teaspoons dried basil or 2 tablespoons finely chopped fresh

2 teaspoons dried dill weed or 2 tablespoons finely chopped fresh

1 teaspoon salt

¼ teaspoon baking soda

2 tablespoons evaporated cane juice

1 envelope (2¼ teaspoons) rapid rise yeast

1 cup low-fat plain yogurt

¼ cup water

1 tablespoon grapeseed oil

1 large egg, lightly beaten

1 In a large bowl, combine the spelt flour, whole wheat flour, onion (if desired), basil, dill, salt, baking soda, cane juice, and yeast. Set aside.

2 In a microwaveable medium bowl, stir together the yogurt, water, and oil. Heat in the microwave until warm, 45 seconds to 1 minute. Stir in the egg.

3 Using an electric mixer with a dough hook on medium speed, slowly mix the yogurt mixture into the flour mixture. Mix until well blended, about 3 minutes. The dough will be stiff. Cover and let rise until doubled in size, 45 minutes to 1 hour.

4 Preheat the oven to 375°F. Lightly grease a 9" x 5" loaf pan.

5 Transfer the dough to the pan. Bake until golden brown, 25 to 30 minutes. Let the bread cool for 5 minutes. Remove from the pan and let cool for another 5 minutes before slicing.

NUTRITION (PER SERVING): 150 calories, 6 g protein, 26 g carbohydrates, 4 g fiber, 4 g sugars, 3 g fat, 1 g saturated fat, 208 mg sodium

NOTE: If you don't have an electric mixer, stir together the yogurt mixture and flour mixture by hand until the flour is incorporated and then knead until smooth, about 5 minutes.

DESSERTS

ROASTED STRAWBERRIES WITH CHOCOLATE SAUCE

PREP TIME: 5 MINUTES / TOTAL TIME: 25 MINUTES / MAKES 2 SERVINGS

Shown in photo insert pages.

I   cup whole strawberries, hulled

2   teaspoons coconut oil

I   tablespoon pure maple syrup

I   tablespoon unsweetened cocoa powder

½   cup plain Greek yogurt

I   tablespoon sliced almonds

1 Preheat the oven to 350°F. On a baking sheet, coat the strawberries lightly with cooking spray. Roast until softened, about 20 minutes.

2 Meanwhile, in a small microwaveable bowl, combine the oil and maple syrup. Microwave on high until the oil is melted, about 30 seconds. Add the cocoa and stir until smooth.

3 Serve the strawberries over the Greek yogurt. Drizzle with the chocolate sauce and top with the almonds.

NUTRITION (PER SERVING): 195 calories, 6 g protein, 17 g carbohydrates, 3 g fiber, 12 g sugars, 13 g fat, 9 g saturated fat, 19 mg sodium

CREAMY COCONUT RICE PUDDING

PREP TIME: 10 MINUTES / TOTAL TIME: 40 MINUTES / MAKES 4 SERVINGS

½ cup brown basmati rice

¾ cup water

¾ cup coconut milk

¼ cup sugar

2 teaspoons pure vanilla extract

3 tablespoons chia seeds

Sliced mango or other fruit (optional)

1 In a medium saucepan over high heat, combine the rice, water, coconut milk, sugar, and vanilla and bring to a boil. Reduce the heat to low, cover, and simmer, stirring occasionally, until the liquid is absorbed and the rice is tender, 40 minutes.

2 Fold in the chia seeds, remove from the heat, and let stand, covered, until all the liquid is absorbed, 10 minutes. Serve with sliced mango or other fruit, if desired.

NUTRITION (PER SERVING): 247 calories, 4 g protein, 33 g carbohydrates, 4 g fiber, 13 g sugars, 12 g fat, 8 g saturated fat, 7 mg sodium

HEALTHY HINT

It's actually supereasy to make your own nondairy nut milk. Soak I cup of raw almonds or walnuts in enough water to cover for 4 hours, or as long as overnight. Drain the nuts and puree them in a blender with 4 cups of water until smooth, about I minute. Strain the mixture through cheesecloth. Refrigerate the milk in a covered container for up to 3 days.

CHOCOLATE ESPRESSO MOUSSE

PREP TIME: 5 MINUTES / TOTAL TIME: 10 MINUTES / MAKES 2 SERVINGS

Shown in photo insert pages.

¼ cup (about I ounce) dark chocolate pieces (at least 80% cacao)

I avocado, halved, peeled, and pitted

I tablespoon unsweetened vanilla almond milk

I tablespoon unsweetened cocoa powder

I tablespoon honey

¼ teaspoon pure vanilla extract

3 teaspoons espresso

¼ teaspoon salt

1 In a microwaveable bowl, microwave the dark chocolate until smooth, stirring every 15 seconds, 2 minutes. Set aside to cool slightly.

2 In a food processor, combine the melted chocolate, avocado, almond milk, cocoa, honey, vanilla, espresso, and salt. Process until creamy, 2 minutes.

3 Refrigerate for at least 1 hour before serving.

NUTRITION (PER SERVING): 287 calories, 4 g protein, 26 g carbohydrates, 9 g fiber, 13 g sugars, 21 g fat, 6 g saturated fat, 95 mg sodium

HEALTHY HINT

Cold-brew coffee has become immensely popular over the last few years, and if you haven't tried it yet, it may be worth the venture. Cold brew tends to be less acidic than regular coffee, so it's gentler on your stomach. Less bite also means it generally needs less milk and sweetener, so if you use either, going cold could help you cut down on calories.

ORANGE–DARK CHOCOLATE CHUNK COOKIES

PREP TIME: 15 MINUTES / TOTAL TIME: 1 HOUR / **MAKES 15 COOKIES**

1   cup almond meal/flour

2   tablespoons raw sugar

1½   teaspoons baking powder

¼   teaspoon salt

½   pound Medjool dates, pitted

1   egg

2   tablespoons coconut oil, melted

1   tablespoon pure vanilla extract

1½   teaspoons grated orange zest

¼   cup chopped pecans

¼   cup unsweetened coconut flakes

¼   cup + 2 tablespoons chopped dark chocolate (at least 80% cacao)

1 Preheat the oven to 375°F. Line a baking sheet with parchment paper.

2 In a medium bowl, combine the almond meal, sugar, baking powder, and salt.

3 In a food processor, process the dates for 2 minutes, scraping down the sides frequently. Add the egg, oil, vanilla, and orange zest and process until a smooth puree is formed, 2 minutes.

4 Add the puree to the dry ingredients, stirring until combined. Stir in the pecans, coconut flakes, and chocolate.

5 Use a 1½-tablespoon cookie scoop to measure the cookie dough onto the prepared baking sheet, spacing 2" apart.

6 Bake until the edges begin to brown, 15 minutes. Cool on a wire rack. Store cooled cookies in an airtight container.

NUTRITION (PER COOKIE): 160 calories, 3 g protein, 18 g carbohydrates, 2 g fiber, 14 g sugars, 10 g fat, 4 g saturated fat, 90 mg sodium

STEEL-CUT OATMEAL RAISIN COOKIES

PREP TIME: 25 MINUTES / TOTAL TIME: 45 MINUTES / **MAKES 24 COOKIES**

3   tablespoons water

I   tablespoon ground flaxseed

1⅓ cups cooked steel-cut oats

¾   cup whole wheat flour

1½ teaspoons ground cinnamon

¾   teaspoon baking powder

¼   cup + 2 tablespoons coconut oil

¼   cup + I tablespoon brown sugar

2   teaspoons pure vanilla extract

½   cup chopped walnuts

½   cup raisins, lightly chopped

1 Preheat the oven to 300°F. Coat a baking sheet with coconut oil. In a small bowl, stir together the water and flaxseed. Set aside.

2 Spread the cooked oats on the prepared baking sheet. Bake, stirring every 10 minutes, until the oats are dry, 30 minutes. Cool on a wire rack.

3 Increase the oven temperature to 375°F.

4 In a medium bowl, combine the flour, cinnamon, baking powder, and cooled oats.

5 In a large bowl, beat the oil and sugar until combined and lightened in color. Add the flaxseed mixture and vanilla and beat to combine completely. Stir in the flour mixture until incorporated. Stir in the walnuts and raisins.

6 On a baking sheet, place heaping tablespoonfuls of the dough 2" apart. Flatten slightly and bake until golden brown, about 15 minutes. Store cooled cookies in an airtight container.

NUTRITION (PER COOKIE): 112 calories, 2 g protein, 15 g carbohydrates, 2 g fiber, 5 g sugars, 6 g fat, 3 g saturated fat, 17 mg sodium

DARK CHOCOLATE CRACKLE COOKIES

PREP TIME: 15 MINUTES / TOTAL TIME: 23 MINUTES + CHILLING TIME / **MAKES 32 COOKIES**

6   tablespoons butter, melted

¼   cup + 2 tablespoons unsweetened cocoa
      powder

2   teaspoons almond extract

¾   cup light brown sugar

¼   cup + 2 tablespoons unsweetened
      applesauce

2   tablespoons honey

1¼ cups white whole wheat flour
      Pinch of salt

4   teaspoons granulated sugar

1 In a large bowl, combine the butter, cocoa, and almond extract. Stir until smooth. Add the brown sugar, applesauce, and honey. Stir until smooth. Stir in the flour and salt until well blended.

2 Cover the bowl with plastic wrap and refrigerate until the dough is very stiff, several hours or overnight.

3 Preheat the oven to 350°F. Coat several baking sheets with cooking spray.

4 Place the granulated sugar in a small dish or plate. Scoop out a scant tablespoonful of the dough. Roll into a ball between your palms, flattening slightly. Dip 1 side into the sugar and place, sugar side up, on a prepared baking sheet.

5 Bake until the surface is set but still soft to the touch, 7 minutes. Cool on a wire rack. Store cooled cookies in an airtight container.

NUTRITION (PER COOKIE): 129 calories, 2 g protein, 23 g carbohydrates, 2 g fiber, 14 g sugars, 4 g fat, 1 g saturated fat, 51 mg sodium

GOOEY DATE BARS

PREP TIME: 15 MINUTES / TOTAL TIME: 40 MINUTES / MAKES 16 BARS

½ cup honey

⅓ cup fat-free plain yogurt

3 tablespoons canola oil

1 omega-3-enriched egg

1½ teaspoons pure vanilla extract

1 cup chopped, pitted dates

1¾ cups old-fashioned oats

½ cup white whole wheat flour

¼ cup ground flaxseeds

¼ cup chopped walnuts

½ teaspoon baking soda

⅛ teaspoon salt

Confectioners' sugar

1 Preheat the oven to 350°F. Coat an 8" x 8" baking pan with cooking spray.

2 In a large mixing bowl, whisk together the honey, yogurt, oil, egg, and vanilla until smooth. In a medium bowl, toss the dates, oats, flour, flaxseeds, walnuts, baking soda, and salt. Stir into the batter until well blended.

3 Spread into the prepared pan.

4 Bake until the top is browned and moist crumbs cling to a wooden pick inserted into the center, 25 minutes. Cool on a wire rack. Cut into 16 squares. Dust lightly with the confectioners' sugar. Store cooled bars in an airtight container.

NUTRITION (PER BAR): 147 calories, 3 g protein, 23 g carbohydrates, 2 g fiber, 15 g sugars, 5 g fat, 1 g saturated fat, 66 mg sodium

FRUIT AND NUT COOKIE BARS

PREP TIME: 10 MINUTES / TOTAL TIME: 1 HOUR 10 MINUTES / **MAKES 10 BARS**

I cup cashews

¾ cup pitted dates

½ cup dried cherries

2 tablespoons unsweetened cocoa powder

½ teaspoon sea salt

1 In a food processor or high-powered blender, combine the cashews, dates, cherries, cocoa, and salt. Pulse, scraping down the sides as needed, until well combined, about 5 minutes.

2 On a piece of parchment paper or a cutting board, spread into an 8" square about ½" thick. Cut into 10 rectangular bars.

3 Refrigerate for 1 hour to set.

4 Store between layers of parchment paper or in individual bags in an airtight container in the refrigerator.

NUTRITION (PER BAR): 137 calories, 3 g protein, 19 g carbohydrates, 2 g fiber, 11 g sugars, 7 g fat, 1 g saturated fat, 100 mg sodium

RICH BROWNIES

PREP TIME: 20 MINUTES / TOTAL TIME: 1 HOUR / **MAKES 16 BROWNIES**

I   can (15.5 ounces) black beans, rinsed and drained

½   cup unsweetened cocoa powder

½   cup 100% pumpkin puree

½   cup honey

¼   cup ground flaxseeds

4   eggs

2   teaspoons pure vanilla extract

I   cup chopped walnuts

I   cup 60% cocoa bittersweet chocolate chips

1 Preheat the oven to 350°F. Coat an 8" x 8" baking pan with cooking spray.

2 In a food processor, combine the beans, cocoa, pumpkin, honey, flaxseeds, eggs, and vanilla. Blend until smooth. Pour into the prepared pan and sprinkle with the walnuts and chocolate chips.

3 Bake until the top springs back when touched lightly in the center, 30 minutes. Cool on a wire rack. Store cooled brownies in an airtight container.

NUTRITION (PER BROWNIE): 188 calories, 5 g protein, 23 g carbohydrates, 4 g fiber, 16 g sugars, 11 g fat, 3 g saturated fat, 87 mg sodium

PEANUT BUTTER BANANA BLONDIES

PREP TIME: 5 MINUTES / TOTAL TIME: 30 MINUTES / MAKES 9 SERVINGS

Shown in photo insert pages.

1 can (15 ounces) low- or no-sodium chickpeas, rinsed and drained

¼ cup all-natural creamy peanut butter

¼ cup pure maple syrup

1 medium ripe banana

1 large egg

1 teaspoon pure vanilla extract

¼ cup whole wheat flour

½ teaspoon baking powder

1 Preheat the oven to 350°F. Coat an 8" x 8" baking pan with cooking spray.

2 In a food processor, combine the chickpeas, peanut butter, maple syrup, banana, egg, and vanilla. Process until smooth. Stir in the flour and baking powder; pulse until combined.

3 Spread evenly in the prepared pan and bake until a toothpick inserted in the center comes out clean, 20 minutes. Cool on a wire rack. Store cooled blondies in an airtight container.

NUTRITION (PER BLONDIE): 137 calories, 4 g protein, 20 g carbohydrates, 2 g fiber, 8 g sugars, 5 g fat, 1 g saturated fat, 100 mg sodium

FRUIT 'N' NUT BARK

½ cup 60% cocoa bittersweet chocolate chips

½ cup chopped walnuts

¼ cup dried cranberries

1 Line a baking sheet with parchment or waxed paper.

2 In a medium microwavable bowl, microwave the baking chips on medium, stirring twice, until just melted, 2 minutes. Stir in the walnuts and cranberries.

3 On the prepared baking sheet, spread the mixture into a 10" x 8" rectangle. Refrigerate until set, 1 hour. Cut or break the bark into 8 pieces.

NUTRITION (PER SERVING): 110 calories, 2 g protein, 11 g carbohydrates, 1 g fiber, 8 g sugars, 8 g fat, 2 g saturated fat, 1 mg sodium

DARK CHOCOLATE–SEA SALT TRUFFLES

PREP TIME: 10 MINUTES / TOTAL TIME: 10 MINUTES + 1 HOUR CHILLING / **MAKES 15 TRUFFLES**

4   ounces chopped dark chocolate (at least 80% cacao)

¼   cup + 2 tablespoons canned lite coconut milk

1   tablespoon coconut oil

2   teaspoons pure vanilla extract

⅛   teaspoon sea salt

⅓   cup unsweetened shredded coconut

1 In a medium microwaveable bowl, combine the chocolate, coconut milk, and coconut oil. Microwave on medium, stirring twice, until just melted, 2 minutes. Stir in the vanilla and salt. Cover the bowl and refrigerate until firm, about 1 hour.

2 Place the shredded coconut in a shallow dish or pie plate. Roll 1 teaspoon of the chilled chocolate mixture between your palms to form a ball. Drop the ball into the bowl of coconut and roll around until entirely coated. Set in a parchment paper-lined airtight container.

NUTRITION (PER TRUFFLE): 73 calories, 1 g protein, 4 g carbohydrates, 1 g fiber, 2 g sugars, 6 g fat, 4 g saturated fat, 20 mg sodium

RICH CHOCOLATE TORTE

PREP TIME: 22 MINUTES / TOTAL TIME: 1 HOUR 7 MINUTES / **MAKES 16 SERVINGS**

1   tablespoon + ¼ cup cocoa powder, divided

1   cup walnuts

¾   cup sugar, divided

5   omega-3-enriched eggs, separated

½   teaspoon cream of tartar

½   cup reduced-fat sour cream

5   ounces bittersweet chocolate (60% cocoa or higher), melted

1   teaspoon ground cinnamon

1 Preheat the oven to 350°F. Coat an 8" or 9" springform pan with cooking spray and dust with 1 tablespoon of the cocoa.

2 In a blender or food processor, combine the walnuts and ¼ cup of the sugar. Pulse until finely ground.

3 In a large bowl, with an electric mixer on high, beat the egg whites and cream of tartar until foamy. Gradually add the remaining ½ cup sugar, beating until stiff peaks form.

4 In another large bowl, with the same beaters, beat the egg yolks until thick. Add the sour cream, chocolate, cinnamon, and the remaining ¼ cup cocoa. Beat to blend well. Fold in the walnut mixture. Stir one-quarter of the egg whites into the chocolate mixture. Fold in the remaining whites in 2 batches.

5 Pour into the prepared pan and bake until a knife inserted in the center comes out clean, 45 minutes. Place the pan on a rack and cool completely, at least 4 hours. (The cake is best made a day ahead and stored covered in the pan until serving.) Release the sides of the pan and cut into 16 slices.

NUTRITION (PER SERVING): 158 calories, 4 g protein, 17 g carbohydrates, 2 g fiber, 13 g sugars, 10 g fat, 4 g saturated fat, 24 mg sodium

CHOCOLATE CREAM PIE

PREP TIME: 15 MINUTES / TOTAL TIME: 3 HOURS 55 MINUTES / MAKES 8 SERVINGS

Shown in photo insert pages.

CRUST

10 whole low-fat graham crackers

¼   cup walnuts

3   tablespoons sugar

2   tablespoons unsalted butter, melted

FILLING

2¾ cups milk

1   cup sugar

1   large egg

¼   cup unsweetened cocoa powder

¼   cup cornstarch

¼   teaspoon salt

1   teaspoon unsalted butter

1 Preheat the oven to 350°F. Coat a 9" pie plate with cooking spray.

2 *To make the crust:* In a food processor, combine the graham crackers, walnuts, and sugar. Process until fine crumbs form. Add the butter and pulse just until blended. Press the mixture into the bottom and up the sides of the prepared pie plate. Bake until lightly browned, 10 minutes. Cool on a wire rack.

3 *Meanwhile, to make the filling:* In a large saucepan, whisk together the milk, sugar, egg, cocoa, cornstarch, and salt until well combined. Over medium heat, cook, whisking constantly, until the mixture comes to a boil. Cook, whisking frequently, until thickened, 5 minutes. Remove from the heat and whisk in the butter until melted.

4 Press a piece of plastic wrap directly onto the surface of the filling and let cool for 20 minutes. Chill in the refrigerator until completely cooled, 1 hour. Remove the plastic wrap and spread the filling into the crust. Refrigerate for at least 2 hours before serving.

NUTRITION (PER SERVING): 250 calories, 5 g protein, 44 g carbohydrates, 1 g fiber, 36 g sugars, 7 g fat, 3 g saturated fat, 152 mg sodium

CINNAMON APPLE PIE

PREP TIME: 25 MINUTES / TOTAL TIME: 1 HOUR 25 MINUTES / MAKES 10 SERVINGS

DOUGH

- ¾ cup rolled oats
- ½ cup chopped walnuts
- 2 tablespoons pure maple syrup
- ¼ cup coconut oil
- Pinch of salt
- 1 tablespoon water

FILLING

- 2 tablespoons coconut oil, divided
- 6 Pink Lady apples, cored and sliced
- 8 pitted Medjool dates, soaked in warm water for 30 minutes
- 2 tablespoons ground cinnamon
- Pinch of ground nutmeg
- Pinch of ground cloves
- 1 teaspoon fresh lemon juice
- 2 tablespoons orange juice
- 3 tablespoons water

1 Preheat the oven to 350°F.

2 *To make the crust:* In a blender or food processor, combine the oats, walnuts, maple syrup, oil, and salt. Pulse until the oats are broken up but not powdery. Add the water and pulse a few times, just until the dough sticks together. Press the mixture into the bottom and up the sides of an 8" or 9" pie plate.

3 Bake the crust until light brown, about 25 minutes.

4 Raise the oven temperature to 375°F.

5 *To make the filling:* In a large skillet over medium heat, heat 1 tablespoon of the oil. Add the apples and cook until golden and just soft, about 15 minutes.

6 Drain the dates. In a blender, combine the dates, cinnamon, nutmeg, cloves, lemon juice, orange juice, water, and the remaining 1 tablespoon oil. (You may add up to 1 additional tablespoon of water if needed to achieve a smooth consistency.) Process until smooth. Pour over the apples and gently toss to coat.

7 Pour the apple mixture into the pie shell and bake until golden, about 40 minutes. Cool on a wire rack.

NUTRITION (PER SERVING): 258 calories, 3 g protein, 38 g carbohydrates, 6 g fiber, 27 g sugars, 13 g fat, 7 g saturated fat, 18 mg sodium

CHERRY, PEAR, AND PECAN CRISP

PREP TIME: 10 MINUTES / TOTAL TIME: 40 MINUTES / **MAKES 4 SERVINGS**

2   Medjool dates, pitted and finely chopped

¼   cup chopped pecans

1   tablespoon coconut oil, melted

1   tablespoon unsweetened plain almond milk or milk of your choice

1   tablespoon whole wheat flour

½   cup rolled oats, divided

1   cup chopped pears

1   cup pitted dark sweet cherries

¼   teaspoon ground cardamom

1   teaspoon pure vanilla extract

1   tablespoon pure maple syrup

1 Preheat the oven to 400°F. Lightly coat two 8-ounce ramekins with coconut oil.

2 In a food processor, combine the dates, pecans, oil, milk, flour, and ¼ cup of the oats. Process until crumbly, 1 to 2 minutes. Set aside.

3 In a medium bowl, combine the pears, cherries, cardamom, and the remaining ¼ cup oats. Drizzle the vanilla and maple syrup over the mixture and stir to combine. Divide among the ramekins. Sprinkle with the pecan topping mixture.

4 Cover each ramekin with foil and bake for 15 minutes. Remove the foil and bake until the topping is lightly browned and the mixture is bubbling, 10 minutes.

NUTRITION (PER SERVING): 230 calories, 3 g protein, 34 g carbohydrates, 5 g fiber, 21 g sugars, 10 g fat, 4 g saturated fat, 4 mg sodium

HEALTHY HINT

Sure, buying nuts in bulk is cost effective, but their high fat content means that they'll go rancid if you don't eat them up within a few weeks. Foresee yourself taking longer? Store nuts in an airtight container in the fridge for up to a year or in the freezer for up to 2 years. To liven up the flavor before you eat them, spread them on a baking sheet and toast at 350°F for 10 minutes

FRESH AND DRIED FRUIT CRISP

PREP TIME: 20 MINUTES / TOTAL TIME: 1 HOUR / **MAKES 8 SERVINGS**

Shown in photo insert pages.

1½ **pounds peaches, pitted and sliced**

3 **cups blueberries**

1 **cup dried apricots, sliced**

1 **cup packed light brown sugar, divided**

1 **tablespoon cornstarch**

1 **teaspoon pure vanilla extract**

¾ **teaspoon ground ginger**

½ **cup quick-cooking oats**

½ **cup whole grain pastry flour**

½ **cup sliced almonds**

3 **tablespoons unsalted butter**

1 Preheat the oven to 375°F. Coat a 2-quart baking dish with cooking spray.

2 In a large bowl, toss the peaches, blueberries, apricots, ½ cup of the sugar, the cornstarch, vanilla, and ginger. Pour into the prepared baking dish.

3 In another bowl, combine the oats, flour, almonds, butter, and the remaining ½ cup sugar. Rub together with fingers until the mixture resembles coarse crumbs and begins to form clumps when squeezed. Sprinkle over the peach mixture. Bake until the filling is thick and bubbling and the top is lightly golden, 35 minutes.

NUTRITION (PER SERVING): 313 calories, 5 g protein, 61 g carbohydrates, 5 g fiber, 46 g sugars, 8 g fat, 1 g saturated fat, 3 mg sodium

LEMON-RASPBERRY CHEESECAKE

PREP TIME: 15 MINUTES / TOTAL TIME: 2 HOURS + CHILLING TIME / **MAKES 8 SERVINGS**

Shown in photo insert pages.

¼ cup oat bran

¼ cup ground golden flaxseeds

½ teaspoon ground cinnamon

1½ cups 1% cottage cheese

¼ cup buttermilk

3 tablespoons whole grain flour

6 tablespoons honey

2 tablespoons fresh lemon juice

1½ teaspoons grated lemon zest

1 tablespoon pure vanilla extract

4 eggs, separated

1 pint raspberries

½ cup raspberry all-fruit spread

1. Preheat the oven to 350°F. Butter the bottom and sides of an 8" springform pan.

2. In a medium bowl, combine the oat bran, flaxseeds, and cinnamon and sprinkle the mixture into the pan, tilting the pan to lightly coat the sides. Press the crumbs into the bottom of the pan.

3. In a food processor, combine the cottage cheese, buttermilk, flour, honey, lemon juice, lemon zest, and vanilla and puree until smooth. Add the egg yolks and pulse to combine. Transfer to a large bowl.

4. In another large bowl, with an electric mixer on high speed, beat the egg whites until stiff peaks form. Gently fold the egg whites and raspberries into the cottage cheese mixture.

5. Pour the batter into the prepared pan. Drop the fruit spread by tablespoons onto the top of the batter. With a knife, swirl the spread into the batter. Bake until puffed and set, 40 minutes. Turn off the oven and open the door for 1 minute to reduce the heat. Close the door and let the cheesecake remain in the oven for 1 hour.

6. Refrigerate for 4 hours or overnight. Remove the pan sides before serving.

NUTRITION (PER SERVING): 225 calories, 11 g protein, 38g carbohydrates, 6 g fiber, 25 g sugars, 5 g fat, 1g saturated fat, 214 mg sodium

POMEGRANATE GREEN TEA ICE POPS

PREP TIME: 5 MINUTES / TOTAL TIME: 5 MINUTES + FREEZING TIME / MAKES 6 SERVINGS

½ cup pomegranate seeds

1½ cups unsweetened iced green tea

1½ cups pomegranate juice

1 In a medium bowl, combine the pomegranate seeds, tea, and juice.

2 Pour the mixture into six 4-ounce ice pop molds. Freeze for 4 hours or overnight.

NUTRITION (PER SERVING): 55 calories, 1 g protein, 13 g carbohydrates, 1 g fiber, 12 g sugars, 0 g fat, 0 g saturated fat, 8 mg sodium

HEALTHY HINT

What's more important, clean eating or exercise? A proper diet and regular exercise are the two pillars of a healthy lifestyle, but that doesn't mean they're equally important when it comes to your weight, your disease risk, or how long you'll live. An editorial in the medical journal *BMJ* suggests that what you eat trumps how much you move. Why? Researchers point to the fact that during the past 30 years, physical activity rates haven't changed even as obesity and diabetes rates have skyrocketed. Sugar and refined carbohydrates, they say, are the biggest drivers of poor health and obesity. That said, regular exercise is extremely important if you want to live a long, healthy life. Many studies have shown that physical activity helps safeguard your heart and brain from disease, including Alzheimer's; protects your joints; and even makes you more likely to stick to dietary changes.

OLIVE OIL ICE CREAM

PREP TIME: 30 MINUTES / TOTAL TIME: 30 MINUTES + CHILL TIME / **MAKES 4 SERVINGS**

1 cup 2% milk

1 cup heavy cream

4 tablespoons sugar, divided

1 egg yolk

2 tablespoons olive oil

1 In a saucepan over medium-low heat, bring the milk, cream, and 2 tablespoons of the sugar to a simmer. Turn off the heat and stir until the sugar is dissolved.

2 In a small bowl, whisk together the egg yolk and the remaining 2 tablespoons sugar until light in color, 1 minute.

3 Whisk 1 tablespoon of the warm milk mixture into the egg yolk mixture. Slowly whisk in another 3 tablespoons of the milk mixture.

4 Whisk the egg yolk mixture into the remaining milk mixture in the saucepan. Over medium heat, cook, stirring constantly, until the mixture coats the back of a spoon, about 3 minutes.

5 Whisk in the olive oil. Pour the mixture into a large bowl, cover with plastic wrap, and refrigerate until cooled, 4 hours or overnight. Process in an ice cream maker according to directions.

6 Transfer the ice cream to an airtight container and store in the freezer for at least 2 hours before serving.

NUTRITION (PER SERVING): 360 calories, 4 g protein, 17 g carbohydrates, 0 g fiber, 16 g sugars, 31 g fat, 16 g saturated fat, 54 mg sodium

CREPES WITH COCOA-HAZELNUT BUTTER AND BANANAS

PREP TIME: 15 MINUTES / TOTAL TIME: 1 HOUR 20 MINUTES / MAKES 4 SERVINGS

¼ cup water

I large egg, lightly beaten

¼ cup + 2 tablespoons 1% milk

I teaspoon pure vanilla extract

½ cup whole wheat flour

I tablespoon confectioners' sugar

¼ teaspoon ground cinnamon

Pinch of ground nutmeg

Pinch of salt

1½ tablespoons + I teaspoon unsalted butter, melted, divided

2 tablespoons Homemade Cocoa-Hazelnut Butter (page 278)

2 bananas, sliced

1 In a blender, combine the water, egg, milk, vanilla, flour, sugar, cinnamon, nutmeg, salt, and 1½ tablespoons of the melted butter. Pulse until blended and smooth, about 30 seconds. Refrigerate for at least 1 hour or up to 2 days.

2 Heat a nonstick medium skillet over medium-high heat. Add ¼ teaspoon of the melted butter to the pan. Pour ⅓ cup batter into the pan and swirl to spread evenly. Cook for 30 seconds on one side and 10 seconds on the other side. Set aside on a plate or cutting board. Repeat to make 4 crepes.

3 Spread ½ tablespoon of the Homemade Cocoa-Hazelnut Butter down the center of each crepe. Top with the banana slices. Roll the crepes around the filling.

NUTRITION (PER SERVING): 330 calories, 6 g protein, 31 g carbohydrates, 4 g fiber, 12 g sugars, 22 g fat, 11 g saturated fat, 77 mg sodium

APPETIZERS AND SNACKS

"PIGS" IN A BLANKET

PREP TIME: 15 MINUTES / TOTAL TIME: 25 MINUTES / **MAKES 6 SERVINGS**

Shown in photo insert pages.

I   tablespoon whole wheat flour, for dusting

½   pound store-bought whole wheat pizza dough

3   extra-lean, nitrate-free, 100% beef hot dogs, each cut into 4 pieces

I   tablespoon olive oil

4   tablespoons unsalted stone-ground mustard

1 Preheat the oven to 375°F. Line a baking sheet with parchment paper.

2 Lightly dust a clean work surface with the flour. Using a rolling pin, roll the dough into a circle about 12" in diameter. Using a pizza cutter, slice the dough into 12 wedges.

3 Beginning at the wide end of each slice, add 1 piece of hot dog and roll up each triangle to the opposite point. Place on the prepared baking sheet. (The ends of the hot dog pieces may or may not be covered, depending on the size of each piece of dough.) Brush the dough with the oil.

4 Bake until the dough is golden brown and the hot dog is heated through, 12 minutes. Serve with the mustard for dipping.

NUTRITION (PER SERVING): 166 calories, 5 g protein, 19 g carbohydrate, 1 g fiber, 1 g sugars, 7 g fat, 2 g sat fat, 502 mg sodium

CRAB CAKES WITH LEMON-DIJON SAUCE

PREP TIME: 20 MINUTES / TOTAL TIME: 30 MINUTES / **MAKES 4 SERVINGS**

2 tablespoons canola oil mayonnaise

1 tablespoon Dijon mustard

3 tablespoons fresh lemon juice, divided

1 clove garlic, minced

12 ounces lump crabmeat

2 scallions, finely chopped

½ red bell pepper, finely chopped

¼ cup plain 0% Greek yogurt

1 egg, lightly beaten

¼ teaspoon crab-boil seasoning

½ cup whole wheat panko bread crumbs, divided

1 In a small bowl, whisk together the mayonnaise, mustard, 1 tablespoon of the lemon juice, and garlic. Refrigerate until ready to serve.

2 Preheat the oven to 425°F. Coat a baking sheet with cooking spray.

3 In a large bowl, combine the crabmeat, scallions, pepper, yogurt, egg, the remaining 2 tablespoons lemon juice, seasoning, and ¼ cup of the bread crumbs. With your hands, loosely form the crab mixture into 8 cakes.

4 Spread the remaining ¼ cup bread crumbs on a plate and roll each crab cake in the crumbs to lightly coat. As the cakes are formed, place on the prepared baking sheet. If the patties are misshapen, use the palm of your hand to shape into a circle the size of a small hockey puck.

5 Bake, turning once, until golden brown, about 15 minutes. Serve the cakes with the mayonnaise mixture.

NUTRITION (PER SERVING): 196 calories, 20 g protein, 11 g carbohydrate, 2 g fiber, 2 g sugars, 8 g fat, 1 g sat fat, 514 mg sodium

BUFFALO CHICKEN QUESADILLAS

PREP TIME: 10 MINUTES / TOTAL TIME: 25 MINUTES / MAKES 4 SERVINGS

1   cooked boneless, skinless chicken breast (6 ounces), finely shredded or chopped

1   cup no-salt-added canned black beans, rinsed and drained

½   cup reduced-fat Cheddar Jack cheese

¼   cup reduced-fat blue cheese crumbles

2   scallions, thinly sliced

1   rib celery, finely chopped

½   to 1 tablespoon hot red-pepper sauce

4   whole wheat tortillas (8" diameter)

1   In a small bowl, combine the chicken, beans, Cheddar Jack cheese, blue cheese, scallions, celery, and red-pepper sauce.

2   Arrange the tortillas on a work surface. Divide the chicken mixture among the tortillas, spreading over the lower half of each tortilla. Fold the top half over the filling to form a semicircle.

3   Heat a large nonstick skillet over medium heat. Cook 2 tortillas at a time, turning once, until lightly browned and heated through, 5 minutes. Transfer to a cutting board and cook the remaining tortillas. Cut each into 3 pieces.

NUTRITION (PER SERVING): 159 calories, 15 g protein, 21 g carbohydrates, 4 g fiber, 1 g sugars, 4 g fat, 2 g saturated fat, 483 mg sodium

SPINACH-ARTICHOKE DIP

PREP TIME: 20 MINUTES / TOTAL TIME: 40 MINUTES / **MAKES 12 SERVINGS**

Shown in photo insert pages.

1	cup plain Greek yogurt
¾	package (6 ounces) Neufchâtel cheese, softened
3	cloves garlic, minced
2	tablespoons stone-ground mustard
⅛	teaspoon paprika
¼	cup grated Parmesan cheese, divided
1	small red onion, finely chopped
1	package (9 ounces) frozen artichoke hearts, thawed, squeezed dry, and chopped
1	package (10 ounces) frozen chopped spinach, thawed and squeezed dry
	Veggies or unsalted tortilla chips (for serving)

1 Preheat the oven to 350°F.

2 In a large bowl, stir together the yogurt, Neufchâtel cheese, garlic, mustard, paprika, and ⅛ cup of the Parmesan cheese. Add the onion, artichoke hearts, and spinach, and stir to combine.

3 Pour into an 8" x 8" baking dish. Top with the remaining ⅛ cup Parmesan cheese.

4 Bake until bubbling hot, 20 minutes. Serve with the veggies or unsalted tortilla chips.

NUTRITION (PER SERVING): 78 calories, 5 g protein, 5 g carbohydrates, 2 g fiber, 2 g sugars, 4 g fat, 2 g saturated fat, 189 mg sodium

LEMONY ROSEMARY WHITE BEAN DIP

PREP TIME: 5 MINUTES / TOTAL TIME: 5 MINUTES / MAKES 8 SERVINGS (2 TABLESPOONS EACH)

Shown in photo insert pages.

- 1 can (15 ounces) low- or no-sodium white beans, rinsed and drained
- 1 clove garlic, roughly chopped
- 1 tablespoon water
- 2 teaspoons fresh lemon juice
- 1 teaspoon lemon zest
- ¼ teaspoon salt
- 1 tablespoon + ¼ teaspoon extra-virgin olive oil or walnut oil, divided
- 1 teaspoon finely chopped fresh rosemary

1 In a food processor, combine the beans, garlic, water, lemon juice, lemon zest, salt, and 1 tablespoon of the oil. Process until smooth.

2 Add the rosemary to the food processor and pulse to combine.

3 Transfer to a serving dish and drizzle with the remaining ¼ teaspoon oil. Store in an airtight container in the refrigerator for up to 5 days.

NUTRITION (PER SERVING): 64 calories, 3 g protein, 9 g carbohydrates, 2 g fiber, 0 g sugars, 2 g fat, 0 g saturated fat, 51 mg sodium

CHANGE IT UP! Use the dip as a sandwich spread, or toss it with whole grain pasta, using a little of the pasta cooking water to thin it.

SPICED SWEET POTATO CHIPS

PREP TIME: 5 MINUTES / TOTAL TIME: 25 MINUTES / **MAKES 4 SERVINGS**

1 tablespoon olive oil

1 tablespoon pure maple syrup

1 teaspoon ground cumin

½ teaspoon black pepper

¼ teaspoon salt

2 sweet potatoes, cut into ⅛" slices

1 Preheat the oven to 375°F. Line 2 large baking sheets with parchment paper.

2 In a large bowl, whisk together the oil, maple syrup, cumin, pepper, and salt. Add the sweet potatoes and toss to coat.

3 Arrange the potatoes in a single layer on the prepared baking sheets. Bake, turning once, until golden and crisp, 20 minutes.

NUTRITION (PER SERVING): 101 calories, 1 g protein, 17 g carbohydrates, 2 g fiber, 6 g sugars, 4 g fat, 1 g saturated fat, 110 mg sodium

SALT-N-VINEGAR POTATO CHIPS

PREP TIME: 20 MINUTES / TOTAL TIME: 1 HOUR 25 MINUTES / MAKES 4 SERVINGS

2　russet (baking) potatoes, thinly sliced using a mandoline or vegetable peeler

2½　cups white vinegar

1　tablespoon olive oil

½　teaspoon salt

1　In a large bowl, combine the potatoes and vinegar and cover for 1 hour. Drain.

2　Preheat the oven to 400°F. Lightly coat 2 large baking sheets with cooking spray.

3　Arrange the potatoes in a single layer on the prepared baking sheets. Drizzle the potato slices with the oil and toss to coat. Arrange in a single layer. Sprinkle with the salt. Bake, turning once, until the chips are golden and crisp, 8 minutes.

NUTRITION (PER SERVING): 116 calories, 2 g protein, 19 g carbohydrates, 1 g fiber, 1 g sugars, 4 g fat, 1 g saturated fat, 202 mg sodium

CHILI-LIME KALE CHIPS

PREP TIME: 10 MINUTES / TOTAL TIME: 25 MINUTES / **MAKES 2 SERVINGS**

6   cups fresh kale roughly torn into 1" pieces
    (tough ribs removed)

1   tablespoon grapeseed oil

⅛   teaspoon salt

⅛   teaspoon chili powder

1   teaspoon grated lime zest

1 Preheat the oven to 350°F. Lightly oil a baking sheet or line with parchment paper.

2 In a large bowl, combine the kale, oil, and salt. With your hands, massage the oil and salt into the kale until evenly coated.

3 Arrange the kale in a single layer on the prepared baking sheet. Bake until crispy, 15 minutes.

4 Sprinkle with the chili powder and lime zest. If desired, season with additional salt and chili powder to taste.

NUTRITION (PER SERVING): 160 calories, 9 g protein, 18 g carbohydrates, 4 g fiber, 0 g sugars, 9 g fat, 1 g saturated fat, 197 mg sodium

HEALTHY HINT

With a dehydrator, you can morph any veggie into a "chip" without the need for loads of added oil. A food dehydrator with adjustable temperature control (which is what you want) will run you around $80, but with quality veggie chips going for around $8 per pound at Whole Foods Market and similar stores, that will pay for itself quickly.

SALT AND PEPPER KALE CHIPS

PREP TIME: 10 MINUTES / TOTAL TIME: 25 MINUTES / MAKES 2 SERVINGS

6 cups fresh kale roughly torn into I" pieces (tough ribs removed)

I tablespoon grapeseed oil

⅛ teaspoon salt

⅛ teaspoon black pepper

1 Preheat the oven to 350°F. Lightly oil a baking sheet or line with parchment paper.

2 In a large bowl, combine the kale, oil, and salt. With your hands, massage the oil and salt into the kale until evenly coated.

3 Arrange the kale in a single layer on the prepared baking sheet. Bake until crispy, 15 minutes.

4 Sprinkle with the pepper.

NUTRITION (PER SERVING): 159 calories, 9 g protein, 18 g carbohydrates, 4 g fiber, 0 g sugars, 9 g fat, 1 g saturated fat, 196 mg sodium

HEALTHY HINT

Spot sneaky trans fats. The label on your box of multigrain crackers may claim to have 0 grams of trans fats, but don't be fooled—read the ingredient list. This lab-made fat that's been linked to diabetes and heart disease is still found in I in I0 packaged foods, according to recent research, even if the label says it doesn't contain any. How can that be? Companies are allowed to say a food has 0 grams if it contains less than 0.5 gram per serving. Until 2018—when companies and restaurants will no longer be able to use trans fats in their foods—avoid products with "partially hydrogenated oils" in the ingredient list.

CINNAMON-SUGAR PITA CHIPS

PREP TIME: 5 MINUTES / TOTAL TIME: 20 MINUTES / **MAKES 2 SERVINGS**

2 teaspoons grapeseed oil

1 teaspoon unsalted butter, melted

1 teaspoon light brown sugar

¼ teaspoon ground cinnamon

⅛ teaspoon salt

1 large whole wheat pita (6" to 7"), cut into 8 wedges

1 Preheat the oven to 350°F.

2 In a small bowl, combine the oil, butter, sugar, cinnamon, and salt.

3 Gently split each pita wedge into 2 triangles.

4 Brush both sides of each triangle with the oil mixture. Spread in a single layer on a baking sheet. Bake, turning once, until the chips are lightly browned and crisp, 15 minutes.

NUTRITION (PER SERVING): 152 calories, 3 g protein, 20 g carbohydrates, 3 g fiber, 3 g sugars, 7 g fat, 2 g saturated fat, 241 mg sodium

PITA CHIPS WITH OLIVE OIL AND SEA SALT

PREP TIME: 5 MINUTES / TOTAL TIME: 20 MINUTES / **MAKES 2 SERVINGS**

I   tablespoon olive oil

⅛   teaspoon garlic powder

I   large whole wheat pita (6" to 7"), cut into 8 wedges

¼   teaspoon sea salt

1 Preheat the oven to 350°F.

2 In a small bowl, combine the oil and garlic powder.

3 Gently split each pita wedge into 2 triangles.

4 Brush both sides of the triangles with the oil mixture. Spread in a single layer on a baking sheet. Sprinkle with the sea salt. Bake, turning once, until the chips are lightly browned and crisp, 15 to 20 minutes.

NUTRITION (PER SERVING): 145 calories, 3 g protein, 18 g carbohydrates, 2 g fiber, 0 g sugars, 8 g fat, 1 g saturated fat, 339 mg sodium

SWEET CHILI PITA CHIPS

PREP TIME: 5 MINUTES / TOTAL TIME: 35 MINUTES / MAKES 2 SERVINGS

2   teaspoons olive oil

¼   teaspoon light brown sugar

¼   teaspoon ground cumin

¼   teaspoon chili powder

¼   teaspoon garlic powder

⅛   teaspoon salt

l   large whole wheat pita (6" to 7"), cut into 8 wedges

1 Preheat the oven to 350°F.

2 In a small bowl, combine the oil, sugar, cumin, chili powder, garlic powder, and salt.

3 Gently split each pita wedge into 2 triangles.

4 Brush both sides of the triangles with the oil mixture. Spread in a single layer on a baking sheet. Bake, turning once, until the chips are lightly browned and crisp, 15 minutes.

NUTRITION (PER SERVING): 131 calories, 3 g protein, 19 g carbohydrates, 3 g fiber, 1 g sugars, 6 g fat, 1 g saturated fat, 263 mg sodium

HEALTHY HINT

Try to always pair pita chips with a healthy dip, such as guacamole or hummus. Both have either protein or fat and fiber—nutrients that can help stabilize the blood sugar spike you can get by eating the carbs in chips, and thus help minimize subsequent cravings.

GREMOLATA PARMESAN POPCORN

PREP TIME: 5 MINUTES / TOTAL TIME: 10 MINUTES / MAKES 2 SERVINGS

½   cup popcorn kernels (or 10 cups clean, store-bought, plain air-popped popcorn)

¼   cup chopped fresh parsley

1   small clove garlic, minced

½   teaspoon lemon zest

1   tablespoon finely grated Parmesan cheese

1   teaspoon grapeseed oil

½   teaspoon salt

1 If you're popping your own popcorn with an air popper, pop the kernels per the machine directions.

2 If you're popping your own popcorn in the microwave oven, pop the kernels in a 2- to 3-quart microwaveable bowl. Completely cover the bowl with a microwaveable plate. Microwave on high until the popping slows down to 3 to 4 seconds between each pop, about 4 minutes. Using a pot holder, carefully remove the plate, avoiding the steam escaping from the bowl. Remove the bowl from the microwave and let cool slightly.

3 On a cutting board, pile the parsley, garlic, lemon zest, and cheese on top of each other and finely chop together to make the gremolata.

4 Toss the popcorn with the oil. Add the gremolata and salt, and toss until coated.

NUTRITION (PER SERVING): 41 calories, 1 g protein, 2 g carbohydrates, 1 g fiber, 0 g sugars, 3 g fat, 1 g saturated fat, 333 mg sodium

Savory Variations

Toss the popcorn with the grapeseed oil and try one of the following flavor combinations for a tasty alternative.

Chive and Cheese: Snipped chives, garlic powder, Parmesan (or some other clean cheese)

Lemon-Dill: Dried dill, grated lemon zest

Chili Lime: Chili powder, lime zest

Sweet Variations

Toss the popcorn with the grapeseed oil and try one of the following flavor combinations for a tasty alternative.

Sweet Popcorn: Either cocoa powder or cocoa nibs, drizzle of honey

Bombay Blend: Garam masala, toasted coconut flakes

Maple Cracker Jack: Peanuts, pumpkin pie spice, drizzle of pure maple syrup

ROSEMARY AND SUNFLOWER SEED OAT CRACKERS

PREP TIME: 5 MINUTES / TOTAL TIME: 15 MINUTES / **MAKES 50 CRACKERS**

⅓ cup whole wheat flour

⅓ cup rolled oats

¼ teaspoon salt

½ teaspoon dried rosemary, divided

1 tablespoon sunflower oil

½ teaspoon honey

3 tablespoons water

¼ cup + 1 tablespoon sunflower seeds, divided

1 Preheat the oven to 425°F.

2 In a medium bowl, combine the flour, oats, salt, and ¼ teaspoon of the rosemary.

3 Stir in the oil, honey, and water. Mix with your hands until a sticky dough forms. Knead in ¼ cup of the sunflower seeds. Form the dough into a ball, adding more flour if needed to make the dough dry enough to handle.

4 Lightly flour a work surface, and with a rolling pin, roll out the dough as thin as possible. (Aim for the thickness of a tortilla.)

5 Brush the surface lightly with water and sprinkle on the remaining 1 tablespoon sunflower seeds and ¼ teaspoon rosemary. Cut into 1" squares. Prick the center of each cracker with a skewer to make one or more holes, if desired.

6 Bake the crackers on a baking sheet until crisp and golden, 8 minutes. Cool on a wire rack.

NUTRITION (PER SERVING): 13 calories, 0 g protein, 1 g carbohydrates, 0 g fiber, 0 g sugars, 1 g fat, 0 g saturated fat, 8 mg sodium

PUMPKIN SEED, CHERRY, AND PECAN GRANOLA BARS

PREP TIME: 10 MINUTES / TOTAL TIME: 35 MINUTES + 30 MINUTES COOLING TIME / **MAKES 10 SERVINGS**

- 2 cups rolled oats
- ⅓ cup pumpkin seeds
- ⅓ cup chopped pecans
- ¼ cup unsweetened shredded coconut
- ½ cup dried cherries
- 2 tablespoons hemp seeds
- ¾ teaspoon ground cinnamon
- ¼ teaspoon salt
- ⅓ cup honey
- ¼ cup almond butter
- 3 tablespoons coconut oil
- I teaspoon pure vanilla extract

1 Preheat the oven to 350°F. Lightly coat an 8" x 8" baking pan with oil and line the bottom with parchment paper.

2 On a large rimmed baking sheet, combine the oats, pumpkin seeds, pecans, and coconut. Toast, stirring twice, until lightly browned and fragrant, 5 minutes.

3 Meanwhile, in a large bowl, stir together the cherries, hemp seeds, cinnamon, and salt. Stir in the toasted oats, nuts, and seeds.

4 In a small microwaveable bowl, combine the honey, almond butter, oil, and vanilla. Microwave to warm the mixture, 30 seconds. Stir to blend and pour over the dry ingredients, tossing to coat.

5 Spread the mixture in the prepared pan and bake until the bars are lightly golden on top, 20 minutes.

6 Cool on a wire rack. Cut into 10 rectangular bars.

NUTRITION (PER SERVING): 212 calories, 4 g protein, 18 g carbohydrates, 2 g fiber, 14 g sugars, 14 g fat, 6 g saturated fat, 65 mg sodium

PEANUT BUTTER BARS

PREP TIME: 5 MINUTES / TOTAL TIME: 10 MINUTES + CHILLING / **MAKES 8 SERVINGS**

¼ cup creamy peanut butter

3 tablespoons honey

2 teaspoons pure vanilla extract

1½ cups whole grain O's cereal

1 Line an 8" x 8" baking pan with parchment paper.

2 In a medium saucepan over medium heat, combine the peanut butter, honey, and vanilla. Cook, stirring, until well combined, 3 minutes. Remove from the heat and gently stir in the cereal, tossing until well coated.

3 Spread the mixture into the prepared pan, pressing to smooth.

4 Chill for at least 1 hour before cutting into 8 bars. Store in an airtight container.

NUTRITION (PER SERVING): 89 calories, 2 g protein, 12 g carbohydrates, 1 g fiber, 8 g sugars, 4 g fat, 1 g saturated fat, 59 mg sodium

CHOCOLATE CHIP COOKIE DOUGH ENERGY BITES

PREP TIME: 10 MINUTES / TOTAL TIME: 1 HOUR 10 MINUTES / **MAKES 10 SERVINGS**

I   cup rolled oats

¼   cup unsweetened shredded coconut

⅓   cup chopped dates

¼   cup pure maple syrup

¼   cup cashew butter

3   tablespoons unsweetened vanilla almond milk

I   teaspoon pure vanilla extract

½   cup mini chocolate chips

1 In a blender or food processor, pulse the oats and coconut until ground. Add the dates, maple syrup, cashew butter, almond milk, and vanilla, and pulse until combined.

2 Stir in the chocolate chips.

3 Line a plate with parchment paper. Roll the dough into 10 balls and place the balls on the plate.

4 Chill for 1 hour before serving. Store in an airtight container in the refrigerator.

NUTRITION (PER SERVING): 164 calories, 3 g protein, 22 g carbohydrates, 2 g fiber, 14 g sugars, 8 g fat, 3 g saturated fat, 32 mg sodium

MEXICAN CHOCOLATE POPCORN BALLS

PREP TIME: 5 MINUTES / TOTAL TIME: 30 MINUTES / MAKES 4 SERVINGS

Shown in photo insert pages.

⅓   **cup honey**

2   **tablespoons light brown sugar**

2½   **tablespoons unsweetened cocoa powder**

½   **teaspoon ground cinnamon**

1¼   **teaspoons ground red pepper**

    Pinch of salt

5   **cups stove-top popped popcorn**

1 In a small saucepan over medium heat, cook the honey, sugar, cocoa, cinnamon, ground red pepper, and salt until simmering. Reduce the heat to low. Simmer, uncovered, until the mixture darkens and thickens, about 2 minutes.

2 In a large bowl, place the popcorn. Pour the honey mixture over the popcorn, tossing with a rubber spatula to coat well.

3 With hands coated with olive oil, form the mixture into 4 balls, pressing gently to stick. Let stand for at least 20 minutes to firm up.

NUTRITION (PER BALL): 180 calories, 2 g protein, 38 g carbohydrates, 2 g fiber, 30 g sugars, 4 g fat, 1 g saturated fat, 43 mg sodium

HEALTHY HINT

Next time you want to add some cheesy flavor to your popcorn, skip the Parmesan and try sprinkling your snack with nutritional yeast. This gluten- and dairy-free powder, which is simply vitamin-fortified inactive yeast made from cane or beet molasses, is packed with B vitamins and 6 grams of protein in every 45-calorie ¼ cup. (Compare that to the 110 calories in the same amount of Parmesan.)

DRESSINGS, SAUCES, SPREADS, AND BROTHS

CILANTRO-PEAR VINAIGRETTE

PREP TIME: 5 MINUTES / TOTAL TIME: 5 MINUTES / **MAKES 6 SERVINGS**

½   **cup fresh cilantro**

I   **small pear, cored and quartered**

I   **clove garlic, peeled**

    Juice of I lemon

2   **tablespoons white wine vinegar**

¼   **teaspoon salt**

½   **cup extra-virgin olive oil**

1 In a blender or food processor, combine the cilantro, pear, garlic, lemon juice, vinegar, and salt. Puree until smooth.

2 With the machine running on low speed, drizzle in the oil until well blended and thickened. Store in an airtight container in the refrigerator for up to 4 days. Shake to blend, if settling occurs.

NUTRITION (PER SERVING): 185 calories, 0 g protein, 5 g carbohydrates, 1 g fiber, 3 g sugars, 19 g fat, 3 g saturated fat, 66 mg sodium

HEALTHY HINT

Stuck in a rut and always reaching for olive oil when you make a dressing or marinade? One of the simplest ways to mix up the flavor and nutrition profile of any dressing is by switching up the oils. Some of the most flavorful (and healthiest) options include avocado, walnut, flax, and safflower.

ORANGE-MISO SALAD DRESSING

¼ cup fresh orange juice

1 tablespoon sunflower seed oil

1 tablespoon gluten-free, reduced-sodium tamari

1 tablespoon rice wine vinegar

2 teaspoons white miso paste

1 teaspoon toasted sesame oil

½ teaspoon minced garlic

In a jar with tight-fitting lid, combine the orange juice, sunflower seed oil, tamari, vinegar, miso, sesame oil, and garlic. Shake to blend. Store in an airtight container in the refrigerator for up to 1 week.

NUTRITION (PER SERVING): 35 calories, 1 g protein, 1 g carbohydrates, 0 g fiber, 1 g sugars, 3 g fat, 0 g saturated fat, 167 mg sodium

HEALTHY HINT

Ever wonder what that "No HPP" label on your juice bottle means? It means that drink hasn't been subjected to high pressure processing (HPP), a cold pasteurization technique that prevents bacterial growth and extends shelf life. Some juice brands claim that HPP makes a product less fresh and causes beneficial enzymes and nutrients to degrade. Right now, you'll only see this label on superfresh juices sold in juice bars or the stores where they're made.

CREAMY GREEN GODDESS DRESSING

PREP TIME: 5 MINUTES / TOTAL TIME: 5 MINUTES / MAKES 8 SERVINGS

½ avocado, pitted and peeled

½ cup scallion greens

½ cup fresh parsley

½ cup fresh dill

½ cup cilantro

½ cup water

¼ cup rice wine vinegar

¼ cup olive oil

2 tablespoons mayonnaise

I clove garlic, peeled

½ teaspoon salt

In a blender or food processor, combine the avocado, scallion greens, parsley, dill, cilantro, water, vinegar, oil, mayonnaise, garlic, and salt. Process until smooth. Store in an airtight container in the refrigerator for up to 4 days.

NUTRITION (PER SERVING): 107 calories, 1 g protein, 2 g carbohydrates, 1 g fiber, 0 g sugars, 11 g fat, 2 g saturated fat, 146 mg sodium

> **CHANGE IT UP!** Serve over salad or use for dipping vegetables.

HEALTHY HINT

For an even healthier sandwich, consider spreading your bread with hummus or guacamole. Either spread will increase your protein and fiber intake while adding a bit of Mediterranean or Mexican flair.

GARLIC AND ONION SANDWICH SPREAD

PREP TIME: 5 MINUTES / TOTAL TIME: 5 MINUTES / MAKES 2 SERVINGS

2   tablespoons mayonnaise

2   tablespoons 2% plain Greek yogurt

I   teaspoon dried or fresh chives

¼   teaspoon garlic powder

¼   teaspoon onion powder

⅛   teaspoon salt

In a small bowl, stir together the mayonnaise, yogurt, chives, garlic powder, onion powder, and salt. Store leftovers in an airtight container in the refrigerator for 4 days.

NUTRITION (PER SERVING): 106 calories, 1 g protein, 1 g carbohydrates, 0 g fiber, 1 g sugars, 11 g fat, 2 g saturated fat, 213 mg sodium

CHANGE IT UP! Spread on a sandwich or use as a dipping sauce for veggies.

HEALTHY HINT

Canola oil has gotten a bad rap over the years, but it is actually one of the most heart-healthy oils out there. Canola oil is actually higher in anti-inflammatory omega-3s than most vegetable oils (including olive oil!), which may help reduce your risk of inflammatory illnesses such as heart disease and cancer. The reason it's misunderstood is that much of it is produced from genetically modified plants, and it's extracted with the chemical solvent hexane. You can avoid these questionable practices and reap canola's benefits by buying organic expeller-pressed canola oil.

OLIVE OIL MAYO

PREP TIME: 5 MINUTES / TOTAL TIME: 5 MINUTES / MAKES 6 SERVINGS (1 TABLESPOON EACH)

I   large egg, at room temperature

I   tablespoon fresh lemon juice

I   teaspoon stone-ground mustard

¼   teaspoon salt

¼   teaspoon garlic powder

¼   cup extra-virgin olive oil

1 In a food processor, combine the egg, lemon juice, mustard, salt, and garlic powder. Pulse on high for 10 seconds.

2 With the machine running, drizzle in the oil and blend for 30 seconds. Refrigerate to set and store in a sealed container in the refrigerator for up to 1 week.

NUTRITION (PER SERVING): 16 calories, 1 g protein, 1 g carbohydrates, 0 g fiber, 0 g sugars, 1 g fat, 0 g saturated fat, 112 mg sodium

NOTE: Alternatively, you could place all of the ingredients in a cup or narrow bowl and use an immersion blender. Or whisk by hand in a bowl until thick and creamy.

CITRUS GARLIC AIOLI

PREP TIME: 5 MINUTES / TOTAL TIME: 5 MINUTES / MAKES 6 SERVINGS

½ **cup unsalted raw cashews**

½ **cup low-fat plain yogurt**

1 **tablespoon minced garlic**

1 **teaspoon fresh lemon juice**

1 **teaspoon fresh lime juice**

½ **teaspoon grated lemon zest**

1 In a food processor, process the cashews until they start to form a paste, scraping down the sides every few minutes.

2 Add the yogurt, garlic, lemon juice, lime juice, and lemon zest. Season with salt and pepper to taste. Process until thoroughly combined and smooth. Store in an airtight container in the refrigerator for up to 1 week.

NUTRITION (PER SERVING): 82 calories, 3 g protein, 6 g carbohydrates, 1 g fiber, 2 g sugars, 6 g fat, 1 g saturated fat, 57 mg sodium

CHANGE IT UP! Use as a sandwich spread or dipping sauce.

SPICY GINGER-SOY BBQ SAUCE

PREP TIME: 5 MINUTES / TOTAL TIME: 5 MINUTES / MAKES 8 SERVINGS (3 TABLESPOONS EACH)

1   cup canned tomato sauce

¼   cup gluten-free, reduced-sodium tamari

2   tablespoons honey

1   tablespoon fresh lime juice

1   teaspoon smoked paprika

1   teaspoon onion powder

1   teaspoon garlic powder

1   teaspoon ground red pepper

1" piece fresh ginger, grated

In a medium bowl, whisk together the tomato sauce, tamari, honey, lime juice, paprika, onion powder, garlic powder, ground red pepper, and ginger until well blended. Store in an airtight container in the refrigerator for up to 1 week.

NUTRITION (PER SERVING): 36 calories, 2 g protein, 8 g carbohydrates, 1 g fiber, 6 g sugars, 0 g fat, 0 g saturated fat, 512 mg sodium

SPICY GINGER-ALMOND SAUCE

PREP TIME: 5 MINUTES / TOTAL TIME: 5 MINUTES / MAKES 5 SERVINGS (2 TABLESPOONS EACH)

¼ cup almond butter

3 tablespoons canned lite coconut milk

2 tablespoons gluten-free, reduced-sodium tamari

1 teaspoon honey

½ teaspoon minced fresh ginger

¼ teaspoon minced garlic

¼ teaspoon Sriracha sauce

¼ teaspoon toasted sesame oil

In a small bowl, whisk together the almond butter, coconut milk, tamari, honey, ginger, garlic, Sriracha, and oil. Store in an airtight container in the refrigerator for up to 1 week.

NUTRITION (PER SERVING): 93 calories, 3 g protein, 4 g carbohydrates, 1 g fiber, 2 g sugars, 8 g fat, 1 g saturated fat, 414 mg sodium

CHANGE IT UP! Serve as a sauce, dip, or sandwich spread.

KALE PESTO

PREP TIME: 10 MINUTES / TOTAL TIME: 10 MINUTES / **MAKES 12 SERVINGS**

½ cup slivered almonds

I clove garlic

10 ounces roughly chopped and stemmed fresh kale

½ cup loosely packed fresh basil leaves

½ cup grated Parmesan cheese

¾ cup extra-virgin olive oil

¼ cup water

1 In a blender or food processor, pulse the almonds and garlic to make small, even, crumb-size pieces.

2 Add the kale, basil, and cheese. Pulse until thoroughly combined.

3 With the machine running, drizzle in the oil and water. Process until well blended and light green. Store in an airtight container in the refrigerator for up to 1 week.

NUTRITION (PER SERVING): 132 calories, 3 g protein, 3 g carbohydrates, 1 g fiber, 0 g sugars, 13 g fat, 2 g saturated fat, 60 mg sodium

NOTE: Serve this over zucchini noodles, spaghetti squash, or pasta.

TOMATO-BASIL MARINARA

PREP TIME: 10 MINUTES / TOTAL TIME: 40 MINUTES / MAKES 4 SERVINGS

1½ tablespoons olive oil

1½ cups diced onion

3 cloves garlic, chopped

¼ teaspoon dried oregano

½ teaspoon salt

½ teaspoon black pepper

1 can (28 ounces) whole peeled tomatoes

¼ teaspoon red-pepper flakes

½ cup fresh basil leaves, roughly torn

1 In a medium saucepan over medium heat, warm the olive oil. Cook the onion until soft, 15 minutes.

2 Stir in the garlic, oregano, salt, and black pepper. Cook until the garlic is fragrant, 1 minute.

3 Add the tomatoes and, using a potato masher, gently crush the tomatoes. Add the red-pepper flakes and basil leaves, and stir to combine. Let simmer, partially covered, until the sauce thickens, 25 minutes.

4 With an immersion blender, blend the sauce to your desired consistency in the saucepan.

NUTRITION (PER SERVING): 114 calories, 3 g protein, 16 g carbohydrates, 3 g fiber, 7 g sugars, 6 g fat, 1 g saturated fat, 528 mg sodium

NOTE: If you don't have an immersion blender, use a blender or food processor and work in batches.

CHANGE IT UP! Make a quick and super healthy "cream" sauce by using pureed avocado instead of dairy products. Simply combine 1 large avocado, 4 teaspoons lemon juice, and ¼ cup hot water in a blender or food processor. Puree until smooth, toss with pasta, and enjoy!

HOMEMADE COCOA-HAZELNUT BUTTER

PREP TIME: 15 MINUTES / TOTAL TIME: 15 MINUTES / MAKES 6 SERVINGS

1 cup unsalted, dry-roasted, skinned hazelnuts

2 tablespoons honey

1 tablespoon pure vanilla extract

1 teaspoon coconut or grapeseed oil

¼ cup + 2 tablespoons soy or nut milk

3 tablespoons unsweetened cocoa powder

Pinch of salt

1 In a food processor, grind the hazelnuts to a fine powder, scraping down the sides every few minutes, about 5 minutes. With the processor running, slowly add the honey, vanilla, and oil, and process for 5 minutes, scraping down the sides frequently.

2 Add the milk and process until smooth, 2 minutes. Add the cocoa and salt. Process until creamy, 5 minutes. Store in a glass jar in the refrigerator for up to 1 week.

NUTRITION (PER 2-TABLESPOON SERVING): 193 calories, 4 g protein, 12 g carbohydrates, 3 g fiber, 8 g sugars, 15 g fat, 2 g saturated fat, 28 mg sodium

HEALTHY HINT

Enjoying nut butters such as peanut, almond, or this delicious one on your whole grain English muffin in the morning is a great way to curb cravings throughout the day. Research has found that consuming nut butters at breakfast has a profound impact on your blood sugar, keeping it stable past lunch and achieving what's called the "second meal effect."

SPICED PEACH BUTTER

PREP TIME: 35 MINUTES / TOTAL TIME: 2 HOURS 35 MINUTES / **MAKES 12 SERVINGS**

2 **pounds frozen sliced peaches**
¼ **cup + 2 tablespoons water**
½ **cup honey**
1½ **teaspoons ground cinnamon**
¼ **teaspoon ground nutmeg**
¼ **teaspoon ground ginger**

1 In a medium saucepan over medium heat, combine the peaches and water. Bring to a boil, stirring occasionally. Reduce the heat to low. Cover and simmer until the peaches are soft, about 20 minutes. Stir in the honey, cinnamon, nutmeg, and ginger.

2 In a food processor or blender, process or blend the peach mixture until smooth.

3 Return to the saucepan over very low heat and cook, stirring frequently, until thick enough to cling to a spoon when the spoon is turned upside down, up to 2 hours. Store in an airtight container in the refrigerator for up to 2 weeks.

NUTRITION (PER SERVING): 71 calories, 1 g protein, 19 g carbohydrates, 1 g fiber, 18 g sugars, 0 g fat, 0 g saturated fat, 0 mg sodium

HEALTHY HINT

Want to eat fresh peaches year-round without leaving a big carbon footprint? Freeze 'em yourself when they're in season! Simply halve, pit, and slice them into wedges. Place them on a parchment-lined baking sheet, freeze until firm, transfer to a freezer bag, and label. Voilà! Your summer's bounty, preserved at its peak.

RASPBERRY CHIA JAM

PREP TIME: 5 MINUTES / TOTAL TIME: 35 MINUTES / MAKES 8 SERVINGS

3 cups fresh or frozen raspberries

3 tablespoons orange juice

2 tablespoons chia seeds

½ teaspoon pure vanilla extract

1 In a medium saucepan, combine the raspberries, orange juice, and chia seeds. Bring to a boil over medium heat. Reduce the heat to low and simmer, uncovered, until the raspberries break down and the mixture thickens, 10 minutes.

2 Remove from the heat and stir in the vanilla. Let cool for 20 minutes. (The jam will thicken as it cools.) If you prefer a smoother jam, use an immersion blender to puree the mixture to the desired consistency. Store in an airtight container in the refrigerator for up to 2 weeks.

NUTRITION (PER SERVING): 40 calories, 1 g protein, 7 g carbohydrates, 4 g fiber, 3 g sugars, 1 g fat, 0 g saturated fat, 1 mg sodium

HEALTHY HINT

Since sugar acts as a preservative, spreads made from fruit only will spoil more quickly than jams and jellies that include sweeteners. Most fruit-only spreads include expiration dates on the jars and recommend using within I month of opening. To prevent early spoilage, keep your spreads in the back of the refrigerator, where it's colder, not in a door shelves compartment.

HOMEMADE BONE BROTH

PREP TIME: 10 MINUTES / TOTAL TIME: 6 HOURS / MAKES 6 CUPS

Bones from I whole roasted chicken
2   carrots, coarsely chopped
2   ribs celery, coarsely chopped
I   onion, coarsely chopped
2   cloves garlic, crushed
I   bay leaf
¾   teaspoon salt
¼   teaspoon dried rosemary
¼   teaspoon dried thyme
IO cups water

1. In a large stockpot or Dutch over, combine the bones, carrots, celery, onion, garlic, bay leaf, salt, rosemary, thyme, and water. Bring to a boil over high heat. Reduce the heat to low, cover, and simmer for 6 hours.

2. Place a sieve or colander over a large bowl. Pour the broth through the sieve or colander. Discard the solids.

NUTRITION (PER I CUP): 86 calories, 6 g protein, 8 g carbohydrates, 0 g fiber, 4 g sugars, 3 g fat, 1 g saturated fat, 343 mg sodium

HOMEMADE VEGETABLE BROTH

PREP TIME: 10 MINUTES / TOTAL TIME: 4 HOURS / MAKES 6 CUPS

2   ribs celery, coarsely chopped

I   carrot, coarsely chopped

I   onion, coarsely chopped

I   small sweet potato, coarsely chopped

5   cremini mushrooms, halved

I   cloves garlic, crushed

I   tablespoon tomato paste

I   bay leaf

¾   teaspoon salt

¼   teaspoon black pepper

10   cups water

1. In a large stockpot or Dutch oven, combine the celery, carrot, onion, sweet potato, mushrooms, garlic, tomato paste, bay leaf, salt, pepper, and water. Bring to a boil over high heat. Reduce the heat to low, cover, and simmer for 6 hours.

2. Place a sieve or colander over a large bowl. Pour the broth through the sieve or colander. Discard the solids.

NUTRITION (PER I CUP): 21 calories, 1 g protein, 4 g carbohydrates, 0 g fiber, 2 g sugars, 0 g fat, 0 g saturated fat, 324 mg sodium

MEAL PLANS

NOW THAT YOU UNDERSTAND HOW clean eating can boost your metabolism and help you reach your weight-loss goals and you've seen the delicious recipes, discover how to include clean eating into your everyday meals with these sample meal plans.

SUNDAY

BREAKFAST	Hash Brown Frittata (page 104)
LUNCH	Fruit and Walnut Spinach Salad with Lemon-Shallot Vinaigrette (page 146)
	3 ounces cooked chicken breast
SNACK	3 ribs celery, cut into sticks
	1 tablespoon nut butter
DINNER	Traditional Slow-Cooker Pot Roast (page 153)
SNACK	1 ounce cashews
	1 banana

MONDAY

BREAKFAST	2 scrambled eggs
	1 slice whole grain bread
LUNCH	Leftover Traditional Slow-Cooker Pot Roast (page 153)
SNACK	1 cup baby carrots
	2 tablespoons hummus
DINNER	Chicken Cacciatore (page 172)
	Tossed salad
SNACK	1 Peanut Butter Bar (page 263)

TUESDAY

BREAKFAST   1 cup Greek yogurt
Cocoa Granola (page 111)

LUNCH   Chilled Cilantro–Soba Noodle Salad (page 144)
3 ounces roasted salmon

SNACK   1 Peanut Butter Bar (page 263)

DINNER   4 ounces roasted fish
1 cup steamed asparagus
½ cup cooked brown rice

SNACK   1 apple
1 string cheese

WEDNESDAY

BREAKFAST   Zesty Breakfast Pizza (page 101)
1 medium orange

LUNCH   4 ounces cooked shrimp
Tossed salad

SNACK   1 apple
1 ounce cashews

DINNER   Shrimp Scampi Fettuccine (page 190)
1 cup steamed broccoli
1 piece crusty whole wheat bread

SNACK   10 whole grain tortilla chips
¼ cup guacamole

THURSDAY

BREAKFAST Blueberry Protein Pancakes (page 106)

LUNCH Shrimp Scampi Fettuccine (page 190)

SNACK Spinach-Artichoke Dip (page 251)
1 cup baby carrots

DINNER Bean Enchiladas (page 199)

SNACK 1 sliced apple
1 tablespoon nut butter

FRIDAY

BREAKFAST 1 scrambled egg
3 ounces smoked salmon
1 slice whole grain toast

LUNCH Shaved Salad (page 147)
3 ounces cooked chicken breast
½ cup fresh pineapple

SNACK Gremolata Parmesan Popcorn (page 260)
1 string cheese

DINNER Leftover Bean Enchiladas (page 199)
1 cup sautéed green beans

SNACK 1 Peanut Butter Banana Blondie (page 235)

SATURDAY

BREAKFAST 1 cup Greek yogurt topped with
1 cup blueberries

LUNCH Sweet Potato Lentil Burgers (page 192)
Whole wheat roll

SNACK 1 Pumpkin Seed, Cherry, and Pecan Granola Bar (page 262)

DINNER Baked Chicken with Mustard Sauce (page 175)
½ cup cooked quinoa
Tossed salad

SNACK 1 cup red grapes

SUNDAY

BREAKFAST   Chocolate-Banana Stuffed French Toast (page 108)
1 ounce almonds

LUNCH   Leftover Baked Chicken with Mustard Sauce (page 175)
½ cup cooked quinoa
1 pear

SNACK   Lemony Rosemary White Bean Dip (page 252)
3 ribs celery, cut into sticks

DINNER   Chicken Pot Pie (page 174)
Tossed salad

SNACK   1 Pumpkin Seed, Cherry, and Pecan Granola Bar (page 262)

MONDAY

BREAKFAST   1 cup steel-cut oats
2 tablespoons almond butter
1 banana, sliced

LUNCH   Tuna and Cannellini Salad (page 139)
½ avocado, sliced

SNACK   1 cup Greek yogurt
½ cup cantaloupe

DINNER   Lamb Burgers with Lemon-Yogurt Sauce (page 163)
½ cup cooked bulgur

SNACK   1 Mexican Chocolate Popcorn Ball (page 265)

TUESDAY

BREAKFAST   Salmon Breakfast Burrito (page 103)

LUNCH   Hamburger with ½ roll
Tossed salad
1 apple

SNACK   1 cup strawberries
1 ounce dark chocolate (70% or higher)

DINNER   Vegetable Lo Mein (page 197)
3 ounces cooked boneless pork chop

SNACK   1 Fruit and Nut Cookie Bar (page 233)

WEDNESDAY

BREAKFAST   Peach Smoothie (page 118)
1 slice whole grain toast

LUNCH   Leftover Vegetable Lo Mein (page 197)
4 ounces cooked shrimp

SNACK   1 Chocolate Chip Cookie Dough Energy Bite (page 264)

DINNER   1 Mediterranean Chicken Wrap (page 170)
Tossed salad

SNACK   1 ounce almonds
1 medium apple

THURSDAY

BREAKFAST Simple Overnight Steel-Cut Oats (page 112)
1 hard-cooked egg

LUNCH 2 slices whole grain bread
6 ounces canned wild salmon
1 tablespoon organic mayonnaise
½ cup spinach
2 slices tomato
2 slices red onion

SNACK 1 Chocolate Chip Cookie Dough Energy Bite (page 264)

DINNER Orange-Sage Braised Chicken Thighs (page 179)
½ cup brown rice

SNACK 1 Mexican Chocolate Popcorn Ball (page 265)

FRIDAY

BREAKFAST 2 eggs scrambled with spinach and tomato
1 slice whole grain toast

LUNCH Beef Barley Soup (page 122)
Tossed salad

SNACK 1 Dark Chocolate Crackle Cookie (page 231)

DINNER Leftover Orange-Sage Braised Chicken Thighs (page 179)

SNACK Cinnamon-Sugar Pita Chips (page 257)
1 ounce walnuts

SATURDAY

BREAKFAST 1 Warm Berry Breakfast Bar (page 113)
2 hard-cooked eggs

LUNCH Creamy Chicken, Green Grape, and Farro Salad (page 137)

SNACK 1 ounce pistachios
1 pear

DINNER 3 ounces grilled steak
1 cup steamed asparagus
1 small baked potato

SNACK 1 Dark Chocolate Crackle Cookie (page 231)

SUNDAY

BREAKFAST 1 leftover Warm Berry Breakfast Bar (page 113)
1 grapefruit

LUNCH Vegetarian Chili (page 194)
Tossed salad

SNACK Homemade Cocoa-Hazelnut Butter (page 278)
10 whole wheat crackers

DINNER Beef Stroganoff (page 155)
1 cup steamed cauliflower

SNACK 1 cup baby carrots
2 tablespoons hummus

MONDAY

BREAKFAST Mocha Peanut Butter Smoothie (page 117)
2 hard-cooked eggs

LUNCH ½ cup cooked quinoa
¼ cup chickpeas
1 cup packed baby kale
3 ounces cooked turkey breast

SNACK 1 slice whole grain toast
½ avocado, mashed

DINNER Salmon Pasta Casserole (page 186)

SNACK ½ red bell pepper, sliced into strips
2 tablespoons hummus

TUESDAY

BREAKFAST Green Ginger Smoothie (page 119)
1 ounce almonds

LUNCH Leftover Salmon Pasta Casserole (page 186)

SNACK 2 ounces organic deli turkey
1 cup carrots

DINNER Slow-Cooker BBQ Pulled Chicken Flatbreads
(page 171)

SNACK 1 Rich Brownie (page 238)

WEDNESDAY

BREAKFAST Mushroom Omelet (page 105)
1 slice whole grain toast

LUNCH 2 cups salad greens
5 ounces water-packed tuna, drained
½ avocado
½ cup cherry tomatoes
2 tablespoons dressing (from pages 268–270)

SNACK ½ cup Greek yogurt
½ cup strawberries, sliced

DINNER Mom's Meat Loaf (page 158)
1 cup steamed broccoli
½ cup mashed sweet potatoes

SNACK 1 Orange–Dark Chocolate Chunk Cookie
(page 229)

THURSDAY

BREAKFAST   2 scrambled eggs
2 tablespoons salsa
¼ cup shredded Cheddar cheese

LUNCH   4 ounces water-packed sardines, drained
Tossed salad
1 cup roasted vegetables

SNACK   2 ounces organic deli turkey
1 cup carrots

DINNER   Pork Tenderloin with Roasted Vegetables and
Apples (page 165)

SNACK   1 Dark Chocolate–Sea Salt Truffle (page 237)

FRIDAY

BREAKFAST   2 fried eggs
1 slice whole grain toast spread with
¼ avocado

LUNCH   Leftover Pork Tenderloin with Roasted Vegetables
and Apples (page 165)

SNACK   1 cup papaya
1 ounce walnuts

DINNER   Sweet and Sour Shrimp (page 189)
½ cup cooked brown rice

SNACK   Roasted Strawberries with Chocolate Sauce (page 226)

SATURDAY

BREAKFAST   Apple Pie Parfait (page 109)
1 scrambled egg

LUNCH   1 Salmon Salad Lettuce Wrap (page 184)

SNACK   10 Rosemary and Sunflower Seed Oat Crackers (page 261)
2 tablespoons hummus

DINNER   3 ounces grilled wild salmon
½ cup quinoa
1 cup roasted Brussels sprouts

SNACK   1 cup cherry tomatoes
2 tablespoons dressing (from pages 268–270)

Endnotes

CHAPTER 1

1   P. Møller, "Gastrophysics and the Brain and Body," *Flavour* 2, no. 8 (January 9, 2013). Accessed July 11, 2016, doi: 10.11186/2044=7248=2=8.

2   D. Stern et al., "The Nutrient Content of U.S. Household Food Purchases by Store Type," *American Journal of Preventive Medicine*, 50, no. 2 (February 2016): 180–90.

3   M. Jeltema et al., "Model for Understanding Consumer Textural Food Choice," *Food Science & Nutrition* 3, no. 3 (2015): 202–12.

4   P. Rada et al., "Daily Bingeing on Sugar Repeatedly Releases Dopamine in the Accumbens Shell," *Neuroscience* 134, no. 3 (2005): 737–44; E. M. Schulte et al., "Which Foods May Be Addictive? The Roles of Processing, Fat Content, and Glycemic Load," *PLoS One* 10, no. 2 (2015): e0117959; M. J. Morris et al., "Salt Craving: The Psychobiology of Pathogenic Sodium Intake," *Physiology and Behavior* 94, no. 5 (August 2008): 709–21.

5   K. Blum et al., "Dopamine and Glucose, Obesity, and Reward Deficiency Syndrome," *Frontiers in Psychology* 5, no. 919 (2014): 1–11.

6   D. Ludwig et al., "High Glycemic Index Foods, Overeating, and Obesity," *Pediatrics* 103, no. 3 (March 1999): E26.

7   Center for Science in the Public Interest, "Sugar: Too Much of a Sweet Thing," https://cspinet.org/new/pdf/combined_infographic.pdf. Accessed August 1, 2016.

8   Ibid.

9   R. Bethene Ervin et al., "Consumption of Added Sugars among U.S. Adults, 2005–2010," NCHS Data Brief No. 122.

10 A. Pan et al., "Effects of Carbohydrates on Satiety: Differences between Liquid and Solid Food," *Current Opinion in Clinical Nutrition & Metabolic Care* 14 (2011): 385–90.

11 See previous note 9.

12 Corn Refiners Association, "Questions & Answers about High Fructose
    Corn Syrup," https://www.cargillfoods.com/wcm/groups/public
    /@cseg/@food/@all/documents/document/na3047237.pdf. Accessed
    July 28, 2016.

13 G. A. Bray, "Consumption of High-Fructose Corn Syrup in Beverages May
    Play a Role in the Epidemic of Obesity," *American Journal of Clinical
    Nutrition* 79, no. 4 (2004): 537–43.

14 K. L. Teff, "Dietary Fructose Reduces Circulating Insulin and Leptin,
    Attenuates Postprandial Suppression of Ghrelin, and Increases
    Triglycerides in Women," *Journal of Clinical Endocrinology &
    Metabolism* 89, no. 6 (June 2004): 2963–72.

15 F. Rosvquist et al., "Overfeeding Polyunsaturated and Saturated Fat
    Causes Distinct Effects on Liver and Visceral Fat Accumulation in
    Humans," *Diabetes* 63, no. 7 (July 2014): 2356–68.

16 D. P. Bolhuis et al., "Salt Promotes Passive Overconsumption of Dietary
    Fat in Humans," *Journal of Nutrition* 146, no. 4 (April 2016): 838–45.

17 Y. S. Yoon et al., "Sodium Density and Obesity; the Korea National Health
    and Nutrition Examination Survey 2007–2010," *European Journal of
    Clinical Nutrition* 67, no. 2 (February 2013): 141–46.

18 "Get the Facts: Sodium's Role in Processed Food, Centers for Disease
    Control and Prevention, last modified June 2012. Accessed November
    2016, https://www.cdc.gov/salt/pdfs/sodium_role_processed.pdf.

19 S. Fowler et al., "Diet Soda Intake Is Associated with Long-Term Increases
    in Waist Circumference in a Biethnic Cohort of Older Adults: The
    San Antonio Longitudinal Study of Aging," *Journal of the American
    Geriatric Society* 63 (2015): 708–15.

20 S. P. Fowler et al., "Fueling the Obesity Epidemic? Artificially Sweetened
    Beverage Use and Long-Term Weight Gain," *Obesity* 16, no. 8 (2008):
    1894–900.

21 J. Suez et al., "Artificial Sweeteners Induce Glucose Intolerance by
    Altering the Gut Microbiota," *Nature* 514 (2014): 181–86.

22 S. P. Fowler, "Low-Calorie Sweetener Use and Energy Balance: Results from
    Experimental Studies in Animals, and Large-Scale Prospective Studies in
    Humans," *Physiology & Behavior* 164, PT. B (April 2016): 517–23.

23 B. Chaissing et al., "Dietary Emulsifiers Impact the Mouse Gut Microbiota Promoting Colitis and Metabolic Syndrome," *Nature* 519 (2015): 92–96.

24 C. Ciardi et al., "Food Additives Such as Sodium Sulphite, Sodium Benzoate, and Curcumin Inhibit Leptin Release in Lipopolysaccharide-Treated Murine Adipocytes in Vitro," *British Journal of Nutrition* 107, no. 6 (March 2012): 826–33.

25 V. Brown et al, "Potential Obesogen Identified: Fungicide Triflumizole Is Associated with Increased Adipogenesis in Mice," *Environmental Health Perspectives* 120, no. 12 (2012): A474.

26 X. Li et al., "Triflumizole Is an Obesogen in Mice That Acts through Peroxisome Proliferator Activated Receptor Gamma (PPARy)," *Environmental Health Perspectives* 120, no. 12 (December 2012): 1720–26.

27 K. A. Thayer et al., "Role of Environmental Chemicals in Diabetes and Obesity: A National Toxicology Program Workshop Review," *Environmental Health Perspectives* 120, no. 6 (June 2012): 779–89.

28 D. K. Layman, "Dietary Guidelines Should Reflect New Understandings about Adult Protein Needs," *Nutrition and Metabolism (Lond)* 6 (2009): 12; B. J. Brehm et al., "Benefits of High-Protein Weight Loss Diets: Enough Evidence for Practice?," *Current Opinion in Endocrinology, Diabetes, and Obesity* 15, no. 5 (2008): 416–21; D. Paddon-Jones et al., "Protein, Weight Management, and Satiety," *American Journal of Clinical Nutrition* 87, no. 5 (2008): 1558S-1561S; H. J. Leidy et al., "The Effects of Consuming Frequent, Higher Protein Meals on Appetite and Satiety During Weight Loss in Overweight/Obese Men," *Obesity* 19, no. 4 (2011): 818–24; M. S. Westerterp-Plantenga, "Dietary Protein, Weight Loss, and Weight Maintenance," *Annual Review of Nutrition* 29 (2009): 21–41.

29 C. S. Johnson et al., "Postprandial Thermogenesis Is Increased 100% on a High-Protein, Low-Fat Diet versus a High-Carbohydrate, Low-Fat Diet in Healthy, Young Women," *Journal of the American College of Nutrition* 21, no. 1 (February 2002): 55–61.

30 N. Tentolouris et al., "Diet-Induced Thermogenesis and Substrate Oxidation Are Not Different between Lean and Obese Women after Two Different Isocaloric Meals, One Rich in Protein and One Rich in Fat," *Metabolism* 57, no. 3 (March 2008): 313–20.

31 W. Westcott, "ACSM Strength Training Guidelines: Role in Body Composition and Health Enhancement," *ACSM's Health & Fitness Journal* 13, no. 4 (July 2009): 14–22.

32 S. Devkota, "Protein Metabolic Roles in Treatment of Obesity," *Current Opinion in Clinical Nutrition and Metabolic Care* 13, no. 14 (2010): 403–7.

33 R. D. Mattes et al., "Impact of Peanuts and Tree Nuts on Body Weight and Healthy Weight Loss in Adults," *Journal of Nutrition* 138 (2008): 1741S–1745S.

34 C. S. Johnston, "Strategies for Healthy Weight Loss: From Vitamin C to the Glycemic Response," *Journal of the American College of Nutrition* 24, no. 3 (2005): 158–65.

35 M. Bertoia et al., "Dietary Flavonoid Intake and Weight Maintenance: Three Prospective Cohorts of 124,086 US Men and Women Followed for up to 24 Years," *British Medical Journal* 352, no. 17 (2016): i17. doi:http://dx.doi.org/10.1136/bmj.i17; N. R. Stendell-Hollis et al., "Green Tea Improves Metabolic Biomarkers, Not Weight or Body Composition: A Pilot Study in Overweight Breast Cancer Survivors," *Journal of Human Nutrition and Dietetics* 23, no. 6 (December 2010): 590–600; L. Josic et al., "Does Green Tea Affect Postprandial Glucose, Insulin, and Satiety in Healthy Subjects: A Randomized Controlled Trial," *Nutrition Journal* 9, no. 63 (November 2010). doi: 10.1186/1475-2891-63; B. E. Carter and A. Drewnowski, "Beverages Containing Soluble Fiber, Caffeine, and Green Tea Catechins Suppress Hunger and Lead to Less Energy Consumption at the Next Meal," *Appetite* 59, no. 3 (December 2012): 755–61; H. Badshah et al., "Anthocyanins Attenuate Body Weight Gain via Modulating Neuropeptide Y and GABAB1 Receptor in Rats Hypothalamus," *Neuropeptides* 47, no. 5 (October 2013): 347–53; M. S. Westerterp-Plantenga et al., "Body Weight Loss and Weight Maintenance in Relation to Habitual Caffeine Intake and Green Tea Supplementation," *Obesity Research* 13, no. 7 (July 2005): 1195–204; T. Komatsu et al., "Oolong Tea Increases Energy Metabolism in Japanese Females," *Journal of Medical Investigation* 0, no. 3–4 (August 2003): 170–75; J. J. Choo, "Green Tea Reduces Body Fat Accretion Caused by High-Fat Diet in Rats through Beta-Adrenoceptor Activation of Thermogenesis in Brown Adipose Tissue," *Journal of Nutritional Biochemistry* 14, no. 11 (November 2003): 671–76; P. Auvichayapat et al., "Effectiveness of Green Tea on Weight Reduction

in Obese Thais: A Randomized, Controlled Trial," *Physiology & Behavior* 93, no. 3 (February 2008): 486–91.

36 C. B. Ebbeling et al., "Effects of Dietary Composition on Energy Expenditure during Weight-Loss Maintenance," *JAMA* 307, no. 24 (June 2012): 2627–34; M. A. Pereira, "Effects of a Low-Glycemic Load Diet on Resting Energy Expenditure and Heart Disease Risk Factors during Weight Loss," *JAMA* 292, no. 20 (November 2004): 2482–90.

37 M. J. Ludy et al., "The Effects of Capsaicin and Capsiate on Energy Balance: Critical Review and Meta-Analyses of Studies in Humans," *Chemical Senses* 37 (2012): 103–21.

38 M. Lee et al., "Reduction of Body Weight by Dietary Garlic Is Associated with an Increase in Uncoupling Protein mRNA Expression and Activation of AMP-Activated Protein Kinase in Diet-Induced Obese Mice," *Journal of Nutrition* 141 (2011): 1947–53.

39 A. L. Brown et al., "Health Effects of Green Tea Catechins in Overweight and Obese Men: A Randomised Controlled Cross-Over Trial," *British Journal of Nutrition* 106, no. 12 (December 2011): 1880–89.

40 A. M. Dostal et al., "Long-Term Supplementation of Green Tea Extract Does Not Modify Adiposity or Bone Mineral Density in a Randomized Trial of Overweight and Obese Postmenopausal Women," *Journal of Nutrition* 146, no. 2 (February 2016): 256–64.

41 R. Hursel et al., "The Effects of Catechin Rich Teas and Caffeine on Energy Expenditure and Fat Oxidation: A Meta-Analysis," *Obesity Reviews* 12, no. 7 (July 2011): e573–81.

42 C. M. Brown et al., "Water-Induced Thermogenesis Reconsidered: The Effects of Osmolality and Water Temperature on Energy Expenditure After Drinking," *Journal of Clinical Endocrinology and Metabolism* 91, no. 9 (September 2006): 3598–602.

43 T. Chang et al., "Inadequate Hydration, BMI, and Obesity among US Adults: NHANES 2009–2012," *Annals of Family Medicine* 14, no. 4 (July/August 2016): 320–24.

44 ConsumerLab.com, "Product Review: Green Tea Supplements, Drinks, Brewable Teas, and Matcha Review," https://www.consumerlab.com/reviews/Green_Tea_Review_Supplements_and_Bottled/Green_Tea/. Accessed August 8, 2016.

45   A. O'Connor, "What's in Your Green Tea?" *New York Times*, May 23, 2013.

46   R. Green et al., "Common Tea Formulations Modulate In Vitro Digestive Recovery of Green Tea Catechins," *Molecular Nutrition & Food Research* 51 (2007): 1152–62.

47   D. K. Layman et al., "A Moderate-Protein Diet Produces Sustained Weight Loss and Long-Term Changes in Body Composition and Blood Lipids in Obese Adults," *Journal of Nutrition* 139, no. 3 (2009): 514–21.

48   S. M. Pasiakos et al., "Higher-Protein Diets Are Associated with Higher HDL Cholesterol and Lower BMI and Waist Circumference in US Adults," *Journal of Nutrition* 145, no. 3 (March 2015): 605–14.

49   D. K. Layman et al., "Dietary Guidelines Should Reflect New Understandings about Adult Protein Needs," *Nutrition & Metabolism (Lond)* 6 (2009): 12; D. K. Layman et al., "Dietary Protein and Exercise Have Additive Effects on Body Composition during Weight Loss in Adult Women," *Journal of Nutrition* 135, no. 8 (2005): 1903–10.

50   J. A. Paniagua a et al., "Monounsaturated Fat-Rich Diet Prevents Central Body Fat Distribution and Decreases Postprandial Adiponectin Expression Induced by a Carbohydrate-Rich Diet in Insulin-Resistant Subjects," *Diabetes Care* 30, no. 7 (July 2007): 1717–23.

51   J. L. Rosenbloom et al., "Calcium and Vitamin D Supplementation Is Associated with Decreased Abdominal Visceral Adipose Tissue in Overweight and Obese Aults." *American Journal of Clinical Nutrition* 95, Jan 2012 (1):101–8.

52   T. E. Lehnen et al., "A Review on Effects of Conjugated Linoleic Fatty Acid (CLA) upon Body Composition and Energetic Metabolism," *Journal of the International Society of Sports Nutrition* 12 (2015): 36.

53   C. A. Daley et al., "A Review of Fatty Acid Profiles and Antioxidant Content in Grass-Fed and Grain-Fed Beef," *Nutrition Journal* 9 (2010): 10.

54   K. Hairston et al., "Lifestyle Factors and 5-Year Abdominal Fat Accumulation in a Minority Cohort: The IRAS Family Study," *Obesity* (Silver Spring) 20, no. 2 (February 2012):421–27.

55   N. M. McKeown et al., "Whole- and Refined-Grain Intakes are Differentially Associated with Abdominal Visceral and Subcutaneous Adiposity in Healthy Adults: The Framingham Heart Study," *American Journal of Clinical Nutrition* 92, no. 5 (November 2010): 1165–71.

56 J. Halkjaer et al., "Intake of Macronutrients as Predictors of 5-y Changes in Waist Circumference," *American Journal of Clinical Nutrition* 84, no. 4 (October 2006): 789–97.

57 H. P. Chang et al., "Antiobesity Activities of Indole-3-Carbinol in High-Fat-Diet-Induced Obese Mice," *Nutrition* 27, no. 4 (April 2011): 463–70.

58 Y. Ma et al., "Single-Component versus Multicomponent Dietary Goals for the Metabolic Syndrome," *Annals of Internal Medicine* 162, no. 4 (February 2015): 248–57.

59 T. F. Turner et al., "Dietary Adherence and Satisfaction with a Bean-Based High-Fiber Weight Loss Diet: A Pilot Study," *ISRN Obesity* (October 2013): 915415.

60 S. J. Kentish, "High-Fat Diet-Induced Obesity Ablates Gastric Vagal Afferent Circadian Rhythms," *Journal of Neuroscience* 36, no. 11 (March 2016): 3199–207.

61 E. Adamska, "The Role of Gastrointestinal Hormones in the Pathogenesis of Obesity and Type 2 Diabetes," *Gastroenterology Review* 9, no. 2 (2014): 69–76; H. Pan, "Advances in Understanding the Interrelations between Leptin Resistance and Obesity," *Physiology & Behavior* 130 (May 2014): 157–69.

62 B. E. Bayham, "A Randomized Trial to Manipulate the Quality Instead of Quantity of Dietary Proteins to Influence the Markers of Satiety," *Journal of Diabetes and Its Complications* 28, no. 4 (July–August 2014): 547–52.

63 H. Leidy et al., "Beneficial Effects of a Higher-Protein Breakfast on the Appetitive, Hormonal, and Neural Signals Controlling Energy Intake Regulation in Overweight/Obese, 'Breakfast-Skipping,' Late-Adolescent Girls," *American Journal of Clinical Nutrition* 97 (2013): 677–88.

64 See note 59 above; N. A. Schwarz, "A Review of Weight Control Strategies and Their Effects on the Regulation of Hormonal Balance," *Journal of Nutrition and Metabolism* (2011): 237932.

65 J. L. Stevenson, "Hunger and Satiety Responses to High-Fat Meals of Varying Fatty Acid Composition in Women with Obesity," *Obesity* (Silver Spring) 23, no. 10 (October 2015): 1980–86.

66 I. Abete, "Specific Insulin Sensitivity and Leptin Responses to a Nutritional Treatment of Obesity via a Combination of Energy Restriction and Fatty Fish Intake," *Journal of Human Nutrition and Dietetics* 21, no. 6 (2008): 591–600.

67 J. Higgins et al., "Resistant Starch Consumption Promotes Lipid Oxidation," *Nutrition & Metabolism* 1, no. 8 (2004). Accessed July 11, 2016, doi: 10.1186/1743-7075-1-8; C. L. Bodinham et al., "Acute Ingestion of Resistant Starch Reduces Food Intake in Healthy Adults," *British Journal of Nutrition* 103, no. 6 (2010): 917–22.

68 A. Kokkinos, "Eating Slowly Increases the Postprandial Response of the Anorexigenic Gut Hormones, Peptide YY and Glucagon-Like Peptide-1," *Journal of Clinical Endocrinology and Metabolism* 95, no. 1 (January 2010): 333–37.

69 M. Shah, "The Effect of Eating Speed at Breakfast on Appetite Hormone Responses and Daily Food Consumption," *Journal of Investigative Medicine* 63, no. 1 (January 2015): 22–28.

70 S. D. Anton, "Diet Type and Changes in Food Cravings following Weight Loss: Findings from the POUNDS LOST Trial," *Eating and Weight Disorders* 17, no. 2 (June 2012): e101–8.

71 M. L. Pelchat and S. Schaefer, "Dietary Monotony and Food Cravings in Young and Elderly Adults," *Physiology & Behavior* 68, no. 3 (January 2000): 353–59; A. J. Hill and L. Heaton-Brown, "The Experience of Food Craving: A Prospective Investigation in Healthy Women," *Journal of Psychosomatic Research* 38, no. 8 (November 1994): 801–14; H. P. Weingarten and D. Elston, "Food Cravings in a College Population," *Appetite* 17, no. 3 (December 1991): 167–74.

72 T. Deckersbach, "Pilot Randomized Trial Demonstrating Reversal of Obesity-Related Abnormalities in Reward System Responsivity to Food Cues with a Behavioral Intervention," *Nutrition & Diabetes* 4 (2014): e129.

73 G. Musso et al., "Interactions between Gut Microbiota and Host Metabolism Predisposing to Obesity and Diabetes," *Annual Review of Medicine* 62 (2011): 361–80.

74 J. Alcock et al., "Is Eating Behavior Manipulated by the Gastrointestinal Microbiota? Evolutionary Pressures and Potential Mechanisms," *BioEssays* 36 (2014): 940–49.

75 P. J. Turnbaugh et al., "The Core Gut Microbiome, Energy Balance and Obesity," *Journal of Physiology* 587, pt. 17 (September 2009): 4153–58.

76 P. J. Turnbaugh et al., "An Obesity-Associated Gut Microbiome with Increased Capacity for Energy Harvest," *Nature* 444, no. 7122 (December 2006): 1027–31.

77 F. Francois et al., "The Effect of *H. pylori* Eradication on Meal-Associated Changes in Plasma Ghrelin and Leptin," *BMC Gastroenterology* 11 (April 2011): 37.

78 R. J. Perry et al., "Acetate Mediates a Microbiome–Brain–β-Cell Axis to Promote Metabolic Syndrome," *Nature* 534 (June 2016): 213.

79 H. D. Holscher et al., "Fiber Supplementation Influences Phylogenetic Structure and Functional Capacity of the Human Intestinal Microbiome: Follow-Up of a Randomized Controlled Trial," *American Journal of Clinical Nutrition* 101, no. 1 (January 2015): 55–64.

80 "Your Gut Bacteria Don't Like Junk Food—Even if You Do," The Conversation, accessed November 16, 2016, http://theconversation.com /your-gut-bacteria-dont-like-junk-food-even-if-you-do-41564.

81 The Conversation, "Your Gut Bacteria Don't Like Junk Food—Even If You Do," by Tim Spector, https://theconversation.com/your-gut-bacteria -dont-like-junk-food-even-if-you-do-41564. Accessed August 2, 2016.

82 Scientific American, "Fiber-Famished Gut Microbes Linked to Poor Health by Katherine Harmon Courage," March 23, 2015. http://www .scientificamerican.com/article/fiber-famished-gut-microbes-linked-to -poor-health1/. Accessed August 2, 2016.

83 F. Guarner, et al., "Studies with Inulin-Type Fructans on Intestinal Infections, Permeability, and Inflammation," *Journal of Nutrition* 137, sup. 11 (November 2007): 2568S–2571S.

84 E. G. Christensen et al., "Bifidogenic Effect of Whole-Grain Wheat During a 12-Week Energy-Restricted Dietary Intervention in Postmenopausal Women," *European Journal of Clinical Nutrition* 67, no. 12 (December 2013): 1316–21.

85 K. Kotzampassi et al., "Bacteria and Obesity: The Proportion Makes the Difference," *Surgery: Current Research* 3:152.

86 M. A. Ciorba, "A Gastroenterologist's Guide to Probiotics," Clinical *Gastroenterology and Hepatology* 10, no. 9 (September 2012): 960–68.

87 R. Caesar et al., "Crosstalk between Gut Microbiota and Dietary Lipids Aggravates WAT Inflammation through TLR Signaling," *Cell Metabolism* 22, no. 4 (October 2015): 658–68.

88 J. Suez et al., "Artificial Sweeteners Induce Glucose Intolerance by Altering the Gut Microbiota," *Nature* 514, no. 7521 (October 2014): 181–86.

89 J. Suez et al., "Non-Caloric Artificial Sweeteners and the Microbiome: Findings and Challenges," *Gut Microbes* 6, no. 2 (2015): 149–55.

90 F. R. Reichert, "The Role of Perceived Personal Barriers to Engagement in Leisure-Time Physical Activity," *American Journal of Public Health* 97, no. 3 (March 2007): 515–19; J. H. Leslie, "Factors Affecting Healthy Eating and Physical Activity Behaviors among Multiethnic Blue- and White-Collar Workers: A Case Study of One Healthcare Institution," *Hawai'i Journal of Medicine and Public Health* 72, no. 9 (September 2013): 300–6.

91 American Academy of Sleep Medicine, "Study Links Diet with Daytime Sleepiness and Alertness in Healthy Adults." Presented at 2013 Sleep conference of American Academy of Sleep Medicine. http://www.aasmnet.org/articles.aspx?id=3869. Accessed July 30, 2016.

92 AS Wells, "Influences of Dietary and Intraduodenal Lipid on Alertness, Mood, and Sustained Concentration," *British Journal of Nutrition* 74, no. 1 (1995): 115–23.

93 A. P. Smith, "Breakfast Cereal, Fibre, Digestive Problems and Well-Being," *Current Topics in Nutraceutical Research* 8, no. 2–3 (2010): 1–10.

94 Y. C. Zeng et al., "Influences of Protein to Energy Ratios in Breakfast on Mood, Alertness, and Attention in the Healthy Undergraduate Students," *Health* 3, no. 6 (2011): 383–93.

CHAPTER 2

1 E. M. Steele et al., "Ultra-Processed Foods and Added Sugars in the US Diet: Evidence from a Nationally Representative Cross-Sectional Study," *BMJ Open* 6, no. 3 (2016): e009892.

2 "Heart Disease Fact Sheet." Centers for Disease Control and Prevention, accessed August 3, 2016, http://www.cdc.gov/dhdsp/data_statistics/fact_sheets/fs_heart_disease.htm.

3 "The Power of Prevention," Centers for Disease Control and Prevention, accessed August 3, 2016, http://www.cdc.gov/chronicdisease/pdf/2009-power-of-prevention.pdf.

4   Y. Li et al., "Saturated Fats Compared with Unsaturated Fats and Sources of Carbohydrates in Relation to Risk of Coronary Heart Disease," *Journal of the American College of Cardiology* 66, no. 14 (October 2015): 1538–48.

5   Harvard T. H. Chan School of Public Health, "Butter Is Not Back: Limiting Saturated Fat Still Best for Heart Health," https://www.hsph.harvard .edu/news/press-releases/butter-is-not-back-limiting-saturated-fat-still -best-for-heart-health/. Accessed August 5, 2016.

6   J. B. Brill, "Lifestyle Intervention Strategies for the Prevention and Treatment of Hypertension: A Review," *American Journal of Lifestyle Medicine* 5 (2011): 346; P. M. Kris-Etherton et al., "Milk Products, Dietary Patterns and Blood Pressure Management," *Journal of the American College of Nutrition* 28, no. 1 (February 2009): 103S–119S.

7   A. J. Viera, "Resistant Hypertension," *Journal of the American Board of Family Medicine* 25, no. 4 (July–August 2012): 487–95.

8   S. Engeli, "Weight Loss and the Renin-Angiotensin-Aldosterone System," http://hyper.ahajournals.org/content/45/3/356.long.

9   J. H. Dwyer et al., "Oxygenated Carotenoid Lutein and Progression of Early Atherosclerosis: The Los Angeles Atherosclerosis Study," *Circulation* 103, no. 24 (June 2001): 2922–27.

10   H. Du et al., "Fresh Fruit Consumption and Major Cardiovascular Disease in China," *New England Journal of Medicine*, 374, no. 14 (2016): 1332.

11   E. Georgousopoulou et al., "Adherence to Mediterranean is the Most Important Protector against the Development of Fatal and Non-Fatal Cardiovascular Event: 10-Year Follow-Up (2002-12) of the Attica Study." Presented at the American College of Cardiology's 64th Annual Scientific Session in San Diego, March 2015.

12   A. Mohebi-Nejad et al., "Omega-3 Supplements and Cardiovascular Diseases," *Tanaffos* 13, no. 1 (2014): 6–14.

13   Vestfold Heartcare Study Group, "Influence on Lifestyle Measures and Five-Year Coronary Risk By a Comprehensive Lifestyle Intervention Programme in Patients with Coronary Heart Disease," *European Journal of Preventive Cardiology* 10, no. 6 (December 2003): 429–37.

14   E. Pimenta et al., "Effects of Dietary Sodium Reduction on Blood Pressure in Subjects with Resistant Hypertension," *Hypertension* 54, no. 3 (September 2009): 475–81.

15 "Statistics About Diabetes," American Diabetes Association, accessed August 4, 2016, http://www.diabetes.org/diabetes-basics/statistics/.

16 P. L. Lutsey et al., "Dietary Intake and the Development of the Metabolic Syndrome," *Circulation* 117, no. 6 (February 2008): 754–61.

17 E. S. Ford et al., "Metabolic Syndrome and Risk of Incident Diabetes: Findings from the European Prospective Investigation into Cancer and Nutrition–Potsdam Study," *Cardiovascular Diabetology* 7 (2008): 35.

18 A. G. Tabak et al., "Prediabetes: A High-Risk State for Developing Diabetes," *Lancet* 379, no. 9833 (June 2012): 2279–90.

19 The Diabetes Prevention Program (DPP) Research Group, "The Diabetes Prevention Program (DPP)," *Diabetes Care* 25, no. 12 (December 2002): 2165–71.

20 R. F. Hamman, et al., "Effect of Weight Loss with Lifestyle Intervention on Risk of Diabetes," *Diabetes Care* 29, no. 9 (2006): 2102–7.

21 P. Carter, "Fruit and Vegetable Intake and Incidence of Type 2 Diabetes Mellitus: Systematic Review and Meta-Analysis," *BMJ* 341 (August 2010): c422.

22 J. De Munter et al., "Whole Grain, Bran, and Germ Intake and Risk of Type 2 Diabetes: A Prospective Cohort Study and Systematic Review," *PLoS Medicine* 4, no. 8 (2007): e261.

23 A. Due et al., "Comparison of the Effects on Insulin Resistance and Glucose Tolerance of 6-mo High-Monounsaturated-Fat, Low-Fat, and Control Diets," *American Journal of Clinical Nutrition* 87, no. 4 (April 2008): 855–62.

24 F. Imamura, "Effects of Saturated Fat, Polyunsaturated Fat, Monounsaturated Fat, and Carbohydrate on Glucose-Insulin Homeostasis: A Systematic Review and Meta-analysis of Randomised Controlled Feeding Trials," *PLoS Medicine* 13, no. 7 (July 2016): e1002087

25 I. Aeberli et al., "Moderate Amounts of Fructose Consumption Impair Insulin Sensitivity in Healthy Young Men: A Randomized Controlled Trial," *Diabetes Care* 36, no. 1 (January 2013): 150–56.

26 J. Suez et al., "Artificial Sweeteners Induce Glucose Intolerance by Altering the Gut Microbiota," *Nature* 514, no. 7521 (October 2014): 181–86.

27 L. O'Connor, "Prospective Associations and Population Impact of Sweet Beverage Intake and Type 2 Diabetes, and Effects of Substitutions with Alternative Beverages," *Diabetologia* 58, no. 7 (July 2015): 1474–83. See Table 3.

28 C. M. Clinton et al., "Whole-Foods, Plant-Based Diet Alleviates the Symptoms of Osteoarthritis," *Arthritis* 2015 (2015): 708152.

29 L. J. Wright et al., "Chronic Pain, Overweight, and Obesity: Findings from a Community-Based Twin Registry," *Journal of Pain* 11, no. 7 (July 2010): 628–35.

30 S. E. Kotowski et al., "Influence of Weight Loss on Musculoskeletal Pain: Potential Short-Term Relevance," *Work* 36, no. 3 (2010): 295–304.

31 A. G. VanDenKerkhof et al., "Diet, Lifestyle, and Chronic Widespread Pain: Results from the 1958 British Birth Cohort Study," *Pain Research and Management* 16, no. 2 (March–April 2011): 87–92.

32 "What America Thinks. MetLife Foundation Alzheimer's Survey," accessed August 4, 2016, https://www.metlife.com/assets/cao/foundation/alzheimers-2011.pdf.

33 "Breast Cancer Risk in American Women," National Cancer Institute, accessed August 4, 2016, http://www.cancer.gov/cancertopics/factsheet/detection/probability-breast-cancer; National Cancer Institute, accessed August 4, 2016, http://seer.cancer.gov/statfacts/html/prost.html.

34 O. Oyebode et al., "Fruit and Vegetable Consumption and All-Cause, Cancer, and CVD Mortality: Analysis of Health Survey for England Data," *Journal of Epidemiology and Community Health* 68, no. 9 (September 2014): 856–62.

35 "What You Need to Know about Obesity and Cancer," American Institute for Cancer Research, accessed August 5, 2016, http://www.aicr.org/learn-more-about-cancer/infographics/infographic-obesity-and-cancer.html.

36 "Isothiocyanates," Linus Pauling Institute, accessed August 4, 2016, http://lpi.oregonstate.edu/mic/dietary-factors/phytochemicals/isothiocyanates.

37 G. DenBesten et al., "The Role of Short-Chain Fatty Acids in the Interplay between Diet, Gut Microbiota, and Host Energy Metabolism," *Journal of Lipid Research* 54, no. 9 (September 2013): 2325–40.

38 S. L. Schmit et al., "Coffee Consumption and the Risk of Colorectal Cancer," *Cancer Epidemiology Biomarkers & Prevention* 25, no. 4 (2016): 634.

39 N. Seeram et al., "Blackberry, Black Raspberry, Blueberry, Cranberry, Red Raspberry, and Strawberry Extracts Inhibit Growth and Stimulate Apoptosis of Human Cancer Cells In Vitro," *Journal of Agricultural and Food Chemistry,* 54, no. 25 (2006): 9329–39.

40 K. Zu et al., "Dietary Lycopene, Angiogenesis, and Prostate Cancer: A Prospective Study in the Prostate-Specific Antigen Era," *Journal of the National Institute* 106, no. 2 (February 2014): djt43.

41 M. K. Sorongon-Legaspi et al., "Blood Level Omega-3 Fatty Acids As Risk Determinant Molecular Biomarker for Prostate Cancer," *Prostate Cancer* 2013 (2013): 875615.

42 J. S. Zheng et al., "Intake of Fish and Marine n-3 Polyunsaturated Fatty Acids and Risk of Breast Cancer: Meta-Analysis of Data from 21 Independent Prospective Cohort Studies," *British Medical Journal* 346 (June 2013): f3706.

43 M. Karnani et al., "Activation of Central Orexin/Hypocretin Neurons by Dietary Amino Acids," *Neuron* 72, no. 4 (2011): 616–29.

44 K. Blum et al., "Dopamine and Glucose, Obesity, and Reward Deficiency Syndrome," *Frontiers in Psychology* 5, no. 919 (2014): 1–11.

45 R. Mujcic, "Are Fruit and Vegetables Good for Our Mental and Physical Health? Panel Data Evidence from Australia," *Munich Personal RePEc Archive* 59149, no. 8 (2014). Accessed July 11, 2016, https://mpra.ub.uni -muenchen.de/59149/1/MPRA_paper_59149.pdf.

46 B. White et al., "Many Apples a Day Keep the Blues Away—Daily Experiences of Negative and Positive Affect and Food Consumption in Young Adults," *British Journal of Health Psychology* 18 (2013): 782–98.

47 F. Jacka et al., "Association of Western and Traditional Diets with Depression and Anxiety in Women," *American Journal of Psychiatry* 167 (2010): 1–7.

48 P. Wirtz et al., "Dark Chocolate Intake Buffers Stress Reactivity in Humans," *Journal of the American College of Cardiology* 63 (2014): 2297–99; D. Taubert et al., "Effects of Low Habitual Cocoa Intake on Blood Pressure and Bioactive Nitric Oxide: A Randomized Controlled Trial," *Journal of the American Medical Association.* 298, no. 1 (2007): 49–60.

49 "Lack of Sleep Is Affecting Americans, Finds the National Sleep Foundation," The National Sleep Foundation, accessed June 7 2016, https://sleepfoundation.org/media-center/press-release/lack-sleep -affecting-americans-finds-the-national-sleep-foundation.

50 S. Patel et al., "Association between Reduced Sleep and Weight Gain in Women," *American Journal of Epidemiology* 164, no. 10 (2006): 947–54.

51 M. St-Onge et al., "Fiber and Saturated Fat Are Associated with Sleep Arousals and Slow Wave Sleep," *Journal of Clinical Sleep Medicine* 12, no. 1 (2016): 19–24.

52 E. Hanlon et al., "Sleep Restriction Enhances the Daily Rhythm of Circulating Levels of Endocannabinoid 2-Arachidonoylglycerol," *SLEEP* 39, no. 3 (2016): 653–64.

53 M. Beydoun et al., "Serum Nutritional Biomarkers and Their Associations with Sleep among US Adults in Recent National Surveys," *PLoS One* 9, no. 8 (2014): e103490. doi: 10.1371/journal.pone.0103490.

54 P. Montgomery et al., "Fatty Acids and Sleep in UK Children: Subjective and Pilot Objective Sleep Results from the DOLAB Study—A Randomized Controlled Trial," *Journal of Sleep Research* 23, no. 4 (2014): 364–88.

55 Paul Montgomery, interviewed by author, June 24, 2014.

56 M. St-Onge et al., "Fiber and Saturated Fat Are Associated with Sleep Arousals and Slow Wave Sleep," *Journal of Clinical Sleep Medicine* 12, no. 1 (2016): 19–24.

57 A. M. Spaeth et al., "Resting Metabolic Rate Varies by Race and by Sleep Duration," *Obesity* 23, no. 12 (2015): 2349–56.

58 A. Liu et al., "Tart Cherry Juice Increases Sleep Time in Older Adults with Insomnia," *FASEB Journal* 28, no. 1, supplement 830.9 (2014): 579–83.

59 R. J. Reiter et al., "Melatonin in Walnuts: Influence on Levels of Melatonin and Total Antioxidant Capacity of Blood," *Nutrition* 21, no. 9 (2005): 920–24.

60 C. Leung et al., "Soda and Cell Aging: Associations between Sugar-Sweetened Beverage Consumption and Leukocyte Telomere Length in Healthy Adults from the National Health and Nutrition Examination Surveys," *American Journal of Public Health* 104, no. 12 (2014): 2425–31.

61 T. Satoh et al., "Effect of *Bifidobacterium breve* B-3 on Skin Photoaging Induced by Chronic UV Irradiation in Mice," *Beneficial Microbes* 6, no. 4 (2015): 497–504; T. Levkovich et al., "Probiotic Bacteria Induce a 'Glow of Health,'" *PLoS One* 8, no. 1 (2013): e53867. doi:10.1371/journal.pone.0053867.

62 R. Whitehead et al., "You Are What You Eat: Within-Subject Increases in Fruit and Vegetable Consumption Confer Beneficial Skin-Color Changes," *PLoS One* 7, no. 3 (2012): e32988. doi:10.1371/journal.pone.0032988.

CHAPTER 3

1 M. Shah et al., "Slower Eating Speed Lowers Energy Intake in Normal-Weight but not Overweight/Obese Subjects," *Journal of the Academy of Nutrition and Dietetics* 114 (2014): 393–402.

2 B. Wansink et al., "Slim by Design: Kitchen Counter Correlates of Obesity," *Health Education & Behavior* (2015) pii: 1090198115610571.

3 B. Wansink et al., "The Clean Plate Club: About 92 Percent of Self-Served Food Is Eaten," *International Journal of Obesity* 39 (2015): 371–74.

4 L. Ledochowski et al., "Acute Effects of Brisk Walking on Sugary Snack Cravings in Overweight People, Affect and Responses to a Manipulated Stress Situation and to a Sugary Snack Cue: A Crossover Study," *PLoS One* 10, no. 3 (2015): e0119278. doi:10.1371/journal.pone.0119278.

5 C. Morewedge et al., "Thought for Food: Imagined Consumption Reduces Actual Consumption," *Science* 330 (2010): 1530–33.

6 E. Van Kleef et al., "Just a Bite: Considerably Smaller Snack Portions Satisfy Delayed Hunger and Craving," *Food Quality and Preference* 27 (2013): 96–100.

CHAPTER 4

1 R. An, "Fast-Food and Full-Service Restaurant Consumption and Daily Energy and Nutrient Intakes in U.S. Adults," *European Journal of Clinical Nutrition* 70, no. 1 (January 2016): 97–103.

2   Brian Wansink, Slim by Design: Mindless Eating Solutions for Everyday Life (New York: William Morrow, 2014), 74–75.

3   N. I. Larson et al., "Food Preparation by Young Adults Is Associated with Better Diet Quality," *Journal of the American Dietetic Association* 106, no. 12 (December 2006): 2001–7.

4   M. A. Pereira et al., "Fast-Food Habits, Weight Gain, and Insulin Resistance (the CARDIA Study): 15-Year Prospective Analysis," *Lancet* 365, no. 9,453 (January 2005): 36–42.

5   S. A. French et al., "Fast Food Restaurant Use among Women in the Pound of Prevention Study: Dietary, Behavioral and Demographic Correlates," *International Journal of Obesity and Related Metabolic Disorders* 24, no. 10 (October 2000): 1,353–59

6   M. Bertoia et al., "Changes in Intake of Fruits and Vegetables and Weight Change in United States Men and Women Followed for up to 24 Years: Analysis from Three Prospective Cohort Studies," *PLoS Medicine* 12, no. 9 (2015): e1001878. doi:10.1371/ journal.pmed.1001878.

7   M. Baranski et al., "Higher Antioxidant and Lower Cadmium Concentrations and Lower Incidence of Pesticide Residues in Organically Grown Crops: A Systematic Literature Review and Meta-Analyses," *British Journal of Nutrition* 112 (2014): 794–811.

8   I. Cho et al., "Antibiotics in Early Life Alter the Murine Colonic Microbiome and Adiposity," *Nature* 488, no. 7413 (2012): 621–26.

9   "PCBs in Farmed Salmon: Wild Versus Farmed," The Environmental Working Group, accessed June 7, 2016, http://www.ewg.org/research/pcbs-farmed-salmon/wild-versus-farmed.

10 World Bank Group, "Fish 2030: Prospects for Fisheries and Aquaculture," Agriculture and Environmental Services Discussion Paper no. 3 (2013), http://documents.worldbank.org/curated/en/458631468152376668/Fish-to-2030-prospects-for-fisheries-and-aquaculture.

11 "Buying Fish? What You Need to Know," Environmental Defense Fund, accessed June 7, 2016, http://seafood.edf.org/buying-fish-what-you-need-know.

12 "Oceana Reveals Mislabeling of America's Favorite Fish: Salmon," Oceana, accessed June 7, 2016, http://usa.oceana.org/press-releases/oceana-reveals-mislabeling-americas-favorite-fish-salmon.

13   L. Yanping et al., "Saturated Fats Compared with Unsaturated Fats and Sources of Carbohydrates in Relation to Risk of Coronary Heart Disease: A Prospective Cohort Study," *Journal of the American College of Cardiology* 66, no. 14 (2015): 1538–48.

14   M. Assuncao et al., "Effects of Dietary Coconut Oil on the Biochemical and Anthropometric Profiles of Women Presenting Abdominal Obesity," *Lipids* 44 (2009): 593–601.

15   A. Albertson et al., "Whole Grain Consumption Trends and Associations with Body Weight Measures in the United States: Results from the Cross Sectional National Health and Nutrition Examination Survey 2001–2012," *Nutrition Journal* 15, no. 8 (2016): doi: 10.1186/s12937 -016-0126-4.

16   "CSPI Downgrades Sucralose from 'Caution' to 'Avoid,'" Center for Science in the Public Interest, accessed June 7, 2016, http://www.cspinet.org /new/201602081.html.

CHAPTER 5

1   Kim, Jung Eun et al. "Effects of Egg Consumption on Carotenoid Absorption from Co-Consumed, Raw Vegetables." *American Journal of Clinical Nutrition* 102.1 (2015): 75–83. *PMC*. Web. 7 Dec. 2016.

Index

Underscored page references indicate boxed text. An asterisk (*) indicates recipe photos are shown in the color-inserts.

Cherries
  benefits of, 50
  Cherry, Pear, and Pecan
    Crisp, 241
  Pumpkin Seed, Cherry, and
    Pecan Granola Bars,
    262
Chia seeds
  complexion, effect on, 51
  Raspberry Chia Jam, 280
Chicken
  Baked Chicken with
    Mustard Sauce, 175
  Broccoli-Chicken Casserole,
    178
  Buffalo Chicken
    Quesadillas, 250
  Chicken, Quinoa, and
    Peach Salad, 138
  Chicken Pad Thai,* 177
  Chicken Pot Pie,* 174
  Chicken Soup with Asian
    Noodles, 123
  Creamy Chicken, Green
    Grape, and Farro
    Salad, 137
  Homemade Bone Broth, 281
  Mediterranean Chicken
    Wraps, 170
  Orange-Sage Braised
    Chicken Thighs, 179
  Panzanella,* 148
  Parmesan Chicken Fingers,
    176
  Quick, Creamy Chicken
    Lasagna, 173
  Slow-Cooker BBQ Pulled
    Chicken Flatbreads,*
    171
Chickpeas
  Minestrone, 124
  Peanut Butter Banana
    Blondies,* 235
Chips
  Chili-Lime Kale Chips, 255
  Cinnamon-Sugar Pita
    Chips, 257

pairing with healthy dips,
  259
Pita Chips with Olive Oil
  and Sea Salt, 258
Salt and Pepper Kale Chips,
  256
Salt-n-Vinegar Potato
  Chips, 254
Spiced Sweet Potato Chips,
  253
Sweet Chili Pita Chips,
  259
Chocolate
  Chocolate Chip Cookie
    Dough Energy Bites,
    264
  Chocolate Cream Pie,*
    239
  Chocolate Espresso
    Mousse,* 228
  Cocoa Granola, 111
  Crepes with
    Cocoa-Hazelnut Butter
    and Bananas, 246
  Dark Chocolate Crackle
    Cookies, 231
  Dark Chocolate–Sea Salt
    Truffles, 237
  Fruit 'n' Nut Bark, 236
  Homemade
    Cocoa-Hazelnut
    Butter, 278
  Mexican Chocolate
    Popcorn Balls,* 265
  Mocha Peanut Butter
    Smoothie, 117
  Orange–Dark Chocolate
    Chunk Cookies, 229
  Rich Brownies, 234
  Rich Chocolate Torte,
    238
  Roasted Strawberries with
    Chocolate Sauce,*
    226
Cholesterol, dietary, 205
Cholesterol, effect of clean
  eating on, 33–34

Cilantro
  Chilled Cilantro–Soba
    Noodle Salad, 144
  Cilantro-Pear Vinaigrette,
    268
Citrus fruits. See also lemon;
  oranges
  calorie burn, increasing
    with, 16
  Citrus Garlic Aioli, 273
CLA, 20
Clean eating, 3–29
  additives and chemicals,
    effect on metabolism,
    13–14
  belly fat, reducing, 18–21
  burning more calories with,
    15–18
  energy level, increasing, 29
  general discussion, 4–8
  gut bacteria, nurturing,
    24–25, 28–29
  love of clean foods,
    developing, 18–19
  overeating and cravings,
    conquering, 21–24
  processed foods, effect on
    metabolism, 9–13
"Clean Fifteen" list, 74–75
Clean foods, identifying,
  71–95
  everyday essentials, 89–90
  fats, 79–81
  packaged foods, 88
  packaging claims,
    deciphering, 85–88
  plant proteins, 78–79
  produce, 73–75
  proteins, 76–78
  sugars, hidden, 82–85
  whole grains, 81–82
CMC, 13–14
Coconut
  Creamy Coconut Rice
    Pudding, 227
  Dark Chocolate–Sea Salt
    Truffles, 237

Dopamine, 9, 42
DPP, 36
Dressings
    Cilantro-Pear Vinaigrette, 268
    Creamy Green Goddess Dressing, 270
    Lemon-Shallot Vinaigrette, 146
    oils for, 268
    Orange-Miso Salad Dressing, 269
Drinks. *See also* coffee; tea
    artificial sweeteners in, 13
    cravings, curbing with, 70
    diabetes risk, lowering, 37
    Green Ginger Smoothie, 119
    Mocha Peanut Butter Smoothie, 117
    Peach Smoothie, 118
    soda, 37, 51
    sugar and carbohydrates in, 11
    water, 11, 17
Dyes, food, 84

E

Eating slowly, 23, 61
EGCG, 17
Eggs
    benefits of, 100
    Hash Brown Frittata, 104
    labels on packages, 85
    Mini Spinach Quiche,* 102
    Mushroom Omelet, 105
    organic, 76
    Salmon Breakfast Burrito, 103
    saturated fats in, 80
    Southwest Skillet Eggs,* 100
    Zesty Breakfast Pizza,* 101
Ellagic acid, 40

Emotions
    effect of food on, 42–43
    food journals, identifying triggers with, 61
    mood swings, 42–43, 42, 45, 52
Emulsifiers, 13–14
Energy bars, 88
Energy level, increasing, 29, 40–42
Enjoying meals, 60–61
Environmental Working Group, 74–75
Epigallocatechin gallate (EGCG), 17
Exercise, 20, 29, 244
Expeller-pressed oils, 80

F

Farmed fish, 76–77
Farmers' markets, 91–92
Farro
    Creamy Chicken, Green Grape, and Farro Salad, 137
Fast food, 73
Fat, belly, 15–18
Fat-free dressings, 140
Fats. *See also* omega-3 fatty acids
    diabetes risk, lowering, 36–37
    in dressings, 140
    gut bacteria, nurturing, 28
    healthy, 79–81
    heart disease risk, lowering, 33
    monounsaturated, 20, 36–37, 80
    polyunsaturated, 12, 23, 80
    satiety hormones, 23
    saturated, 12, 33, 80–81
    sleepiness caused by, 29
    trans, 81, 84, 256
Fermented drinks, 87–88

Fermented foods, 28
Fiber
    blood sugar levels, lowering, 21
    gut bacteria, nurturing, 28
    high-fiber label, 87
    hormone boosting, 23
    LDL cholesterol, lowering, 33–34
    satisfaction from foods with, 22
    soluble, 20
Firmicutes, 24, 25
Fish
    Asian Fish Packets, 187
    buying, 76–78
    farmed, 76–77, 77
    Greek Salad with Salmon, 141
    omega-3 fatty acids in, 28, 40, 80
    Salmon Breakfast Burrito, 103
    Salmon Croquettes, 185
    Salmon Pasta Casserole, 186
    Salmon Salad Lettuce Wraps, 184
    sleep quality and, 49
Flavonoids, 16
Flavor of foods, and satisfaction, 15–18
Flaxseeds, 51
Flours, 23, 113
Focusing on food when eating, 60–61
Food dehydrators, 255
Food dyes, 84
Food journals, 61
Free-range, 85–86
Freezing peaches, 279
French Toast
    Chocolate-Banana Stuffed French Toast, 108
    PB and J Stuffed French Toast,* 107
Fructose, 11–12

burning calories, 15–18, <u>49</u>
processed foods, effect on, 9–13
Microbiome
  artificial sweeteners, effect on, 13
  nurturing, 25, 28–29
  obesity and, 24–25
Milk
  belly fat, reducing, 20
  goat, <u>130</u>
  nut, <u>227</u>
Millet
  Butternut Squash with Millet and Pistachios,* 213
Mindful eating, 55–70, <u>68</u>, <u>194</u>
  benefits of, <u>58</u>
  checklist, 57
  cravings, coping with, 66–70
  focusing on food, 60–61
  general discussion, 56–57
  good and bad foods, concept of, 57–58
  hunger, identifying, 60
  kitchen organization, 64–65
  nonfood rewards, 65–66
  triggers, identifying, 61, 64
Miso
  Orange-Miso Salad Dressing, 269
Monosodium glutamate (MSG), 84
Monounsaturated fats (MUFAs), 20, 36–37, 80
Monterey Bay Aquarium Seafood Watch, 78
Mood swings, 42–43, <u>42</u>, <u>45</u>, <u>52</u>
Mozzarella
  Roasted Tomato and Garlic Soup with Mozzarella Toasts, 132
MSG, 84

MUFAs, 20, 36–37, 80
Muscle density, maintaining, 16
Mushrooms
  Black Bean and Mushroom Burgers, 191
  Creamy Spinach and Mushroom Soup, 131
  Hearty Lentil Mushroom Soup, 126
  immune benefits, <u>131</u>
  Mushroom Omelet, 105
  Stuffed Portobello Mushrooms, 193
  Wheat-Free Pizza,* 199

N

Natural food stores, 91
Natural label, 86
No Hormones label, 86
"No HPP" label, <u>269</u>
Nonfood rewards, 65–66
Non-GMO label, 88
Nut butters, 90, <u>278</u>
Nutrient deficiency, cravings from, <u>67</u>
Nutritional yeast, <u>265</u>
Nuts
  almond butter, 50
  Almond Spice Scones,* 116
  basic staples, 90
  Butternut Squash with Millet and Pistachios,* 213
  calorie burn, increasing with, 16
  Cherry, Pear, and Pecan Crisp, 241
  Crepes with Cocoa-Hazelnut Butter and Bananas, 246
  Fettuccine with Basil-Walnut Sauce, 221

Fruit and Nut Cookie Bars, 233
Fruit 'n' Nut Bark, 236
Homemade Cocoa-Hazelnut Butter, 278
milk from, making, <u>227</u>
Mocha Peanut Butter Smoothie, 117
PB&J Granola, 110
PB and J Stuffed French Toast,* 107
Peanut Butter Balls, 115
Peanut Butter Banana Blondies,* 235
Peanut Butter Bars, 263
protein from, 78–79, <u>79</u>
Pumpkin Seed, Cherry, and Pecan Granola Bars, 259
Spicy Ginger-Almond Sauce, 275
walnuts, 50

O

Oats
  Cocoa Granola, 111
  oatmeal, <u>112</u>
  PB&J Granola, 110
  Pumpkin Seed, Cherry, and Pecan Granola Bars, 262
  Simple Overnight Steel-Cut Oats, 112
  Steel-Cut Oatmeal Raisin Cookies, 230
Obesity
  artificial sweeteners and, 28–29
  cancer risk from, 39
  chemicals linked to, 14
  pain, increase from, 38
  plate size and, 165
Obesogens, 14

Walnuts (*cont.*)
    Fettuccine with
        Basil-Walnut Sauce,
        221
    Fruit 'n' Nut Bark, 236
    skin benefits from, 51
Water, drinking, <u>11</u>, 17
Weight loss, 55–70
    blood pressure, lowering, 34
    cravings, coping with,
        66–70
    diet vs. exercise, <u>244</u>
    focusing on food, 60–61
    good and bad foods,
        concept of, 57–58
    hunger, identifying, 60
    kitchen organization,
        64–65
    mindful eating, 56–57, <u>58</u>
    nonfood rewards, 65–66
    pain, easing through, 38
    sleep and, 48–49, <u>49</u>
    stress from worrying about,
        <u>44</u>
    traveling and, <u>46–47</u>
    triggers, identifying, 61, 64

Whole grains
    breads from, 82
    buying, 81–82
    cancer protection from,
        39
    diabetes risk, lowering, 36
    high-fiber label, 87
    pastas from, 82
    protein in, 78
    storing flour, <u>113</u>
Whole-milk yogurt, <u>193</u>
Wild-caught seafood, 77, <u>77</u>
Wild rice
    Squash Stuffed with Wild
        Rice and Raisins,
        216
    Wild Rice Casserole, 217
Work, balancing clean eating
    and, <u>62</u>, <u>63</u>
Wraps
    Mediterranean Chicken
        Wraps, 170
    Salmon Salad Lettuce
        Wraps, 184
    Turkey Cuban Wrap with
        Black Bean Salad, 180

Y

Yeast, nutritional, <u>265</u>
Yogurt
    Apple Pie Parfait, 109
    Citrus Garlic Aioli, 273
    Dill and Basil Yogurt
        Bread, 223
    gut bacteria, nurturing,
        28
    Lamb Burgers with
        Lemon-Yogurt Sauce,
        163
    whole-milk, <u>193</u>

Z

Zinc, <u>67</u>
Zucchini
    Arugula Salad with
        Zucchini Ribbons,
        145
    Pasta with Summer
        Vegetables, 195
    Shaved Salad,* 147